THE COMPLETE
KETO
AIR FRYER
COOKBOOK
FOR
BEGINNERS

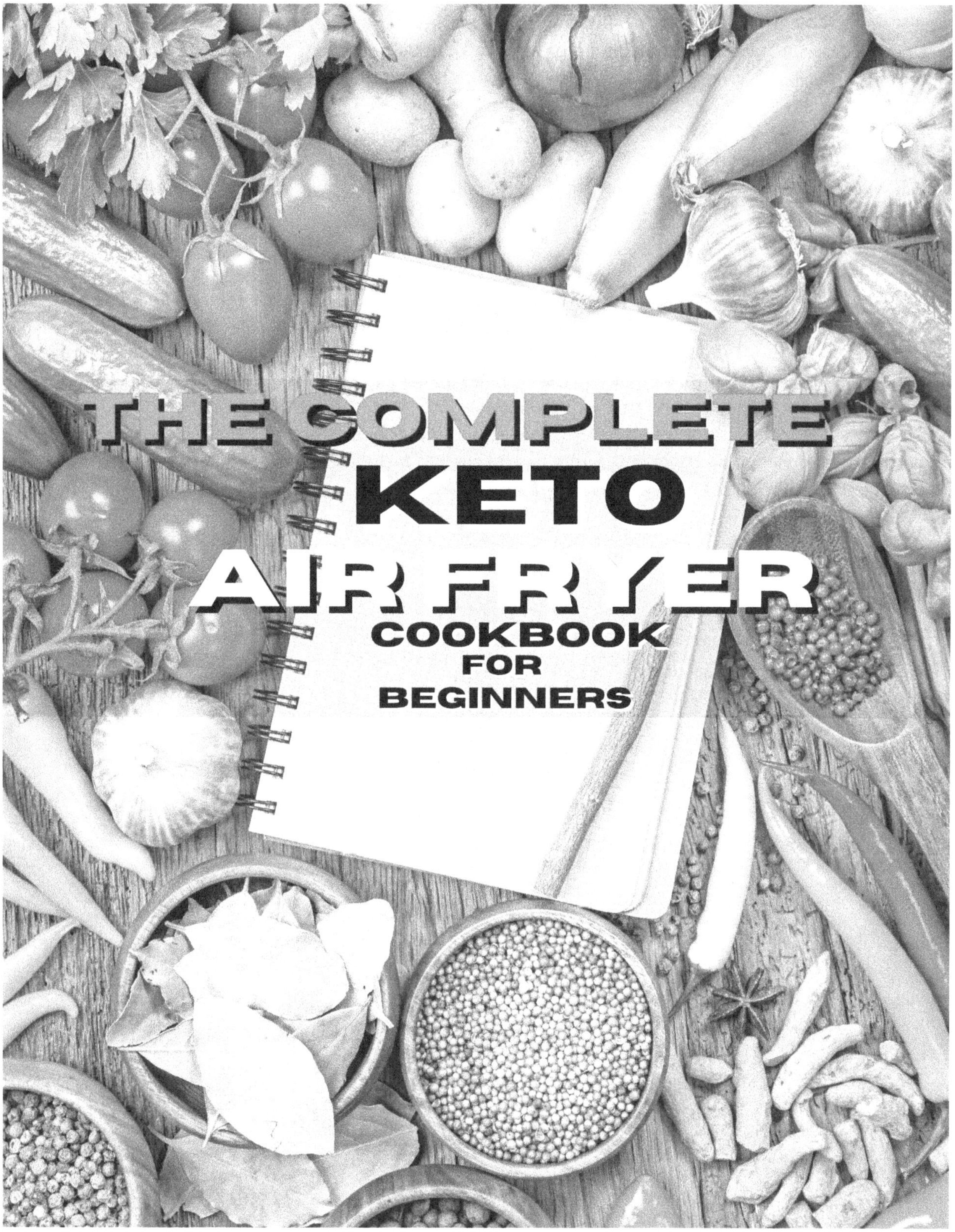

APPETIZERS AND SNACKS................51

CHICKEN MAIN DISHES 118

Lunch Recipes...........210

INTRODUCTION

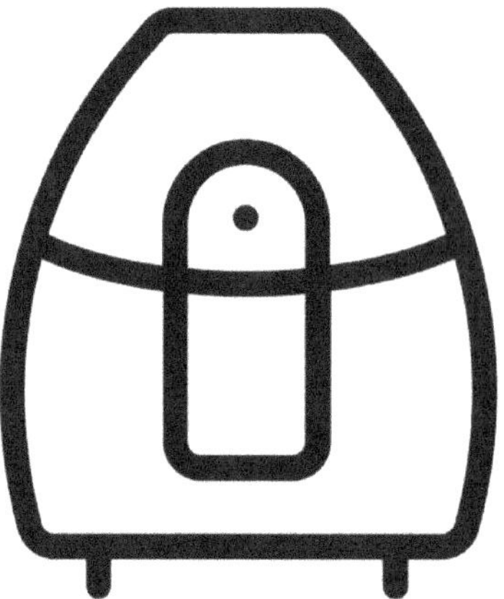

If you have an air fryer, you already know it's a revolutionary appliance meant to save you time and help you live better. If you still haven't leaped, you'll be excited to learn just how quickly you'll be hooked and using your air fryer to prepare nearly every meal. But what's so special about air frying?

The air fryer can replace your oven, your microwave, your deep fryer, and your dehydrator and evenly cook delicious meals in a fraction of the time you're used to. If you're looking to provide your family with healthy meals but don't have a lot of time, the air fryer is a game-changer.

An air fryer can also help with your success on the keto diet. One of the many benefits of air frying is the short cooking times it provides. This is especially beneficial when you are hungry and short on time, a recipe for cheating on your diet. Long-term success on a ketogenic diet is often attributed to the ease of preparing healthy meals. That's why your air fryer will be your best friend throughout your keto journey and help you stay on track, even on the days when you're short on time.

Throughout this book, you'll learn everything you need to know about how and why to use an air fryer, as well as some basics that will help you find success following the ketogenic diet. Let's get cooking!

CHAPTER 1: COOKING WITH AN AIR FRYER

Cooking with an air fryer is as easy as using a microwave. Anybody can do it, and after just a few uses, you'll wish you had switched over to this genius method of cooking earlier. This chapter will introduce you to air frying options, maximize your cooking time and crispness, explain how to keep your air fryer clean and recommend accessories that will make your air frying experience even more comfortable and enjoyable.

While this chapter will cover the basics of using your air fryer, the first step is reading the manual that came with your air fryer. All air fryers are different, and with the recent rise in popularity of the appliance, there are many other models on the market. Learning how to use your specific air fryer thoroughly is the key to success and will familiarize you with troubleshooting issues and safety functions. Reading over the manual and washing all parts with warm, soapy water before first use will help you feel ready to unleash your culinary finesse!

Why air frying?
Air frying is increasingly popular because it allows you to quickly and evenly prepare delicious meals with little oil and little effort. Here are just a few of the reasons you'll want to switch to air frying:

It replaces other cooking appliances. You can use your air fryer in place of your oven, microwave, deep fryer, and dehydrator! In one small device, you can quickly cook up perfect dishes for every meal without sacrificing flavor.

It cooks faster than traditional cooking methods. Air frying works by circulating hot air around the cooking chamber. This results in fast and even cooking, using a fraction of the energy of your oven. Most air fryers can be set to a maximum temperature of 400°F. Because of this, just about anything you can make in a range, you can make in an air fryer.

It uses little to no cooking oil. The main selling point of air fryers is that you can achieve beautifully cooked foods with little to no cooking oil. While that may be attractive to some because it can mean lower fat content, people following the keto diet can rejoice because it means fewer calories, which still matters if you're doing keto for weight loss. It has a fast cleanup. With any cooking method, you're sure to dirty your cooker, but with your air fryer's smaller cooking chamber and removable basket, thorough cleanup is a breeze!

Choosing an air fryer
When choosing an air fryer, the two most important factors to focus on are the size and temperature range. Air fryers are usually measured by quart size and scope from about 1.2 quarts to 10 or more quarts. Suppose you're looking to cook meals to feed a family. In that case, you might be interested in at least a 5.3-quart fryer that can be used to beautifully roast an entire chicken . Still, if you need a small machine because of limited counter space and you're cooking for only one or two, you can crisp up some Jicama Fries with a much smaller air fryer. As for temperature range, some air fryers allow you the ability to dehydrate foods because you can cook them at a shallow temperature, say 120°F, for an extended period. Depending on the functions you need, you'll want to make sure your air fryer has the appropriate cooking capacity and temperature range.

Most air fryers are equipped with buttons to help you prepare anything, such as grilling the perfect salmon, roasting an entire chicken, or even baking a chocolate cake.

These buttons are attached to preset times and temperatures based on your specific air fryer. Because of the wide variety of air fryers on the market, all recipes in this book were created using manual times and temperatures. Every air fryer allows you to set these yourself. Still, it is essential to know how the cooking programs work on your air fryer and when to use them.

While some air fryer recipes call for preheating the appliance, this is more of a personal preference. Some people preheat their air fryers while others just add a few minutes to cooking, which is what is done in these recipes. There's no benefit to preheating in my personal experience, which is why it is not called for in this book.

Essential accessories
Your air fryer's cooking chamber is just a large, open space for the hot air to circulate. This is a massive advantage because it gives you the option to incorporate several different accessories into your cooking. These accessories broaden the number of recipes you can make in your air fryer and open up opportunities you never would've thought were possible. Here are some of the standard accessories.

•   *Metal Holder.*
This circular rack is used to add a second layer to your cooking surface so you can maximize space and cook multiple things at once. This is particularly helpful when you're cooking meat and veggies and don't want to wait for one to finish to get started on the other.

•   *Skewer Rack.*
This is similar to a metal holder, but it has built-in metal skewers that make roasting kebabs a breeze.

•   *Ramekin.*
Small ramekins are great for making mini cakes and quiches. If they're oven-safe, they're safe to use in your air fryer.

•   *Cake Pan.*
You can find specially made cake pans for your air fryer that fit perfectly into the cooking chamber. They also come with a built-in handle, so you can easily pull them out when your cakes are made baking.

•   *Cupcake Pan.*
A cupcake pan usually comes with seven mini cups and takes up the entire chamber of your 5.3-quart air fryer. These versatile cups are perfect for muffins, cupcakes, and even egg cups. If you don't want to go this route, you can also use individual silicone baking cups.

•   *Parchment.*
Specially precut parchment can be helpful to making cleanup even easier when baking with your air fryer. Additionally, you can find parchment paper with precut holes for easy steaming.

•   *Pizza Pan.*
Yes, you can bake a pizza in your air fryer, and this book includes several recipes for different kinds of keto-friendly pizzas. This is an excellent option for quickly getting the perfect shape every time.

Accessory removal
At some point, you will need to get those helpful accessories out of your air fryer without burning yourself. Here are some tools that will allow you to safely and efficiently take items out of your air fryer.

•   *Tongs.*

These will be helpful when lifting meat in and out of the air fryer. Tongs are also useful for removing cooking pans that don't come with handles.

- *Oven Mitts.*

Sometimes simple is best. Your food will be scorching when you remove it, so it's great to have these around to protect your hands.

Cleaning your air fryer

Before cleaning it, first, ensure that your air fryer is entirely chilly and unplugged. To clean the air fryer pan, you'll need to:

1. Remove the air fryer pan from the base. Fill the pan with hot water and dish soap. Let the pan soak with the frying basket inside for 10 minutes.
2. Then, clean the basket thoroughly with a sponge or brush.
3. Remove the fryer basket and scrub the underside and outside walls.
4. Clean the air fryer pan with a sponge or brush.
5. Let everything air-dry and return to the air fryer base.

To clean the outside of your air fryer, simply wipe the outside with a damp cloth. Then, be sure all components are in the correct position before beginning your next cooking adventure.

Chapter 2: What Is Keto?

The ketogenic diet, or keto, is a very low-carb, moderate- protein, and high-fat diet that allows the body to fuel itself without glucose or high levels of carbohydrates.

When the body is in short supply of glucose, ketones are made in the liver from the breakdown of fats through ketosis. (Please note this differs from ketoacidosis.) With careful tracking, creative meals, and self-control, this diet can lead to weight loss, lower blood sugar, regulated insulin levels, and controlled cravings.

When you eat a very high-carb diet (pizza, pasta, pastries), your body takes those carbs and turns them into glucose to power itself. When you cut out the carbs, your metabolism burns fat instead. Typically, a ketogenic diet restricts carbs to 0- 50 grams per day.

What Are Macros?

Macronutrients, or macros, are the three ways your body produces energy. They include carbohydrates, protein, and fat. When you're following keto, it is essential to track how many grams of each macronutrient you consume each day.

- Carbs should be around 5 percent of your daily calories
- Protein should be about 25 percent of your daily calories
- Healthy fats should be about 70 percent of your daily

- *Calories*

Some of the best-quality fats come from natural sources such as fish, avocados, and nuts. These fats can help reduce your cholesterol, keep your heart healthy, and fuel your body throughout the day. You should always beware of unhealthy fats. However, that can come from foods like cookies and French fries. Overconsumption of these, especially in conjunction with a high-carb diet, can contribute to heart disease, low energy, and unwanted weight gain.

- *Net Carbs*

Most people following keto opt to track net carbs instead of total carbs. You can figure out net carbs by subtracting your dietary fiber intake from your total carb intake:

- *Total carbs minus dietary fiber equals net carbs.*

You may also subtract sugar alcohols from the total carb count. Net is generally the preferred method because of how your body reacts to the fiber and sugar alcohols. The grams of dietary fiber and sugar alcohol are already included in the total carb count on nutrition labels. Still, because the fiber and (some) sugar alcohols are carbs that your body can't digest, they do not affect your blood sugar levels and can be subtracted.

Tips to Remember

Keep these tips in mind as you plan your daily meals:

- **Carbs are a limit**: Don't go above your allotted daily net carbs.
- **Protein is a goal**: This is the essential macro to hit. If you're losing weight, you want to make sure you're eating enough protein to keep you from also losing muscle.
- **Fat is a lever**—(you use it to adjust your diet): In this diet, grease is designed to keep you full. If you're hungry, go ahead and eat that healthy fat up to your limit. If you're not hungry, you don't have to hit your fat macros.
- **With the quick and easy recipes** in this book, you should never feel deprived of your keto journey. Just remember, if you fall off the wagon, the most important thing is to get back on as quickly as possible. Allow yourself grace and time, but never give up just because you slipped up.

NOW THAT YOU HAVE A BETTER UNDERSTANDING..

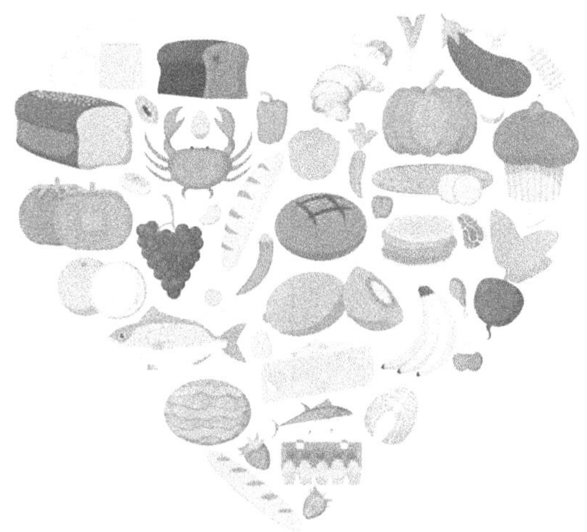

..Of Your Air Fryer And Ketogenic diet, **let's get cooking**! You'll find plenty of recipes for all tastes, for your air fryer, plus other tasty and simple keto recipes.
Use this book as a guide, and always feel free to intuitively season and customize dishes to your liking.

You should never rule out dishes and condiments because they may contain a minimum of sugar/sweeteners, fat, carbs, because what makes you put on weight is **quantity**.
The only real secret that people haven't figured out yet, is that **weekly calorie intake** is what **really makes a difference**!

Remember that a **flexible**, **tasty** and **varied** diet is essential for long-term results.
As you know, most people give up on the stifling diet after a few weeks due to stress (not to mention cortisol damage).

That's exactly why in this book, with my nutritionist colleagues, we decided to provide you with a real "**Air Fryer Bible**" in a compact version.

So you can have 1000 Keto different Ideas for eating healthy and losing weight at your fingertips, and people won't even think you're dieting.

Love,
Mary De Blasio

Quick and delicious low-carb breakfasts will soon be the norm in your household once you put your air fryer to work! These recipes will kick-start your day in a healthy way without depriving you of the savory goodness mornings should be made of! When you're struggling to get out the door in time, it can be really tough to prepare a nourishing meal for yourself or your family. Grabbing a granola bar or toaster pastry may be the easiest option, but it can soon lead to feelings of guilt and serious midday hunger.

The recipes in this chapter are filling and keto-approved, helping you to change your mornings and your entire days. Get ready for nutritious breakfasts that can be made in a flash. With meals you can prepare ahead of time, like Sausage and Cheese Balls, and dishes you can pop in your air fryer to get ready while you get ready, like Quick and Easy Bacon Strips, you'll wish you had started air frying your breakfasts sooner!

CRUNCHY GRANOLA

Missing the crunch of cereal in the morning? This recipe saves the day in a simple way because making it is as easy as mixing all the ingredients together and popping it in your air fryer! Once the granola is done, you can enjoy it in a bowl of unsweetened nut milk or on top of a low-carb, full-fat yogurt!

HandsOn Time: 10 minutes
Cook Time: 5 minutes
Serves 6

- 2 cups pecans, chopped
- 1 cup unsweetened coconut flakes
- 1 cup almond slivers
- 1/3 cup sunflower seeds
- 1/4 cup golden flaxseed
- 1/4 cup low-carb, sugar- free chocolate chips
- 1/4 cup granular erythritol
- 2 tablespoons unsalted butter
- 1 teaspoon ground cinnamon

Directions

- ✓ 1 In a large bowl, mix all ingredients.
- ✓ 2 Place the mixture into a 4-cup round baking dish. Place dish into the air fryer basket.
- ✓ 3 Adjust the temperature to 320°F and set the timer for 5 minutes.
- ✓ 4 Allow to cool completely before serving.

Per serving
Calories: 617 Protein: 10.9 G Fiber: 11.2 G Net Carbohydrates: 6.5 G Sugar Alcohol: 14.7 G Fat: 55.8 G Sodium: 5 Mg

Carbohydrates: 32.4 G Sugar: 2.7 G

WAYS TO ENJOY
You can enjoy this granola with a bowl of unsweetened almond milk, or make it a parfait by mixing up a keto "faux-gurt" made simply of V2 cup sour cream, 1 tablespoon heavy cream, and 1 tablespoon of your favorite low-carb sweetener!

CRISPY SOUTHWESTERN HAM EGG CUPS

This recipe, cooked right in the cups lined with delicious ham, will start your day with a burst of creamy, subtly spicy Southwestern flavor. The sour cream in the dish helps cut the spice and adds fat to your meal that helps keep you full!

HandsOn Time: 5 minutes
Cook Time: 12 minutes
Serves 2

- 4 (1-ounce) slices deli ham 4 large eggs
- 2 tablespoons full-fat sour cream
- 1/4 cup diced green bell pepper 2 tablespoons diced red bell pepper 2 tablespoons diced white onion 1/2 cup shredded medium Cheddar cheese

Directions

- ✓ Place one slice of ham on the bottom of four baking cups.
- ✓ In a large bowl, whisk eggs with sour cream. Stir in green pepper, red pepper, and onion.
- ✓ Pour the egg mixture into ham-lined baking cups.
- ✓ Top with Cheddar. Place cups into the air fryer basket.
- ✓ Adjust the temperature to 320°F and set the timer for 12 minutes or until the tops are browned.
- ✓ Serve warm.

Per serving
Calories: 382 Protein: 29.4 G Fiber: 1.4 G Net Carbohydrates: 4.6 G Fat: 23.6 G Sodium: 977 Mg Carbohydrates: 6.0 G Sugar: 2.1 G

<u>**BUFFALO EGG CUPS**</u>

Looking for a great way to take your morning eggs to the next level while packing in an extra boost of protein? These Buffalo Egg Cups are your answer. The spicy buffalo sauce will satisfy your palate, and the eggs' fat and protein will work together to keep you full!

HandsOn Time: 10 minutes
Cook Time: 15 minutes
Serves 2

- 4 large eggs
- 2 ounces full-fat cream cheese
- 2 tablespoons buffalo sauce
- 1/2 cup shredded sharp Cheddar cheese

Directions
- ✓ Crack eggs into two (4") ramekins.
- ✓ In a small microwave-safe bowl, mix cream cheese, buffalo sauce, and Cheddar. Microwave for 20 seconds and then stir. Place a spoonful into each ramekin on top of the eggs.
- ✓ Place ramekins into the air fryer basket.
- ✓ Adjust the temperature to 320°F and set the timer for 15 minutes.
- ✓ Serve warm.

Per serving
Calories: 354
Protein: 21.0 G Fiber: 0.0 G
Net Carbohydrates: 2.3 G Fat: 22.3 G
Sodium: 886 Mg Carbohydrates: 2.3 G Sugar: 1.4 G

<u>**VEGGIE FRITTATA**</u>

Want to get your day started with a nutritious and filling boost? This breakfast is just what you need to help you get your daily veggies in early! Of course vegetables are packed with nutrients to help keep you healthy and strong, but it's important to keep an eye on the carb counts because vegetables have a huge range.

HandsOn Time: 15 minutes
Cook Time: 12 minutes
Serves: 4

- 6 large eggs
- 1/4 cup heavy whipping cream
- 1/2 cup chopped broccoli
- 1/4 cup chopped yellow onion
- 1/4 cup chopped green bell pepper

Directions
- ✓ In a large bowl, whisk eggs and heavy whipping cream. Mix in broccoli, onion, and bell pepper.
- ✓ Pour into a 6" round oven-safe baking dish. Place baking dish into the air fryer basket.

- ✓ Adjust the temperature to 350°F and set the timer for 12 minutes.
- ✓ Eggs should be firm and cooked fully when the frittata is done. Serve warm.

Per serving
Calories: 168
Protein: 10.2 G Fiber: 0.6 G
Net Carbohydrates: 2.5 G Fat: 11.8 G Sodium: 116
Mg Carbohydrates: 3.1 G Sugar: 1.5 G

<u>**PUMPKIN SPICE MUFFINS**</u>

Who doesn't love the taste of pumpkin on a crisp autumn morning? For most people, pumpkin and fall go hand in hand, and this recipe will be a staple in your breakfast rotation all season long!

HandsOn Time: 10 minutes
Cook Time: 15 minutes
Serves 6

- 1 cup blanched finely ground almond flour
- 1/2 cup granular erythritol
- 1/2 teaspoon baking powder
- 1/4 cup unsalted butter, softened
- 1/4 cup pure pumpkin puree
- 1/2 teaspoon ground cinnamon
- 1/4 teaspoon ground nutmeg
- 1 teaspoon vanilla extract
- 2 large eggs

Directions
- ✓ In a large bowl, mix almond flour, erythritol, baking powder, butter, pumpkin puree, cinnamon, nutmeg, and vanilla.
- ✓ Gently stir in eggs.
- ✓ Evenly pour the batter into six silicone muffin cups. Place muffin cups into the air fryer basket, working in batches if necessary.
- ✓ Adjust the temperature to 300°F and set the timer for 15 minutes.
- ✓ When completely cooked, a toothpick inserted in center will come out mostly clean. Serve warm.

Per serving
Calories: 205 Protein: 6.3 G Fiber: 2.4 G Sodium: 65
Mg Carbohydrates: 17.4 G

Note
Make sure you use regular pumpkin puree instead of pumpkin pie puree! It can be tricky because they're usually right next to each other on store shelves, but the latter has added carbs and sugar that you definitely don't need for this flavorful treat!

QUICK AND EASY BACON STRIPS

What's better than perfectly crisped bacon in the morning? Gone are the days of cautiously standing over a hot pan while grease splatters at you. With your air fryer, you're just minutes away from delicious strips of evenly cooked bacon every time!

HandsOn Time: 5 minutes

Cook Time: 12 minutes

Serves 4

- 8 slices sugar-free bacon

Directions

- ✓ Place bacon strips into the air fryer basket.
- ✓ Adjust the temperature to 400°F and set the timer for 12 minutes.
- ✓ After 6 minutes, flip bacon and continue cooking time. Serve warm.

Per serving

Calories: 88 Protein: 5.8 G Fiber: 0.0 G Net Carbohydrates: 0.2 G Fat: 6.2 G Sodium: 355 Mg Carbohydrates: 0.2 G Sugar: 0.0 G

BANANA NUT CAKE

Even though bananas aren't a great option for keto because of high carb count, you can still enjoy banana nut cake by employing the help of the very low-carb banana extract. You can customize these muffins to your liking by swapping out the walnuts for your favorite nut.

HandsOn Time: 15 minutes

Cook Time: 25 minutes

Serves 6

- 1 cup blanched finely ground almond flour
- 1/2 cup powdered erythritol
- 2 tablespoons ground golden flaxseed
- 2 teaspoons baking powder
- 1/2 teaspoon ground cinnamon
- 1/4 cup unsalted butter, melted
- 21/2 teaspoons banana extract
- 1 teaspoon vanilla extract
- 1/4 cup full-fat sour cream
- 2 large eggs
- 1/4 cup chopped walnuts

Directions

- ✓ In a large bowl, mix almond flour, erythritol, flaxseed, baking powder, and cinnamon.
- ✓ Stir in butter, banana extract, vanilla extract, and sour cream.
- ✓ Add eggs to the mixture and gently stir until fully combined. Stir in the walnuts.
- ✓ Pour into 6" nonstick cake pan and place into the air fryer basket.
- ✓ Adjust the temperature to 300°F and set the timer for 25 minutes.

- ✓ Cake will be golden and a toothpick inserted in center will come out clean when fully cooked. Allow to fully cool to avoid crumbling.

Per serving

Calories: 263 Protein: 7.6 G Fiber: 3.1 G Net Carbohydrates: 3.3 G Sugar Alcohol: 12.0 G Fat: 23.6 G Sodium: 192 Mg Carbs: 18.4 G Sugar: 1.3

WHY NOT REAL BANANAS?

- One medium banana has about 24 grams of net carbohydrates. That's more than you would probably eat in a whole day!
- Banana extract is an excellent replacement that can be found in your local grocery store.

LEMON POPPY SEED CAKE

You can set this cake cooking when you get up in the morning, hop in the shower, and return to a moist and delicious low-carb treat that will be hard to put down! It's a great way to get your day started with a smile on your face!

HandsOn Time: 10 minutes

Cook Time: 14 minutes

Serves 6

- 1 cup b lanched finely ground almond flour
- 1/2 cup powdered erythritol
- 1/2 teaspoon baking powder
- 1/4 cup unsalted butter,
- melted 1/4 cup unsweetened almond milk
- 2 large eggs
- 1 teaspoon vanilla extract
- 1 medium lemon
- 1 teaspoon poppy seeds

Directions

- ✓ In a large bowl, mix almond flour, erythritol, baking powder, butter, almond milk, eggs, and vanilla.
- ✓ Slice the lemon in half and s◻ueeze the juice into a small bowl, then add to the batter.
- ✓ Using a fine grater, zest the lemon and add 1 tablespoon zest to the batter and stir. Add poppy seeds to batter.
- ✓ Pour batter into nonstick 6" round cake pan. Place pan into the air fryer basket.
- ✓ Adjust the temperature to 300°F and set the timer for 14 minutes.
- ✓ When fully cooked, a toothpick inserted in center will come out mostly clean. The cake will finish cooking and firm up as it cools. Serve at room temperature.

Calories: 204 Protein: 6.3 G Fiber: 2.4 G
Net Carbohydrates: 2.5 G Sugar Alcohol: 12.0 G Fat:
18.2 G Sodium: 72 Mg
Carbohydrates: 16.9 G Sugar: 0.9 G

PANCAKE CAKE

This bakes up ☐uick for a fluffy and delicious
breakfast for the whole family. It's a treat that the
kids will love, and you'll love how simple it is to
make! For added fun, you can throw in a handful of
low-carb chocolate chips! Serve this with low-carb
syrup or sugar-free whipped cream and low-carb
berries such as strawberries or blackberries.

HandsOn Time: 10 minutes
Cook Time: 7 minutes
Serves 4

- 1/2 cup blanched finely ground almond flour
- 1/4 cup powdered erythritol
- 1/2 teaspoon baking powder
- 2 tablespoons unsalted butter,
- softened 1 large egg
- 1/2 teaspoon unflavored gelatin
- 1/2 teaspoon vanilla extract
- 1/2 teaspoon ground cinnamon

Directions
- ✓ In a large bowl, mix almond flour, erythritol, and baking powder. Add butter, egg, gelatin, vanilla, and cinnamon. Pour into 6" round baking pan.
- ✓ Place pan into the air fryer basket.
- ✓ Adjust the temperature to 300°F and set the timer for 7 minutes.
- ✓ When the cake is completely cooked, a toothpick will come out clean. Cut cake into four and serve.

Per serving
Calories: 153 Protein: 5.4 G Fiber: 1.7 G Net
Carbohydrates Sodium: 80 Mg
Carbohydrates: 12.6 G Sugar

BACON, EGG, AND CHEESE ROLL UPS

This is the tastiest spin on a breakfast burrito you've
ever tried! With all of the carbs in a regular tortilla,
why not just replace the wrap altogether with crispy
and savory bacon? Load your burrito up with all the
goods, and pick it up just like the classic version!

HandsOn Time: 15 minutes
Cook Time: 15 minutes
Serves 4

- 2 tablespoons unsalted butter
- 1/4 cup chopped onion
- 1/2 medium green bell pepper, seeded and chopped
- 6 large eggs
- 12 slices sugar-free bacon
- 1 cup shredded sharp Cheddar cheese
- 1/2 cup mild salsa, for dipping

Directions
- ✓ In a medium skillet over medium heat, melt butter. Add onion and pepper to the skillet and saute until fragrant and onions are translucent, about 3 minutes.
- ✓ Whisk eggs in a small bowl and pour into skillet. Scramble eggs with onions and peppers until fluffy and fully cooked, about 5 minutes. Remove from heat and set aside.
- ✓ On work surface, place three slices of bacon side by side, overlapping about V4". Place V4 cup scrambled eggs in a heap on the side closest to you and sprinkle V4 cup cheese on top of the eggs.
- ✓ Tightly roll the bacon around the eggs and secure the seam with a toothpick if necessary. Place each roll into the air fryer basket.
- ✓   Adjust the temperature to 350°F and set the timer for 15 minutes. Rotate the rolls halfway through the cooking time.
- ✓   Bacon will be brown and crispy when completely cooked. Serve immediately with salsa for dipping.

Per serving
Calories: 460 Protein: 28.2 G Fiber: 0.8 G
Net Carbohydrates: 5.3 G Fat: 31.7 G Sodium: 1,100
Mg Carbohydrates: 6.1 G Sugar: 3.1 G

MAKE IT YOUR OWN!
- Customize this dish with your favorite egg add-ins! Chopped onions, mushrooms, or spinach are all great low-carb options. If you're extra hungry, adding some cooked crumbled breakfast sausage will make this even more filling!

CHEESY CAULIFLOWER HASH BROWNS

Because high-carb potatoes aren't a good option for keto, cauliflower makes a great nutrient-dense, low-carb substitute for hash browns. And with the help of your air fryer, you can get them perfectly crispy in no time at all! The cheese in this recipe helps bind the cauliflower together and adds an irresistible flavor that your whole family will love!

HandsOn Time: 20 minutes
Cook Time: 12 minutes
Serves 4

- 1 (12-ounce) steamer bag cauliflower
- 1 large egg
- 1 cup shredded sharp Cheddar cheese

Directions

- ✓ Place bag in microwave and cook according to package instructions. Allow to cool completely and put cauliflower into a cheesecloth or kitchen towel and squeeze to remove excess moisture.
- ✓ Mash cauliflower with a fork and add egg and cheese.
- ✓ Cut a piece of parchment to fit your air fryer basket. Take V4 of the mixture and form it into a hash brown patty shape. Place it onto the parchment and into the air fryer basket, working in batches if necessary.
- ✓ Adjust the temperature to 400°F and set the timer for 12 minutes.
- ✓ Flip the hash browns halfway through the cooking time. When completely cooked, they will be golden brown. Serve immediately.

Per serving
Calories: 153 Protein: 10.0 G Fiber: 1.7 G Net Carbohydrates: 3.0 G Fat: 9.5 G Sodium: 225 Mg Carbohydrates: 4.7 G Sugar: 1.8 G

BREAKFAST STUFFED POBLANOS

Get ready for a brand-new breakfast in your weekly rotation. This morning spin on jalapeno poppers will give you the kick you need to start your day. Crisped perfectly in your air fryer, this will also become a favorite for those "breakfast for dinner" nights!

HandsOn Time: 15 minutes
Cook Time: 15 minutes
Serves: 4

- 1/2 pound spicy ground pork breakfast sausage
- 4 large eggs
- 4 ounces full-fat cream cheese, softened
- 1/4 cup canned diced tomatoes and green chiles,
- drained 4 large poblano peppers
- 8 tablespoons shredded pepper jack cheese
- 1/2 cup full-fat sour cream

Directions

- ✓ In a medium skillet over medium heat, crumble and brown the ground sausage until no pink remains. Remove sausage and drain the fat from the pan. Crack eggs into the pan, scramble, and cook until no longer runny.
- ✓ Place cooked sausage in a large bowl and fold in cream cheese. Mix in diced tomatoes and chiles. Gently fold in eggs.
- ✓ Cut a 4"-5" slit in the top of each poblano, removing the seeds and white membrane with a small knife. Separate the filling into four servings and spoon carefully into each pepper. Top each with 2 tablespoons pepper jack cheese.
- ✓ Place each pepper into the air fryer basket.
- ✓ Adjust the temperature to 350°F and set the timer for 15 minutes.
- ✓ Peppers will be soft and cheese will be browned when ready. Serve immediately with sour cream on top.

Per serving
Calories: 489 Protein: 22.8 G
Fiber: 3.8 G Net Carbohydrates: 8.8 G Fat: 35.6 G
Sodium: 746 Mg Carbohydrates: 12.6 G Sugar: 2.9 G

AIR FRYER "HARD-BOILED" EGGS

Yes, it is possible to "hard-boil" whole eggs in your air fryer! This method may seem a bit out of the ordinary, but it's a great way to achieve the same results you're used to without having to boil a pot of water on the stove! This is the perfect way to prepare several grab-and-go snacks to support your ketogenic lifestyle.

HandsOn Time: 2 minutes
Cook Time: 18 minutes
Serves 4

- 4 large eggs
- 1 cup water

Directions

- ✓ Place eggs into a 4-cup round baking-safe dish and pour water over eggs. Place dish into the air fryer basket.
- ✓ Adjust the temperature to 300°F and set the timer for 18 minutes.
- ✓ Store cooked eggs in the refrigerator until ready to use or peel and eat warm.

Per serving

Calories: 77 Protein: 6.3 G Fiber: 0.0 G Net Carbohydrates: 0.6 G Fat: 4.4 G Sodium: 62 Mg Carbohydrates: 0.6 G Sugar: 0.6 G

SCRAMBLED EGGS

Sometimes you just don't want to turn on your stove, or you don't have access to it for whatever reason. When you're in a pinch, you can still get classic moist Scrambled Eggs from your air fryer!

HandsOn Time: 5 minutes

Cook Time: 15 minutes

Serves 2

- 4 large eggs
- 2 tablespoons unsalted butter,
- Melted1/2 cup shredded sharp Cheddar cheese

Directions

- ✓ Crack eggs into 2-cup round baking dish and whisk. Place dish into the air fryer basket.
- ✓ Adjust the temperature to 400°F and set the timer for 10 minutes.
- ✓ After 5 minutes, stir the eggs and add the butter and cheese. Let cook 3 more minutes and stir again.
- ✓ Allow eggs to finish cooking an additional 2 minutes or remove if they are to your desired liking.
- ✓ Use a fork to fluff. Serve warm.

Per serving

Calories: 359 Protein: 19.5 G Fiber: 0.0 G Net Carbohydrates: 1.1 G Fat: 27.6 G Sodium: 325 Mg Carbohydrates: 1.1 G Sugar: 0.5 G

LOADED CAULIFLOWER BREAKFAST BAKE

Casseroles aren't just for dinnertime! This is the perfect option for busy weekday mornings, giving you lots of classic breakfast flavor and swapping in cauliflower where potatoes might usually be. Add a dash of hot sauce for some kick if you really want to wake up!

HandsOn Time: 15 minutes

Cook Time: 20 minutes

Serves: 4

- 6 large eggs
- 1/4 cup heavy whipping cream
- 11/2 cups chopped cauliflower
- 1 cup shredded medium Cheddar cheese
- 1 medium avocado, peeled and pitted

- 8 tablespoons full-fat sour cream 2 scallions, sliced on the bias
- 12 slices sugar-free bacon, cooked and crumbled

Directions

- ✓ In a medium bowl, whisk eggs and cream together. Pour into a 4-cup round baking dish.
- ✓ Add cauliflower and mix, then top with Cheddar. Place dish into the air fryer basket.
- ✓ Adjust the temperature to 320°F and set the timer for 20 minutes.
- ✓ When completely cooked, eggs will be firm and cheese will be browned. Slice into four pieces.
- ✓ Slice avocado and divide evenly among pieces. Top each piece with 2 tablespoons sour cream, sliced scallions, and crumbled bacon.

Per serving

Calories: 512 Protein: 27.1 G Fiber: 3.2 G Net Carbohydrates: 4.3 G Fat: 38.3 G Sodium: 865 Mg Carbohydrates: 7.5 G Sugar: 2.3 G

CINNAMON ROLL STICKS

With sweet and gooey cinnamon perfection, you'll have a rich start to your morning and guaranteed trouble sharing these Cinnamon Roll Sticks!

HandsOn Time: 10 minutes

Cook Time: 7 minutes

Serves: 4 (2 sticks per serving)

- 1 cup shredded mozzarella cheese
- 1 ounce full-fat cream cheese
- 1/3 cup blanched finely ground almond flour
- 1/2 teaspoon baking soda
- 1/2 cup granular erythritol, divided 1 teaspoon vanilla extract
- 1 large egg
- 2 tablespoons unsalted butter, melted
- 1/2 teaspoon ground cinnamon
- 3 tablespoons powdered erythritol
- 2 teaspoons unsweetened vanilla almond milk

Directions

- ✓ Place mozzarella in a large microwave-safe bowl and break cream cheese into small pieces and place into bowl. Microwave for 45 seconds.
- ✓ Stir in almond flour, baking soda, V4 cup granular erythritol, and vanilla. A soft dough should form. Microwave the mix for additional 15 seconds if it becomes too stiff.

- ✓ Mix egg into the dough, using your hands if necessary.
- ✓ Cut a piece of parchment to fit your air fryer basket. Press the dough into an 8" x 5" rectangle on the parchment and cut into eight (1") sticks.
- ✓ In a small bowl, mix butter, cinnamon, and remaining granular erythritol. Brush half the mixture over the top of the sticks and place them into the air fryer basket.
- ✓ Adjust the temperature to 400°F and set the timer for 7 minutes.
- ✓ Halfway through the cooking time, flip the sticks and brush with remaining butter mixture. When done, sticks should be crispy.
- ✓ To make glaze, whisk powdered erythritol and almond milk in a small bowl. Drizzle over cinnamon sticks. Serve warm.

Per serving
Calories: 233 Protein: 10.3 G Fiber: 1.2 G
Net Carbohydrates: 2.2 G Sugar Alcohol: 36.8 G Fat: 19.0 G Sodium: 378 Mg CarbS: 40.2 G Sugar: 1.0 G

BREAKFAST CALZONE

This is a great, and portable, way to start your morning! You can customize the filling with all of your favorites, freeze it the night before, and warm it up in your air fryer before taking it with you on your morning commute!
HandsOn Time: 15 minutes
Cook Time: 15 minutes
Serves 4
- 11/2 cups shredded mozzarella cheese
- 1/2 cup blanched finely ground almond flour
- 1 ounce full-fat cream cheese 1 large whole egg
- 4 large eggs, scrambled
- 1/2 pound cooked breakfast sausage,
- crumbled 8 tablespoons shredded mild Cheddar cheese

Directions
- ✓ 1 In a large microwave-safe bowl, add mozzarella, almond flour, and cream cheese. Microwave for 1 minute. Stir until the mixture is smooth and forms a ball. Add the egg and stir until dough forms.
- ✓ 2 Place dough between two sheets of parchment and roll out to V4" thickness. Cut the dough into four rectangles.
- ✓ 3 Mix scrambled eggs and cooked sausage together in a large bowl. Divide the mixture evenly among each piece of dough, placing it on the lower half of the rectangle. Sprinkle each with 2 tablespoons Cheddar.
- ✓ 4 Fold over the rectangle to cover the egg and meat mixture. Pinch, roll, or use a wet fork to close the edges completely.
- ✓ 5 Cut a piece of parchment to fit your air fryer basket and place the calzones onto the parchment. Place parchment into the air fryer basket.
- ✓ 6 Adjust the temperature to 380°F and set the timer for 15 minutes.
- ✓ 7 Flip the calzones halfway through the cooking time. When done, calzones should be golden in color. Serve immediately.

Per serving
Calories: 560 Protein: 34.5 G Fiber: 1.5 G
Net Carbohydrates: 4.2 G Fat: 41.7 G
Sodium: 930 Mg Carbohydrates: 5.7 G Sugar: 2.1 G

CAULIFLOWER AVOCADO TOAST

Disappointed you can't keep up with the trend of avocado toast? Have no fear, this swap is a tasty, crunchy nutrient-rich breakfast that's full of healthy fats to help keep you full and focused throughout the day!
HandsOn Time: 15 minutes
Cook Time: 8 minutes
Serves 2
- 1 (12-ounce) steamer bag cauliflower
- 1 large egg
- 1/2 cup shredded mozzarella cheese
- 1 ripe medium avocado
- 1/2 teaspoon garlic powder
- 1/4 teaspoon ground black pepper

Directions
- ✓ Cook cauliflower according to package instructions. Remove from bag and place into cheesecloth or clean towel to remove excess moisture.
- ✓ Place cauliflower into a large bowl and mix in egg and mozzarella. Cut a piece of parchment to fit your air fryer basket. Separate the cauliflower mixture into two, and place it on the parchment in two mounds. Press out the cauliflower mounds into a 1/4"-thick rectangle. Place the parchment into the air fryer basket.
- ✓ Adjust the temperature to 400°F and set the timer for 8 minutes.
- ✓ Flip the cauliflower halfway through the cooking time.
- ✓ When the timer beeps, remove the

parchment and allow the cauliflower to cool 5 minutes.

- ✓ Cut open the avocado and remove the pit. Scoop out the inside, place it in a medium bowl, and mash it with garlic powder and pepper. Spread onto the cauliflower. Serve immediately.

Per serving
Calories: 278
Protein: 14.1 G Fiber: 8.2 G
Net Carbohydrates: 7.7 G Fat: 15.6 G
Sodium: 267 Mg Carbohydrates: 15.9 G Sugar: 3.9 G

SAUSAGE AND CHEESE BALLS

These breakfast-style meatballs make for a flavorful, protein- filled breakfast that you can make ahead of time, freeze, and pop into your air fryer when you're ready so your busy mornings are easy and delicious!
HandsOn Time: 10 minutes
Cook Time: 12 minutes
Yields 16 balls (4 per serving)

- 1 pound pork breakfast sausage
- 1/2 cup shredded Cheddar cheese
- 1 ounce full-fat cream cheese, softened 1 large egg

Directions
- ✓ Mix all ingredients in a large bowl. Form into sixteen (1") balls. Place the balls into the air fryer basket.
- ✓ Adjust the temperature to 400°F and set the timer for 12 minutes.
- ✓ Shake the basket two or three times during cooking. Sausage balls will be browned on the outside and have an internal temperature of at least 145°F when completely cooked.
- ✓ Serve warm.

Per serving
Calories: 424
Protein: 22.8 G Fiber: 0.0 G
Net Carbohydrates: 1.6 G Fat: 32.2 G
Sodium: 973 Mg Carbohydrates: 1.6 G Sugar: 1.4 G

FREEZER FRIENDLY!
These cheese balls are a great make-ahead item. If you want to freeze them, place cooked balls on a large cookie sheet and freeze for 1 hour. Then place in a freezer-safe storage bag.

CHEESY BELL PEPPER EGGS

Bell peppers are a great source of vitamins A and C, two vitamins that are important for the strength of your immune system. This easy breakfast also gives you some protein from the ham and an extra boost of flavor from the onion. Altogether, you have a nutritious, well-rounded breakfast!
HandsOn Time: 10 minutes
Cook Time: 15 minutes
Serves: 4

- 4 medium green bell peppers
- 3 ounces cooked ham, chopped
- 1/4 medium onion, peeled and chopped 8 large eggs
- 1 cup mild Cheddar cheese

Directions
- ✓ Cut the tops off each bell pepper. Remove the seeds and the white membranes with a small knife. Place ham and onion into each pepper.
- ✓ Crack 2 eggs into each pepper. Top with V4 cup cheese per pepper. Place into the air fryer basket.
- ✓ Adjust the temperature to 390°F and set the timer for 15 minutes.
- ✓ When fully cooked, peppers will be tender and eggs will be firm. Serve immediately.

Per serving
Calories: 314
Protein: 24.9 g fiber: 1.7 g
Net carbohydrates: 4.6 g fat: 18.6 g
Sodium: 621 mg carbohydrates: 6.3 g sugar: 3.0 g

SPAGHETTI SQUASH FRITTERS

Squash is very quick to cook in the air fryer and has so many uses beyond just savory dinners. This dish is surprisingly flavorful and a breeze to make. Feel free to customize to your liking by adding your favorite filling items, such as mushrooms, chopped broccoli, or crumbled sausage.
HandsOn Time: 15 minutes
Cook Time: 8 minutes
Serves 4

- 2 cups cooked spaghetti squash
- 2 tablespoons unsalted butter, softened
- 1 large egg
- 1/4 cup blanched finely ground almond flour
- 2 stalks green onion, sliced
- 1/2 teaspoon garlic powder
- 1 teaspoon dried parsley

Directions
- ✓ Remove excess moisture from the squash using a cheesecloth or kitchen towel.
- ✓ Mix all ingredients in a large bowl. Form into four patties.

✓ Cut a piece of parchment to fit your air fryer basket. Place each patty on the parchment and place into the air fryer basket.
✓ Adjust the temperature to 400°F and set the timer for 8 minutes.
✓ Flip the patties halfway through the cooking time. Serve warm.

Per serving
Calories: 131

EXQUISITE BREAKFAST SAUSAGE

Fixings
- 220g ground chicken
- 220g ground pork
- 1 teaspoon sage
- 1/2 teaspoon salt, thyme, dark pepper
- 1/4 teaspoon celery seed, garlic powder,
- nutmeg, onion powder, paprika
- 1/8 teaspoon cayenne pepper

Guidance
1. Blend the entirety of the **Fixings** in a bowl and manipulate with your hands.
2. Make six cheeseburger patty, envelop them by cling wrap and freeze them. We'll utilize these for the following 6 days so on the off chance that you figure the meat will remain new, you don't need to freeze them, yet I did for good measure. I simply defrost every burger the prior night or defrost them in the microwave the day of.

AVOCADO BUN BREAKFAST BURGER

Fixings
- 1 avocado
- 1 egg
- 1 tablespoon olive oil
- 1 breakfast sausage
- 1 lettuce leaf
- 1 cut tomato
- 1 tablespoon mayo squeeze salt, pepper, sesame seeds

Guidance
1. Lay the avocado on its side, evenly, and cut it directly in the center ensuring you're not cutting it in an abnormal point. Whenever it's cut, cautiously eliminate the seed and cautiously spoon out of the tissue. Cut the lower part of one avocado with the goal that it can remain all alone on the plate.

2. Heat the oil in a non-stick skillet on medium-low heat. Add the breakfast sausage and cook 1-2 minutes on each side until completely cooked. Air out the egg in the skillet, turn the heat to low, cover and concoct bright side. Cook a few minutes until the egg white is completely cooked.
3. Spot the base portion of the avocado on a plate, spoon some mayo in the avocado opening, top with lettuce, the tomato, sausage, cautiously add the egg over and top with the avocado top! Sprinkle some salt, pepper and sesame seeds.

BREAKFAST SAUSAGE, EGGS AND GREENS

Fixings
- 1 breakfast sausage
- 2 eggs
- 4 broccoli florets
- 50g green beans
- 1.5 tablespoon olive oil
- 1 garlic clove squeeze salt, pepper, garlic powder

Guidelines
1. Cut the stems off the green beans. Mince the garlic.
2. Put some water to boil in a pot. Add the broccoli and green beans and cook until delicate. Remove from the water once cooked. Spot the broccoli onto a plate.
3. Add the olive oil to a griddle and add the breakfast sausage. Cook on the two sides until cooked through. Add the eggs and scramble them. Spot the eggs and sausage to the plate.
4. Add the garlic and green beans to the griddle. Fry until the garlic is beginning to fresh up. Sprinkle some salt, pepper and garlic powder over the beans and fried eggs. Spot the beans and eggs onto the plate.

BREAKFAST SAUSAGE AND EGGS

Fixings
- 2 eggs
- 1 breakfast sausage
- 1 tablespoon olive oil
- 2 asparagus
- 3 broccoli
- 3 cherry tomatoes squeeze salt, pepper, parsley

Directions
1. Cut the asparagus in two and remove a gnawed off the stems.

2. Put some water to boil and add the broccoli. Cook until delicate.

3. Add 1/2 tablespoon of olive oil to a non-stick griddle and add the breakfast sausage and asparagus and cook on all sides until cooked through. Move to a plate with the boiled broccoli.

4. Add the other 1/2 tablespoon of olive oil and air out the eggs. Change the heat to low, cover and cook for a couple of moments until the egg whites are completely cooked. Slide to the plate and sprinkle the salt, pepper and parsley over.

SIMPLE WITHOUT DAIRY CAESAR DRESSING

Fixings
- 6 tablespoon mayonnaise
- 2 teaspoon anchovy glue
- 1 garlic clove
- 3 tablespoon unsweetened almond milk
- 1/2 teaspoon lemon juice
- 1.5 teaspoon oregano
- 1/8 teaspoon salt
- 1/4 teaspoon garlic powder

Directions
1. Mince the garlic. Combine the entirety of the **Fixings** as one and keep in a sealed shut holder in the refrigerator. It will save for quite a long time, simply blend it again prior to utilizing.

90 SEC SAUSAGE EGG MCMUFFIN

Fixings
- 1 breakfast sausage
- 1 cut tomato
- 1 egg
- 1 teaspoon olive oil
- 1 teaspoon mayo
- 90 sec bread: blend these
- 1 tablespoon refined coconut oil
- 1 egg
- 1/2 teaspoon salt
- 1/2 teaspoon preparing powder
- 3 tablespoon almond flour

Bearings
1. Consolidate the elements for the 90 second bread into an enormous mug. Blend cautiously and microwave for 90 seconds. Remove it from the mug and cautiously cut down the middle.

2. Heat the olive oil in a griddle and fry the breakfast sausage until cooked. Add the cut bread and flame broil on the two sides until wanted toastness.

3. Utilizing a scaled down egg skillet, cook the egg until the egg whites are completely cooked.

4. Spread the mayo more than one cut of bread, cover with the tomato cut, sausage, egg and last cut of bread. Appreciate!!

BREAKFAST SAUSAGE AND POACHED EGG

Fixings
- 1 breakfast sausage
- 1 tablespoon olive oil
- 1 egg
- 40g new spinach
- 3 cherry tomatoes
- 1/4 avocado
- 1/4 teaspoon salt and pepper
- 1 tablespoon vinegar

Guidelines
1. Put some water to heat in a little pot and add the vinegar. Break the egg inside a little bowl or cup. When the water is stewing, make a flowing movement with a spatula inside the water and drop the egg in the winding. Mood killer the heat, cover for 6 minutes precisely. Remove it from the water once done.

2. Heat the olive oil in a skillet and cook the breakfast sausage on medium-low heat on the two sides until cooked through. Spot the sausage on a plate. Add the new spinach to the griddle with the extra oil from the sausage. Cook until shriveled and move to a plate. Cover with the poached egg.

3. Cut the avocado and put on the plate alongside the cherry tomatoes.

SPINACH AND PORK OMELET

Fixings
- 1 breakfast sausage
- 1 cup new spinach (30g)
- 1/4 red pepper (40g)
- 2 garlic cloves
- 2 tablespoon olive oil
- 1/4 teaspoon salt, pepper, garlic powder, parsley
- 6 eggs

Directions
1. Disintegrate the sausage. Cut the red pepper and mince the garlic.

2. In an enormous non-stick griddle, add the olive oil and cook the sausage. Add the garlic, red pepper and

spinach to the skillet and cook for 1-2 minutes until delicate.
3. Air out the eggs in an enormous bowl, add the flavors and blend in with a race for 2 minutes.
4. Pour the egg player to the skillet, cover and let cook on low heat for 4-5 minutes.
5. At the point when the highest point of the omeltte is cooked through, simply slide the omelet to a plate and cut down the middle. Save half for the following day

SPINACH AND PORK OMELET

Fixings
extras from the past breakfast above

Directions
1. Reheat the breakfast extras.

AVOCADO BOAT, SAUSAGE AND ASPARAGUS

Fixings
- 60g sausage
- 1-2 asparagus
- 1 teaspoon olive oil
- 1/2 avocado
- 70g fish
- 1/4 cup shriveled spinach (50g new)
- 1 tablespoon mayo squeeze salt and pepper

Guidance
1. Heat the olive oil in a little griddle and fry the sausages and asparagus until cooked through. Move to a plate.
2. Scoop within the avocado and spot it in a bowl, alongside the fish, shriveled spinach, mayo and salt and pepper. Stuff the avocado shell with it and spot on the plate.

SOY AND WITHOUT DAIRY CREAMY SESAME DRESSING

Fixings
- 3 tablespoon mayo
- 2.5 tablespoon coconut aminos
- 1 tablespoon sesame oil
- 1 tablespoon tahini
- 1 tablespoon squashed sesame seeds
- 1 tablespoon sesame seeds
- 1 teaspoon vinegar
- 1/16 teaspoon stevia powder

Guidelines

1. Combine the entirety of the **Fixings** as one in a little bowl. Store in an impermeable holder in the ice chest. Only remix with a spoon before utilize each time.

CHICKEN AND VEGETABLE BROCHETTES

Fixings
- 1 boneless chicken leg (300g)
- 4 asparagus
- 1 enormous asian green onion
- 1 tablespoon lemon juice from a lemon
- 1 tablespoon rosemary
- 10 cherry tomatoes
- 1 tablespoon olive oil
- 1 teaspoon salt and pepper
- 5 garlic cloves
- 1/2 teaspoon onion powder

Directions
1. Preheat the stove to 210C/420F.
2. Dice the chicken leg into scaled down pieces. Cut the long green onion into 12-14 pieces. Cut the asparagus into 4.
3. Add the entirety of the **Fixings** to a bowl and combine as one. Stick the veggies and chicken on 9 brochettes.
4. Spot in the stove and heat for 20 minutes.

EGGS, BACON AND TOMATO SALAD

Fixings
- 3 cuts bacon
- 2 eggs
- 1/4 red pepper
- 1/4 zucchini (40g)
- squeeze salt and pepper
- 3 cuts tomato
- 1 basil leaf
- 1 teaspoon olive oil
- 1 garlic clove
- 1/2 teaspoon vinegar
- sprinkle salt and pepper

Guidelines
1. Cut the red pepper and zucchini.
2. Fry the bacon in a little non-stick griddle until fresh. Put the bacon on a plate. Fry the peppers and zucchini in the bacon fat until delicate, air out the eggs and scramble until cooked. Sprinkle the salt and pepper over. Put on the plate with the bacon.
3. Mince the garlic clove and basil leaf. Blend the olive oil, basil, garlic, vinegar, salt and pepper

together in a little bowl. Add the tomato cuts to the plate and pour the dressing over.

BASIL VINAIGRETTE

Fixings
- 3 tablespoon olive oil
- 1 tablespoon white vinegar
- 1 tablespoon lemon juice
- 3 garlic cloves
- 10 basil leaves
- 1/4 teaspoon salt, pepper

Guidance
1. Pound the garlic cloves utilizing a garlic smasher. Mince the basil leaves. Join the entirety of the **Fixings** into a bowl and blend. Refrigerate until later utilized.

AVOCADO BOAT, SAUSAGES AND SCRAMBLED EGGS

Fixings
- 60g sausage
- 2 eggs
- 2 mushrooms
- 1/4 spinach
- 1 tablespoon olive oil
- squeeze salt and pepper
- 1/2 avocado
- 70g fish can
- 1 tablespoon mayo
- 1 teaspoon cut green onion
- squeeze salt and pepper

Guidelines
1. Cut the mushrooms.
2. Heat the oil in a little non stick griddle and fry the sausages. Once cooked, add them to a plate. Fry the mushrooms and new spinach until delicate and add the eggs. Scramble until cooked, sprinkle the salt and pepper, and add to the plate.
3. Scoop out the inner parts of the avocado, and blend in with the green onions, fish, mayo and salt and pepper in a little bowl. Top off the avocado shell with the bowl Fixings and spot on the plate.

FEATHERY OMELET AND VEGGIES

Fixings
- 1/2 red pepper
- 30g swiss chard
- 3 mushrooms

- 1 teaspoon olive oil
- squeeze salt, pepper, garlic powder
- 2 eggs
- 1 teaspoon olive oil

Guidelines
1. Air out the eggs in a bowl and beat with a hand blender for 3 minutes.
2. Add 1 teaspoon of olive oil to a non-stick skillet and pour the whipped eggs in. Cover and cook on low heat for around 2 minutes, or until the eggs are cooked through. This will be a feathery omelet. Overlap fifty-fifty and slide onto a plate.
3. Dice the red pepper, cut the mushrooms and slash the swiss chard. Heat the oil in a non-stick skillet and add the red peppers. Cook briefly, add the mushrooms and swiss chard and cook until shriveled. Sprinkle the salt, pepper and garlic powder. Spot over the collapsed omelet.

BARBECUED VEGGIES AND FLUFFY OMELET

Fixings
- 1/2 red pepper
- 1/2 cup new spinach
- 3 mushrooms
- 2 tablespoon olive oil
- squeeze salt, pepper, garlic powder
- 3 eggs

Guidelines
1. Air out the eggs in a bowl and beat with a hand blender for 3 minutes.
2. Dice the red pepper, cut the mushrooms and cut the mushrooms. Heat 1 tablespoon of olive oil in a nonstick griddle and add the red peppers. Cook briefly, add the mushrooms and spinach and cook until shriveled. Sprinkle the salt, pepper and garlic powder. Put away.
3. Add 1 tablespoon of olive oil to a non-stick dish and pour the whipped eggs in. Cover and cook on low heat for around 2 minutes, or until the eggs are cooked through. This will be a cushy omelet. Spot the cooked veggies on one side of the omelet and crease into equal parts. Cautiously slide onto a plate.

VEGGIE OMELET

Ingredients
- 2 eggs
- 3 broccoli (40g)
- 1 okra (10g)
- 2 mushrooms (20g)
- 1 breakfast sausage (80g)

- 1/4 zucchini (50g)
- 2 cherry tomatoes
- 1 teaspoon olive oil
- squeeze salt and pepper

Guidelines

1. Cut the broccoli, sausages, mushrooms, zucchini and cherry tomatoes in a couple of pieces.

2. Heat the oil in a medium skillet, and fry the sausage, mushrooms and zucchini cuts for 2-3 minutes until cooked through. Set to the side.

3. Put some water to boil and boil the cut broccoli and okra for 2 mintues. Remove from the boiling water, and cut the okra in 6-8 pieces.

4. Break the eggs into a bowl and rush briefly with a whisk. Pour the egg hitter in a skillet and cook on low heat. Top with the entirety of the veggies and meat, cover and cook until the eggs are cooked through. The omelet should simply slide out of the skillet onto a plate.

EGGS IN MINI SKILLET

Fixings

- 2 cuts bacon
- 2 eggs
- 1/2 avocado
- 1 okra
- 1/2 tomato
- 3 boiled broccoli (50g)
- sprinkle salt, pepper, parsley

Guidance

1. Fry the bacon until firm in a 6" small scale skillet. Slash into bits. Dice the tomato and avocado. Cut the okra into a couple of pieces.

2. In similar smaller than usual skillet, rack the eggs open into the bacon oil, cover and cook on low heat until cooked through. Top with the bacon bits, tomato, avocado, okra and broccoli. Sprinkle the salt, pepper and parsley over.

BROCCOLI, BACON AND POACHED EGG

Fixings

- 1 egg
- 140g broccoli (1/3 head)
- 3 cuts bacon (36g cooked)
- 1 segment sesame dressing
- 1 tablespoon white vinegar
- squeeze salt, pepper, parsley

Directions

1. Put the broccoli to boil in a pot of water and cook until delicate. Take the broccoli out and place on a plate.

2. In an alternate pot, add some water and the white vinegar and put to stew. Add the egg in a bowl. Twirl the water with a spatula and add the egg in the whirlpool. Cover and mood killer the heat and cook the egg for 6 minutes precisely. Cautiously assume it out and position over the broccoli.

3. Fry the bacon in a skillet until firm. Cleave it up into a couple of pieces and spot over the broccoli. Sprinkle the sesame dressing over everything. Sprinkle the salt, pepper and parsley.

BREAKFAST EGG BURRITO

Fixings

- 2 eggs
- 1 teaspoon olive oil
- 2 cuts bacon
- 1 lettuce leaf
- 1/2 avocado
- 1 cut tomato
- 1 tablespoon mayo

Guidance

1. In a Japanese rectangular tamagoyaki skillet, heat 1/2 teaspoon of olive oil. In a little bowl, whisk the two eggs together for 20 seconds or somewhere in the vicinity. Empty portion of the eggs into the skillet, spread out equitably and cook on medium-low heat until the egg is cooked through. Cautiously slide onto a plate. Repeat this progression with the extra egg combination.

2. Fry the bacon until fresh.

3. Cut the avocado in a couple of cuts. Cut the tomato in two. Hack the lettuce.

4. On each egg omelet, spread 1/2 tablespoon of mayo. Cover with the lettuce, tomato, avocado and bacon and cautiously move up like a burrito.

CHICKEN AND HERBS MEATBALLS

Fixings

- 3 shiitake mushrooms (60g)
- 1/2 white onion (90g)
- 2 garlic cloves
- 1 teaspoon olive oil
- 650g ground chicken
- 2-3 stems hacked parsley (8g)
- 10 leaves hacked basil (5g)
- 1 teaspoon thyme, sage
- 1/2 teaspoon onion powder, salt, pepper
- 1/4 teaspoon garlic powder

- 1 egg
- 70g whitened almond flour

Directions

1. Preheat the stove to 200C/400F.
2. Mince the garlic, shiitake and onion.
3. Add the olive oil to a skillet and fry the mushrooms, onions and garlic until delicate. Mood killer heat and move to a bowl.
4. Blend the entirety of the leftover **Fixings** into an enormous bowl and blend until very much fused.
5. Spot a material paper over a preparing plate. Make 12 huge meatballs and spot them on the heating plate cautiously making space between every meatball. The blend is somewhat tacky, however that is fine. It'll cook completely in the broiler.
6. Add to the broiler and cook for 25 minutes. Take out and let cool prior to keeping them in the refrigerator.

ASPARAGUS, BACON AND POACHED EGG

Fixings

- 6 asparagus
- 3 cuts bacon
- 1 egg
- 1 tablespoon sesame dressing
- 1 tablespoon white vinegar
- squeeze parsley

Guidelines

1. Add some water to a little pot and the white vinegar and put to stew. Add the egg in a bowl. Twirl the water with a spatula and add the egg inside the center of the whirlpool. Mood killer the heat and cook the egg for 6 minutes precisely. Cautiously take it out.
2. Fry the bacon until firm. Cut the stems off the asparagus and fry into the bacon oil.
3. Spot the asparagus onto a plate, cover with the bacon and poached egg and spoon the sesame dressing over. Add a touch of parlsey over everything.

BACON, SPINACH AND EGGS

Fixings

- 3 cuts bacon (40g cooked)
- 2 eggs
- 30g spinach
- squeeze salt, pepper

Guidance

1. Fry the bacon until fresh.
2. Cleave the spinach and add to the griddle where the bacon was. Cook in the bacon oil until withered. Air out the eggs over the spinach, cover and cook for 2-3 minutes until the whites are completely cooked.
3. Sprinkle the salt and pepper over the eggs. Slide down onto a plate with the bacon.

STEW CON CARNE

Fixings

- 1/4 little white onion (35)
- 1/2 celery stick (5g)
- 50g earthy colored mushrooms
- 1/4 carrot (50g)
- 1 garlic clove
- 2 tablespoon olive oil
- 200g ground hamburger
- 1.5 cups diced tomato can (400g)
- 1/2 cup water
- 1 tablespoon bean stew powder
- 1/2 tablespoon oregano, tomato glue
- 3/4 teaspoon cumin ground
- 1/2 teaspoon thyme
- 1/4 teaspoon salt, pepper
- 1/8 teaspoon cayenne pepper, garlic powder, onion powder

Guidelines

1. Dice the onion, celery and carrot. Cut the mushrooms. Mince the garlic.
2. Add the olive oil to an enormous pot and add the entirety of the veggies. Cook for 3-4 minutes until delicate. Add the ground meat and cook until carmelized. Add the remainder of the **Fixings** and blend to consolidate. Put on low heat and stew for 10-15 minutes until wanted thickness.

BACON, EGGS AND ASPARAGUS

Fixings

- 1/4 avocado
- 3 bacon cuts
- 4 asparagus
- 1 egg
- squeeze salt and pepper

Guidelines

1. Cut the stems off the asparagus. Cut the avocado. Put some water to boil in a pot and add the asparagus. Cook until delicate.
2. Fry the bacon in a skillet until fresh.

3. Break the egg in the bacon oil and cook it until prepared.
4. Add everything to the plate and sprinkle some salt and pepper over everything.

CHICKEN MEATBALLS AND EGGS

Fixings
- 2 chicken meatballs
- 2 eggs
- 3 broccoli (50g)
- 3 cherry tomatoes
- 1 teaspoon olive oil
- squeeze salt, pepper

Guidelines
1. Put some water to boil in a little pot and add the broccoli. Cook until delicate and add to a plate with the cherry tomatoes. Reheat the chicken meatballs and add to the plate.
2. Heat the olive oil in a skillet and scramble the eggs until entirely cooked. Sprinkle some salt and pepper over.

BACON, SPINACH, EGG AND AVOCADO

Fixings
- 3 cuts bacon
- 1 egg
- 30g spinach
- 1/4 avocado
- squeeze salt, pepper

Guidelines
1. Fry the bacon in a skillet until fresh.
2. Add the spinach in a similar skillet and cook in the bacon oil until shriveled, and afterward move to a plate. Break the egg in the bacon oil and cook until the white is cooked.
3. Cut the avocado. Put everything on a plate and sprinkle some salt and pepper over everything.

CHORIZO BREAKFAST PREPARE

Fixings
- 1 tablespoon olive oil
- ½ cup diced red pepper
- ½ cup diced yellow onion
- 4 ounces chorizo sausage
- 2 huge eggs
- Salt and pepper
- 2 cuts thick-cut bacon, cooked

Guidelines

1.Preheat the broiler to 350°F and delicately oil a two ramekins.
2.Heat the oil in a skillet over medium-high heat.
3.Add the peppers and onions and cook for 4 to 5 minutes until carmelized.
4.Split the vegetable blend between the two ramekins.
5.Hack the chorizo and split between the ramekins.
6.Break an egg into every ramekin and season with salt and pepper to taste.
7.Heat for 10 to 12 minutes until the egg is set to the ideal level.
8.Disintegrate the bacon up and over and serve hot. Makes 2 Servings.

HEATED EGGS IN AVOCADO

Fixings
- 1 tablespoon olive oil
- ½ cup diced red pepper
- ½ cup diced yellow onion
- 4 ounces chorizo sausage
- 2 enormous eggs
- Salt and pepper
- 2 cuts thick-cut bacon, cooked

Guidelines
1. Preheat the stove to 350°F and daintily oil a two ramekins.
2. Heat the oil in a skillet over medium-high heat.
3. Add the peppers and onions and cook for 4 to 5 minutes until seared.
4. Split the vegetable blend between the two ramekins.
5. Cleave the chorizo and split between the ramekins.
6. Break an egg into every ramekin and season with salt and pepper to taste.
7. Heat for 10 to 12 minutes until the egg is set to the ideal level.
8. Disintegrate the bacon up and over and serve hot. Makes 2 Servings.

LEMON POPPY RICOTTA HOTCAKES

Fixings
- 1 enormous lemon, squeezed and zested
- 6 ounces entire milk ricotta
- 3 enormous eggs
- 10 to 12 drops fluid stevia
- ¼ cup almond flour
- 1 scoop egg white protein powder
- 1 tablespoon poppy seeds
- ¾ teaspoons heating powder

- ¼ cup powdered erythritol
- 1 tablespoon weighty cream

Guidelines

1. Join the ricotta, eggs, and fluid stevia in a food processor with a large portion of the lemon juice and the lemon zing – mix well at that point fill a bowl.
2. Race in the almond flour, protein powder, poppy seeds, preparing powder, and a touch of salt.
3. Heat an enormous nonstick dish over medium heat.
4. Spoon the player into the dish, utilizing about ¼ cup per flapjack.
5. Cook the hotcakes until bubbles structure in the outside of the hitter at that point flip them.
6. Allow the flapjacks to cook until the base is carmelized then eliminate to a plate.
7. Repeat with the excess hitter.
8. Whisk together the hefty cream, powdered erythritol, and saved lemon squeeze and zing.
9. Serve the flapjacks hot showered with the lemon coat. Makes 2 Servings.

SWEET BLUEBERRY COCONUT PORRIDGE

Fixings
- 1 cup unsweetened almond milk
- ¼ cup canned coconut milk
- ¼ cup coconut flour
- ¼ cup ground flaxseed
- 1 teaspoon ground cinnamon
- ¼ teaspoon ground nutmeg
- Pinch salt
- 60 grams new blueberries
- ¼ cup shaved coconut

Guidelines

1. Warm the almond milk and coconut milk in a pan over low heat.
2. Speed in the coconut flour, flaxseed, cinnamon, nutmeg, and salt.
3. Turn up the heat and cook until the combination bubbles.
4. Mix in the sugar and vanilla concentrate at that point cook until thickened to the ideal level.
5. Spoon into two dishes and top with blueberries and shaved coconut. Makes 2 **Servings**.

SESAME PORK LETTUCE WRAPS

Fixings
- 1 tablespoon olive oil

- ¼ cup diced yellow onion
- ¼ cup diced green pepper
- 2 tablespoons diced celery
- 6 ounces ground pork
- ¼ teaspoon onion powder
- ¼ teaspoon garlic powder
- 2 tablespoons soy sauce
- 1 teaspoon sesame oil
- 4 leaves spread lettuce, isolated
- 1 tablespoon toasted sesame seeds

Guidelines

1. Heat the oil in a skillet over medium heat.
2. Add the onions, peppers, and celery and sauté for 5 minutes until delicate.
3. Mix in the pork and cook until just carmelized.
4. Add the onion powder and garlic powder at that point mix in the soy sauce and sesame oil.
5. Season with salt and pepper to taste at that point eliminate from heat.
6. Spot the lettuce leaves on a plate and spoon the pork blend equally into them.
7. Sprinkle with sesame seeds to serve.

SPICED PUMPKIN SOUP

Fixings
- 2 tablespoons unsalted spread
- 1 little yellow onion, slashed
- 2 cloves minced garlic
- 1 teaspoon minced ginger
- ½ teaspoon ground cinnamon
- ¼ teaspoon ground nutmeg
- Salt and pepper to taste
- ½ cup pumpkin puree
- 1 cup chicken stock
- 3 cuts thick-cut bacon
- ¼ cup weighty cream

Guidelines

1. Soften the margarine in a huge pan over medium heat.
2. Add the onions, garlic and ginger and cook for 3 to 4 minutes until the onions are clear.
3. Mix in the flavors and cook for 1 moment until fragrant. Season with salt and pepper.
4. Add the pumpkin puree and chicken stock at that point heat to the point of boiling.
5. Decrease heat and stew for 20 minutes at that point eliminate from heat.
6. Puree the soup utilizing an inundation blender at that point get back to heat and stew for 20 minutes.
7. Cook the bacon in a skillet until fresh then eliminate to paper towels to deplete.

8. Add the bacon fat to the soup alongside the weighty cream. Disintegrated the bacon over top to serve. Makes 3 **Servings**.

SIMPLE BEEF CURRY

Fixings

- 1 medium yellow onion, cleaved
- 1 tablespoon minced garlic
- 1 tablespoon ground ginger
- 1 ¼ cups canned coconut milk
- 1 pound hamburger toss, cleaved
- 2 tablespoons curry powder
- 1 teaspoon salt
- ½ cup new cleaved cilantro

Directions

1. Consolidate the onion, garlic and ginger in a food processor and mix into a glue.
2. Move the glue to a pot and cook for 3 minutes on medium heat.
3. Mix in the coconut milk at that point stew delicately for 10 minutes.
4. Add the cleaved hamburger alongside the curry powder and salt.
5. Mix well at that point stew, covered, for 20 minutes.
6. Eliminate the top and stew for an additional 20 minutes until the hamburger is cooked through.
7. Change preparing to taste and embellishment with new slashed cilantro. Makes 3 **Servings**.

AVOCADO LIME SALMON

Fixings

- 100 grams hacked cauliflower
- 1 huge avocado
- 1 tablespoon new lime juice
- 2 tablespoons diced red onion
- 2 tablespoons olive oil
- 2 (6-ounce) boneless salmon filets
- Salt and pepper

Guidelines

1. Spot the cauliflower in a food processor and heartbeat into rice-like grains.
2. Oil a skillet with cooking shower and heat over medium heat.
3. Add the cauliflower rice and cook, covered, for 8 minutes until delicate. Put away.
4. Join the avocado, lime juice and red onion in a food processor and mix smooth.

5. Heat the oil in an enormous skillet over medium-high heat.
6. Season the salmon with salt and pepper at that point add to the skillet skin-side down.
7. Cook for 4 to 5 minutes until burned then flip and cook for another 4 to 5 minutes.
8. Serve the salmon over a bed of cauliflower rice finished off with the avocado cream. Makes 2 **Servings**.

ROSEMARY COOKED CHICKEN AND VEGGIES

Fixings

- 4 deboned chicken thighs
- Salt and pepper
- 1 little zucchini, cut
- 2 little carrots, stripped and cut
- 1 little parsnip, stripped and cut
- 2 cloves garlic, cut
- 3 tablespoons olive oil
- 1 tablespoon balsamic vinegar
- 2 teaspoons new hacked rosemary

Directions

1. Preheat the stove to 350°F and gently oil a little rimmed heating sheet with cooking shower.
2. Spot the chicken thighs on the heating sheet and season with salt and pepper.
3. Organize the veggies around the chicken at that point sprinkle with cut garlic.
4. Whisk together the leftover **Fixings** at that point shower over the chicken and veggies.
5. Prepare for 30 minutes at that point broil for 3 to 5 minutes until the skins are fresh. Makes 2 **Servings**.

MESSY SAUSAGE AND MUSHROOM SKILLET

Fixings

- 1 tablespoon coconut oil
- 6 ounces Italian sausage, disintegrated
- 4 ounces cut mushrooms
- 1 little yellow onion, cleaved
- ½ teaspoon dried oregano
- ¼ teaspoon dried thyme
- Salt and pepper
- ¼ cup marinara sauce
- ¼ cup water
- ½ cup destroyed mozzarella cheddar

Guidelines

1. Preheat the broiler to 350°F.

2. Heat the oil in enormous cast-iron skillet over medium heat until smoking.
3. Add the sausages and cook until carmelized and nearly cooked through.
4. Eliminate the sausages to a cutting board and let cool for a couple of moments.
5. Add the mushroom and onion to the skillet and cook for 3 to 4 minutes until carmelized.
6. Cut the sausages and add them back to the skillet.
7. Mix in the oregano, thyme, salt and pepper.
8. Pour in the sauce and water at that point mix well. Move the skillet to the stove and cook for 10 minutes.
9. Sprinkle with mozzarella at that point cook an additional 5 minutes until liquefied. Makes 2 **Servings**.

SHEEP CHOPS WITH ROSEMARY AND GARLIC

Fixings

- 1 tablespoon coconut oil, dissolved
- 1 teaspoon new hacked rosemary
- 1 clove garlic, minced
- 2 bone-in sheep slashes (around 6 ounces meat)
- 1 tablespoon margarine
- Salt and pepper
- ¼ pound new asparagus, managed
- 1 tablespoon olive oil

Guidelines

1. Consolidate the coconut oil, rosemary, and garlic in a shallow dish.
2. Add the sheep slashes at that point go to cover – let marinate in the ice chest short term.
3. Allow the sheep to rest at room temperature for 30 minutes.
4. Heat the spread in a huge skillet over medium-high heat.
5. Add the sheep hacks and cook for 6 minutes at that point season with salt and pepper.
6. Turn the slashes and cook for an additional 6 minutes or until cooked to the ideal level.
7. Let the sheep cleaves rest for 5 minutes prior to serving.
8. Then, throw the asparagus with olive oil, salt and pepper at that point spread on a heating sheet.
9. Broil for 6 to 8 minutes until scorched, shaking once in a while. Serve hot with the sheep hacks.
10.

FAT-BUSTING VANILLA PROTEIN SMOOTHIE

Fixings

- 1 scoop (20g) vanilla egg white protein powder
- ½ cup weighty cream
- ¼ cup vanilla almond milk
- 4 ice blocks
- 1 tablespoon coconut oil
- 1 tablespoon powdered erythritol
- ½ teaspoon vanilla concentrate
- ¼ cup whipped cream

Guidelines

1. Join the entirety of the Fixings aside from the whipped cream in a blender.
2. Mix on fast for 30 to 60 seconds until smooth.
3. Fill a glass and top with whipped cream.

APPETIZING HAM AND CHEDDAR WAFFLES

Fixings

- 4 huge eggs, separated
- 2 scoops (40g) egg white protein powder
- 1 teaspoon preparing powder
- 1/3 cup dissolved margarine
- ½ teaspoon salt
- 1 ounce diced ham
- ¼ cup destroyed cheddar

Directions

1. Separate two of the eggs and put the other two away.
2. Beat 2 of the egg yolks with the protein powder, heating powder, margarine, and salt in a blending bowl.
3. Overlap in the slashed ham and ground cheddar.
4. Whisk the egg whites in a different bowl with a spot of salt until firm pinnacles structure.
5. Overlap the beaten egg whites into the egg yolk combination in two bunches.
6. Oil a preheated waffle producer at that point spoon ¼ cup of the hitter into it and close it.
7. Cook until the waffle is brilliant earthy colored, around 3 to 4 minutes, at that point eliminate.
8. Reheat the waffle iron and repeat with the excess hitter.

9. In the mean time, heat the oil in a skillet and fry the eggs with salt and pepper.

10. Serve the waffles hot, finished off with a singed egg. Makes 2 **Servings**.

MOZZARELLA VEGGIE-STACKED QUICHE

Fixings

- 6 tablespoons almond flour
- 1 tablespoon ground parmesan cheddar
- 2 enormous eggs, partitioned
- 2 cuts thick-cut bacon
- ¼ cup frozen spinach, defrosted and depleted well
- ¼ cup diced zucchini
- ¼ cup destroyed mozzarella cheddar
- 4 cherry tomatoes, split
- 1 tablespoon hefty cream
- 1 teaspoon slashed chives

Guidelines

1. Mix together the almond flour and ground parmesan with one egg and a touch of salt until it shapes a delicate mixture.

2. Press the mixture into the lower part of a little quiche dish as equitably as could be expected.

3. Score the base and sides of the batter at that point prepare for 7 minutes at 325°F and let cool.

4. Cook the bacon in a skillet until sautéed then disintegrate and spread in the quiche container.

5. Sprinkle in the spinach, zucchini, cheddar, and tomatoes.

6. Whisk together the leftover egg with the hefty cream, chives, salt and pepper at that point fill the quiche. Prepare for 22 to 25 minutes until the egg is set at that point serve hot.

PEPPER JACK SAUSAGE EGG MUFFINS

Fixings

- 10 ounces ground breakfast sausage
- ½ cup diced yellow onion
- ¼ teaspoon garlic powder
- Salt and pepper
- 3 huge eggs, whisked
- 2 tablespoons substantial cream
- ½ cup destroyed pepper jack cheddar

Directions

1. Preheat the stove to 350°F and oil three ramekins with cooking splash.

2. Mix together the ground sausage, diced onion, garlic powder, salt and pepper in a blending bowl.

3. Separation the sausage blend equally in the ramekins, squeezing it into the base and sides, leaving the center open.

4. Whisk together the eggs and substantial cream with salt and pepper.

5. Split the egg combination between the sausage cups and top with destroyed cheddar.

6. Heat for 25 to 30 minutes until the eggs are set and the cheddar seared. Makes three Servings.

SIMPLE CHEESEBURGER SALAD

Fixings

- 7 ounces ground hamburger
- Salt and pepper
- 3 tablespoons mayonnaise
- 1 tablespoon diced pickles
- 1 teaspoon mustard
- ½ teaspoon ketchup
- Pinch smoked paprika
- 3 ounces hacked romaine lettuce
- 1/3 cup diced tomatoes
- ¼ cup destroyed cheddar

Directions

1. Earthy colored the ground meat over high heat at that point season with salt and pepper to taste.

2. Channel the fat from the hamburger and eliminate from heat.

3. Join the mayonnaise, pickles, mustard, ketchup, and paprika in a blender.

4. Mix the combination until smooth and very much consolidated.

5. Join the lettuce, tomatoes, and cheddar in a blending bowl.

6. Throw in the ground hamburger and the dressing until equitably covered. Makes 2 Servings.

SEARED PEPPERONI PIZZAS

Fixings

- 6 enormous eggs
- 6 tablespoons ground parmesan cheddar
- 3 tablespoons psyllium husk powder
- 1 ½ teaspoons Italian flavoring
- 3 tablespoons olive oil
- 9 tablespoons low-carb pureed tomatoes, partitioned
- 4 ½ ounces destroyed mozzarella, partitioned
- 1 ½ ounces diced pepperoni, partitioned
- 3 tablespoons new hacked basil

Guidelines

1. Join the eggs, parmesan, and psyllium husk powder with the Italian flavoring and a touch of salt in a blender.
2. Mix until smooth and very much consolidated, around 30 seconds, at that point rest for 5 minutes.
3. Heat 1 tablespoon of oil in a skillet over medium-high heat.
4. Spoon 1/3 of the hitter into the skillet and spread in a circle at that point cook until carmelized underneath.
5. Flip the pizza outside and cook until sautéed on the opposite side.
6. Eliminate the outside to a foil-fixed heating sheet and repeat with the leftover player.
7. Spoon 3 tablespoons of low-carb pureed tomatoes over each outside.
8. Top with diced pepperoni and destroyed cheddar at that point broil until the cheddar is cooked.
9. Sprinkle with new basil at that point cut the pizza to serve. Makes 3 pizzas.

CHICKEN ZOODLE ALFREDO

Fixings
- 2 (6-ounce) chicken bosoms
- 1 tablespoon olive oil
- Salt and pepper
- 2 tablespoons margarine
- ¼ cup weighty cream
- ¼ cup ground parmesan cheddar
- 200 grams zucchini

Guidelines
1. Heat the oil in an enormous skillet over medium-high heat.
2. Season the chicken with salt and pepper to taste at that point add to the skillet.
3. Cook for 6 to 7 minutes on each side until cooked through then cut into strips.
4. Reheat the skillet over medium-low heat and add the spread.
5. Mix in the hefty cream and parmesan cheddar at that point cook until thickened.
6. Spiralize the zucchini at that point throw it into the sauce blend with the chicken.
7. Cook until the zucchini is delicate, around 2 minutes, at that point serve hot. Makes 2 Servings. +

CABBAGE AND SAUSAGE SKILLET

Fixings
- 6 huge Italian sausage joins
- ½ head green cabbage, cut
- 2 tablespoons margarine
- ¼ cup harsh cream
- ¼ cup mayonnaise
- Salt and pepper

Guidelines
1. Cook the sausage in a skillet over medium-high heat until equitably seared then cut them.
2. Reheat the skillet over medium-high heat at that point add the margarine.
3. Throw in the cabbage and cook until shriveled, around 3 to 4 minutes.
4. Mix the cut sausage into the cabbage at that point mix in the acrid cream and mayonnaise.
5. Season with salt and pepper at that point stew for 10 minutes. Makes 4 Servings.

GYRO SALAD WITH AVO-TZATZIKI

Fixings
- 1 tablespoon olive oil
- 1 pound ground sheep meat
- ½ medium yellow onion, diced
- ¼ cup chicken stock
- 4 teaspoons lemon juice, separated
- ½ teaspoon dried oregano
- ½ teaspoon dried thyme
- ½ English cucumber
- 1 medium ready avocado
- 2 teaspoons new slashed mint
- 1 teaspoon new slashed dill
- 6 cups slashed romaine lettuce

Guidelines
1. Heat the oil in an enormous skillet over medium-high heat and add the sheep.
2. Cook for 3 minutes, blending regularly, at that point mix in the onion.
3. Continue to cook until the sheep is cooked through and the onion relaxed then mix in the chicken stock, 2 teaspoons lemon juice, oregano, and thyme.
4. Season with salt and pepper to taste at that point stew for 5 minutes.
5. Mesh the cucumber at that point spread equitably on a clear towel and wring out the dampness.
6. Spot the ground cucumber in a food processor and add the avocado, 2 teaspoons lemon juice, mint and dill with a touch of salt. Mix the combination until smooth.
7. Serve the gyro meat over hacked lettuce with a spoonful of avo-tzatziki. Makes 3 Servings.

SIMPLE CLOUD BUNS

Fixings
- 3 huge eggs, isolated
- 1/8 teaspoon cream of tartar

- 3 ounces cream cheddar, cleaved

Directions

1. Preheat the stove to 300°F and fix a preparing sheet with material.

2. Beat the egg whites until frothy then beat in the cream of tartar until the whites are glossy and obscure with delicate pinnacles.

3. In a different bowl, beat the cream cheddar and egg yolks until all around joined then crease in the egg white combination.

4. Spoon the player onto the preparing sheet in ¼-cup circles around 2 inches separated.

5. Prepare for 30 minutes until the buns are firm to the touch. Makes 10 Servings.

BACON BREAKFAST BOMBS

Fixings

- 4 cuts thick-cut bacon
- 2 huge eggs
- ¼ cup cubed spread
- 2 tablespoons mayonnaise
- Salt and pepper

Directions

1. Cook the bacon in a huge skillet over medium-high heat until fresh.

2. Allow the bacon to cool a little at that point cleave it up and put it away, saving the bacon oil.

3. Fill a pan with water and a spot of salt at that point heat to the point of boiling.

4. Add the eggs and boil them for 10 minutes prior to moving to an ice water shower.

5. Allow the eggs to cool at that point strip them and cleave them coarsely.

6. Squash the hacked eggs with the spread at that point mix in the mayonnaise, salt, and pepper.

7. Mix in the saved bacon oil at that point cover the blend and chill for 30 minutes.

8. Gap the egg combination in six parts and fold them into balls at that point move in the squashed bacon.

9. Serve quickly and store the extras in the ice chest. Makes 2 Servings of 3 bombs.

APPLE DUMPLINGS

Fixings

- 2 Tbsp. raisins
- 2 little apples (stripped—cored)
- 1 Tbsp. earthy colored sugar
- 2 sheets puff baked good
- 2 Tbsp. softened margarine

Guidelines

✓ Preheat the Air Fryer to 356°F.

✓ Blend the sugar and raisins.

✓ Spot every apple on one of the baked good sheets and load up with the raisins/sugar.

✓ Overlap the baked good over until the apple and raisins are completely covered.

✓ Spot them on a piece of foil so they can't fall through the fryer.

✓ Completely brush them with the dissolved margarine.

✓ Set the clock for 25 minutes. It is prepared when the apples are sold and cooked.

Note: Make certain to utilize minuscule apples for this yummy treat.

BANANA BREAKFAST

Fixings

- 8 ready stripped bananas
- 3 Tbsp. corn flour
- One egg white
- 3 Tbsp. vegetable oil
- ¾ cup breadcrumbs

Directions

1) Preheat the fryer at 356°F.

2) In a skillet utilizing the low warmth setting; pour the oil and throw in the breadcrumbs, cooking until brilliant earthy colored.

3) Utilize the flour to cover the bananas; dunk them into the egg white, and coat them with the bread morsels.

4) Spot the bananas on a solitary layer of the bushel and air fry for eight minutes.

5) Eliminate and sit on paper towels.

What a delectable treat to be served warm!

Tip: On the off chance that you have an excessive number of breadcrumbs; you can put them in the ice chest in an impermeable holder to utilize soon.

FRENCH TOAST STICKS

Fixings

- 2 delicately beaten eggs
- 4 cuts of wanted bread
- 2 tablespoons delicate margarine or spread
- Cinnamon
- Salt
- Ground cloves
- Nutmeg
- Topping: Maple syrup

Guidelines

1) Preheat the Air Fryer to 356ºF.

2) Whisk the eggs, a shake of nutmeg, cloves, and cinnamon together in a little bowl.

3) Spread margarine on the two sides of the bread, and cut them into strips.

4) Dig every one of the cuts in the egg blend, and orchestrate in the fryer. (You should make two clusters.)

5) Respite the fryer following two minutes, eliminate the dish, and shower the bread with cooking splash.

6) Flip and shower the opposite side, returning them to the AF for an extra four minutes, igniting sure they don't.

7) It's prepared when it is brilliant earthy colored; serve them right away.

Embellishment with some maple syrup or whipped cream. **Yields**: Two Servings

BACON AND EGGS

Fixings
- 4 eggs
- 12 (1/2-inch thick) cuts of bacon
- Pepper and salt
- 1 Tablespoon margarine
- 2 cut croissants
- 4 Tablespoons relaxed spread

Bar-b-que Sauce Fixings
- 1 C. ketchup
- ¼ C. apple juice vinegar

2 Tablespoons each:
- •Brown sugar
- •Molasses
- ½ teaspoon each:
- Onion powder
- Mustard powder
- 1 Tablespoon Worcestershire sauce
- ½ teaspoon fluid smoke

Directions
1) Preset the temperature Noticeable all around Fryer to 390ºF.

2) On the burner, utilizing medium warmth—blend the molasses, ketchup, earthy colored sugar, vinegar, onion powder, and mustard power utilizing a little saucepot. Whisk the fluid smoke and Worcestershire sauce into the combination to mix altogether. Cook until the sauce thickens. Add extra seasoning as wanted.

3) Spot the bacon on the plate and cook for five minutes. Eliminate and brush the bacon with the grill sauce – flip—and brush the opposite side—get back to the cooker and keep cooking an additional five minutes.

4) Margarine the divided croissant and toast it in the fryer.

5) Meanwhile, utilize a non-stick skillet utilizing the prescription low setting on the burner—dissolve the spread. Add four eggs to the skillet, cooking until the white beginnings setting—flip and cook around thirty additional seconds.

6) Eliminate from the dish, and appreciate with the bacon and croissant.

Yields: Four Servings

MESSY MUSHROOM, HAM, AND EGG

Fixings
- 3 cuts nectar shaved ham
- 1 croissant
- 4 split cherry tomatoes
- 4 little quartered button mushrooms
- 1 egg
- 1.8 ounces mozzarella or cheddar
- Discretionary: ½ generally slashed rosemary branch

Guidelines
1) Softly oil a heating dish with spread to keep the blend from staying.

2) Preset the Air Fryer to 320ºF.

3) Spot the **Fixings** on 2 layers with cheddar in the middle and top layer.

4) Make a space in the focal point of the ham and break the egg.

5) Sprinkle the rosemary and a dab of salt and pepper for seasoning over the combination.

6) Put it into the preheated bin for eight minutes. Remove the croissant from the AF following four minutes to permit more opportunity for the egg to cook.

Yields: One Serving

FRIED EGGS

Fixings
- 2 eggs
- Pepper and salt to taste

Directions
1) Preset the Air Fryer to 284ºF for around five minutes.

2) Put the margarine in the fryer to soften, and spread it out uniformly.

3) Void the eggs and some other **Fixings** like cheddar or tomatoes.

4) Open the AF like clockwork to speed to the ideal

yellow and soft consistency. Make a fried egg sandwich or with toast as an afterthought.

AIR FRYER SPINACH FRITTATA

For a phenomenal feast useful for breakfast, lunch, dinnertime, or whenever; you have discovered it!

Fixings
- 1/3 bundle (or thereabouts) of spinach
- 1 little minced red onion
- Mozzarella cheddar
- 3 eggs

Guidelines
1) Preset the Air Fryer at 356ºF for at any rate three minutes.
2) Add oil to a heating prospect minute.
3) Add the onions and keep cooking for a few minutes; throw in the spinach and cook three to five minutes extra minutes.
4) Race in the eggs, add the flavors, cheddar, and add to the container.
5) Cook for eight minutes. Season with salt and pepper.

BACON WRAPPED POTATO TODDLERS

Fixings
- 3 tablespoons harsh cream
- 1 pound cut bacon (medium)
- 1 enormous sack firm potato toddlers
- 4 scallions
- ½ cup destroyed cheddar

Guidelines
1) Preheat the Air Fryer to 400ºF.
2) Envelop every one of the toddlers by bacon and spot them into the fryer crate. Try not to pack, keep them in a solitary layer.
3) Set the AF clock for 8 minutes.
4) When the clock blares; place the toddlers on a plate.
5) Present with the scallions and cheddar embellish.
6) Add a scramble of harsh cream and appreciate.
Yields: Four Servings

BUTTERMILK ROLLS

These must be considered for breakfast additionally in light of the fact that they are so heavenly!

Fixings
- ½ C. cake flour
- ¾ tsp. salt
- 1-¼ C. generally useful flour
- ¼ tsp. preparing pop
- 1 teaspoon granulated sugar
- ½ tsp. preparing powder
- ¾ C. buttermilk
- 4 Tbsp. unsalted virus spread (cut into solid shapes) + soften 1 Tbsp.

Discretionary for Serving:
- Nectar or jelly
- Spread

Note: Extra flour is required for cleaning the counter or cutting board.

Directions
1. Preheat the Air Fryer to 400ºF.
2. Filter together the generally useful flour, sugar, cake flour, preparing pop, and the salt in a medium blending dish.
3. Utilize a baked good shaper (or your fingers) to mix the **Fixings** into pea-sized consistency. Pour in the buttermilk and mix utilizing an elastic spatula (or your hands), and make a batter ball. Make an effort not to over-blend the mixture.
4. Sprinkle some flour on the counter surface and start to press the batter into about a ½-inch thickness. It ought to be around eight crawls in breadth.
5. Utilize a shaper to cut the mixture into rolls; plunge the tip of the tip of the shaper with the flour making a quick cut. In the event that you turn the mixture; it could keep it from rising.
6. Spot the bread rolls in a container and brush them with the softened spread. Spot the mixture in the bushel of the fryer and set the clock for eight minutes.
7. Appreciate the completed item for certain nectar or your #1 jam, jam, or jam.

VEGGIE LOVER SMALLER THAN EXPECTED BACON WRAPPED BURRITOS

Fixings

- 2 **Servings** Tofu Scramble or Veggie lover Egg
- 2-3 tablespoons tamari
- 2 tablespoons cashew spread
- 1-2 tablespoons water
- 1-2 tablespoons fluid smoke
- 4 bits of rice paper
- Vegetable Add-Ins
- 8 strips broiled red pepper
- 1/3 cup yam broiled shapes
- 1 little sautéed tree broccoli
- Modest bunch of greens (kale, spinach, and so forth)
- 6-8 stalks of new asparagus

Directions

1) Line the container utilized for preparing with material. Preheat the Air Fryer to 350ºF.

2) Whisk the tamari, cashew spread, water, and fluid smoke; set aside.

3) Set up the fillings.

4) Hold a rice paper under cool running water—getting the two sides wet—simply a second. Spot on the plate to fill.

5) Start by filling the **Fixings** – just-off-from the middle—leaving the sides of the paper free.

6) Crease in two of the sides as you would when you make a burrito. Seal them and dunk every one in the fluid smoke blend—covering totally.

7) Cook until fresh; generally around eight to ten minutes.

Yields: Four Small Burritos

PORK HOTDOG PATTIES

It's not difficult to make your own hotdog, yet you can likewise control what goes into the food. This hotdog can be made in bigger bunches and can be handily frozen for future morning suppers!

Involved Time: 10 minutes
Cook Time: 20 minutes
Fixings | **Yields** 8 frankfurter patties

- 12 ounces lean ground pork
- 1 teaspoon new thyme leaves
- 1 tablespoon earthy colored sugar
- Squeeze ground nutmeg
- 1/4 teaspoon salt
- 1/4 teaspoon newly ground dark pepper
- 1 tablespoon water

1. Preheat air fryer at 350°F for 3 minutes.

2. In an enormous bowl, join pork, thyme, sugar, nutmeg, salt, and pepper. Structure into eight patties.

3. Empty water into lower part of air fryer. Spot four patties in fryer container and cook 5 minutes. Flip patties. Cook an extra 5 minutes. Rehash with residual patties.

4. Move to a plate and serve warm.

Per serving Calories: 58 | Fat: 1.6 g | Protein: 8.9 g | Sodium: 97 mg | Fiber: 0.0 g | Starches: 1.2 g | Sugar: 1.1 g

ZESTY SCOTCH EGGS

A Scotch egg is a gastropub exemplary made by framing wiener or meat around a cooked egg, covering it in bread pieces, and afterward profound browning it. With the air fryer, you avoid the shower in hot oil and go straight for the decency without the entirety of the blame.

Active Time: 5 minutes
Cook Time: 12 minutes
Fixings | **Yields** 4 eggs

- 1/2 pound ground chorizo, free or eliminated from housings
- 4 delicate bubbled eggs, stripped
- 1 huge egg
- 1 cup plain bread pieces

1. Preheat air fryer at 375°F for 3 minutes.

2. Tenderly structure chorizo around stripped eggs.

3. In a little bowl, whisk enormous egg. In another little bowl, add bread morsels.

4. Plunge chorizo canvassed eggs in whisked egg and afterward dig in bread scraps.

5. Spot eggs in air fryer bin. Cook 6 minutes. Turn. Cook an extra 6 minutes. Serve warm.

Per serving Calories: 322 | fat: 22.2 g | protein: 19.7 g | sodium: 775 mg | fiber: 0.3 g | carbs: 6.2 g | sugar: 0.7

MAPLE-SAGE BREAKFAST CONNECTIONS

The maple syrup loans a pleasantness against the exquisite flavors and the pinelike kind of the sage. Also, these connections are drained of any additives and fillers that locally acquired partners might be loaded up with.

Involved Time: 10 minutes

Cook Time: 9 minutes

Fixings | **Yields** 8 frankfurter connections

- 12 ounces ground gentle pork hotdog, free or eliminated from housings
- 1 teaspoon scoured sage
- 2 tablespoons unadulterated maple syrup
- Squeeze cayenne pepper
- ¼ teaspoon salt
- ¼ teaspoon newly ground dark pepper
- 1 tablespoon water

1. Preheat air fryer at 350°F for 3 minutes.
2. Join pork, sage, maple syrup, cayenne pepper, salt, and dark pepper. Structure into eight connections.
3. Empty water into lower part of air fryer. Spot joins in air fryer bushel. Cook 9 minutes.
4. Move to a plate and serve warm.

Per serving Calories: 130 | fat: 8.8 g | protein: 6.5 g | sodium: 483 mg | fiber: 0.1 g | starches: 4.9 g | sugar: 3.3 g

AIR-SEARED MAPLE BACON

What's superior to bacon? Maple bacon! This sweet and pungent treat will awaken you cheerfully. It's likewise tasty on breakfast sandwiches, crushed up into your number one **Servings** of mixed greens, and surprisingly plunged in a little chocolate for some bacon candy. Evil, genuinely wicked!

Involved Time: 5 minutes
Cook Time: 12 minutes

Fixings | **Serves:** 4
- 2 tablespoons water
- 4 cuts bacon, divided
- 2 teaspoons maple syrup, isolated

1. Preheat air fryer at 400°F for 3 minutes.
2. Empty water into lower part of air fryer. Spot 4 bacon parts in air fryer container. Cook 3 minutes. Flip bacon. Brush 1 teaspoon maple syrup on bacon. Cook an extra 3 minutes. Move to a paper towel-lined plate.
3. Rehash with residual bacon and serve warm.

Per serving Calories: 51 | fat: 3.0 g | protein: 3.6 g | sodium: 162 mg | fiber: 0.0 g | starches: 2.2 g | sugar: 2.0 g

GARLIC PARMESAN CHICKEN WINGS

Garlic Parmesan is a rich, messy combination that is an ideal sauce for flavorful wings. Regardless of whether they're for game day with your companions or an organization potluck, these wings will be the star of any hors d'oeuvre plate!

Involved Time: 5 minutes
Cook Time: 25 minutes
Serves: 4
Fixings
- 2 pounds crude chicken wings
- 1 teaspoon pink Himalayan salt
- ½ teaspoon garlic powder
- 1 tablespoon heating powder
- 4 tablespoons unsalted margarine, softened
- ⅓ cup ground Parmesan cheddar
- ¼ teaspoon dried parsley

1 In an enormous bowl, place chicken wings, salt, ½ teaspoon garlic powder, and heating powder, at that point throw. Spot wings into the air fryer bin.
2 Change the temperature to 400°F and set the clock for 25 minutes.
3 Throw the bushel a few times during the cooking time.
4 In a little bowl, join spread, Parmesan, and parsley.
5 Eliminate wings from the fryer and spot into a perfect enormous bowl. Pour the spread combination over the wings and throw until covered. Serve warm.

Per serving Calories: 565
Protein: 41.8 g Fiber: 0.1 g
Net sugars: 2.1 g Fat: 42.1 g Sodium: 1,067 mg
Sugars: 2.2 g

FIERY BISON CHICKEN PLUNGE

This game day exemplary packs a lot of protein and genuine warmth. With only a couple basic **Fixings**, you'll have a gooey, delicious plunge to fill in as the ideal ally for establishing in your number one group. Avoid the chips and rather plunge celery sticks for a sublime and nutritious smash in each nibble!

Active Time: 10 minutes
Cook Time: 10 minutes
Serves: 4
- 1 cup cooked, diced chicken bosom
- 8 ounces full-fat cream cheddar, mollified
- ½ cup bison sauce
- ⅓ cup full-fat farm dressing
- ⅓ cup hacked cured jalapeños
- 1½ cups destroyed medium cheddar, separated
- 2 scallions, cut on the predisposition

1. Spot chicken into a huge bowl. Add cream cheddar, bison sauce, and farm dressing. Mix until the sauces are all around blended and generally smooth. Overlap in jalapeños and 1 cup Cheddar.
2. Empty the blend into a 4-cup round preparing dish and spot remaining Cheddar on top. Spot dish into the air fryer crate.
3. Change the temperature to 350°F and set the clock for 10 minutes.
4. At the point when done, the top will be earthy colored and the plunge gurgling. Top with cut scal-lions. Serve warm.

Per serving Calories: 472
Protein: 25.6 g Fiber: 0.6 g Net sugars: 8.5 g
Fat: 32.0 g Sodium: 1,532 mg Sugar: 7.4 g

BACON JALAPEÑO CHEDDAR BREAD

Needing a late-night extravagance that feels like you're undermining your eating routine? Your air fryer can assist with that! This cheddar bread is an appetizing magnum opus that you will not have any desire to share!

Involved Time: 10 minutes
Cook Time: 15 minutes
Yields 8 sticks (2 sticks for every serving)
- 2 cups destroyed mozzarella cheddar
- ¼ cup ground Parmesan cheddar
- ¼ cup cleaved cured jalapeños
- 2 huge eggs
- 4 cuts without sugar bacon, cooked and cleaved

1. Blend all Fixings in a huge bowl. Slice a piece ot material to accommodate your air fryer crate.
2. Hose your hands with a touch of water and press out the blend into a circle. You may have to isolate this into two more modest cheddar breads, contingent upon the size of your fryer.
3. Spot the material and cheddar bread into the air fryer crate.
4. Change the temperature to 320°F and set the clock for 15 minutes.
5. Cautiously flip the bread when 5 minutes remain.
6. When completely cooked, the top will be brilliant earthy colored. Serve warm.

Per serving Calories: 273
Protein: 20.1 g Fiber: 0.1 g Net carbs: 2.1 g
Fat: 18.1 g Sodium: 749 mg Carbs: 2.3 g Sugar: 0.7 g

CHOCOLATE CHIP BISCUITS

These cushy biscuits are an extraordinary method to begin your day with somewhat of a treat. In not more than minutes you'll have a group satisfying, sans sugar keto breakfast without warming up your stove. Biscuits will keep in a canvassed compartment in the fridge for as long as 4 days.

Pantry Staples: Preparing powder
Hands On schedule: 5 minutes
Cook Time: 15 minutes
Yields 6 biscuits

- 1½ cups whitened finely ground almond flour
- ⅓ cup granular earthy colored erythritol
- 4 tablespoons salted spread, softened
- 2 huge eggs, whisked
- 1 tablespoon preparing powder
- ½ cup low-carb chocolate chips

1. In a huge bowl, join all **Fixings** . Equitably empty player into six silicone biscuit cups lubed with cooking splash.
2. Spot biscuit cups into air fryer bushel. Change the temperature to 320°F and set the clock for 15 minutes. Biscuits will be brilliant earthy colored when done.
3. Allow biscuits to cool in cups 15 minutes to abstain from disintegrating. Serve warm.

Per serving (1 biscuit)
Calories: 329 Protein: 10g Fiber: 8g
Net sugars: 4g Sugar liquor: 16g Fat: 29g
Sodium: 328mg Sugars: 28g Sugar: 1g

BLUEBERRY BISCUITS

In case you're searching for the ideal breakfast biscuits made instantly, this formula will get your day going right. Shockingly better, you can make them early, hold up them, and warmth them up in your air fryer for 3 minutes at 350°F when you're prepared to appreciate!
Pantry Staples: Heating powder
Hands On schedule: 5 minutes
Cook Time: 15 minutes
Yields 6 biscuits

- 1½ cups whitened finely ground almond flour
- ½ cup granular erythritol
- 4 tablespoons salted margarine, dissolved
- 2 enormous eggs, whisked

- 2 teaspoons heating powder
- ⅓ cup new blueberries, slashed

1. In an enormous bowl, consolidate all **Fixings** . Equally empty hitter into six silicone biscuit cups lubed with cooking shower.
2. Spot biscuit cups into air fryer container. Change the temperature to 320°F and set the clock for 15 minutes. Biscuits ought to be brilliant earthy colored when done.
3. Allow biscuits to cool in cups 15 minutes to abstain from disintegrating. Serve warm.

Per serving (1 biscuit) Calories: 269
Protein: 8g Fiber: 3g Net carbs: 4g
Sugar liquor: 16g Fat: 24g Sodium: 165mg
Carbs: 23g Sugar: 2g

ZEST BISCUITS

Allspice is a sweet-smelling mix that may help you to remember cloves or cinnamon. On the off chance that you don't have any close by, you can substitute an equivalent measure of pumpkin pie zest. This blend of fall flavors will carry an additional piece of comfort to your day, particularly when served close by a warm mug of espresso or tea.

Pantry Staples: Heating powder
Hands On schedule: 5 minutes
Cook Time: 15 minutes
Yields 6 biscuits
Fixings
- 1 cup whitened finely ground almond flour
- ¼ cup granular erythritol
- 2 tablespoons salted margarine, liquefied
- 1 enormous egg, whisked
- 2 teaspoons heating powder
- 1 teaspoon ground allspice

1. In an enormous bowl, join all **Fixings** . Equally empty player into six silicone biscuit cups lubed with cooking shower.
2. Spot biscuit cups into air fryer bin. Change the temperature to 320°F and set the clock for 15 minutes. Cooked biscuits ought to be brilliant earthy colored.
3. Let biscuits cool in cups 15 minutes to abstain from disintegrating. Serve warm.

Per serving (1 biscuit) Calories: 160
Protein: 5g Fiber: 2g
Net carbs: 2g Sugar liquor: 16g
Fat: 14g Sodium: 123mg Carbs: 20g

BACON, EGG, AND CHEDDAR CALZONES

This straightforward formula is incredible for making ahead and taking in a hurry. These delectable, messy calzones warm well and make for a superfilling and delicious breakfast. The keto "breading" is cushy, which gives it that extreme solace food feel.

Hands On schedule: 15 minutes
Cook Time: 12 minutes
Serves: 4
Fixings
- 2 enormous eggs
- 1 cup whitened finely ground almond flour
- 2 cups destroyed mozzarella cheddar
- 2 ounces cream cheddar, relaxed and broken into little pieces
- 4 cuts cooked sans sugar bacon, disintegrated

1. Beat eggs in a little bowl. Fill a medium nonstick skillet over medium warmth and scramble. Put away.
2. In a huge microwave-safe bowl, blend flour and mozzarella. Add cream cheddar to bowl.
3. Spot bowl in microwave and cook 45 seconds on high to dissolve cheddar, at that point mix with a fork until a delicate mixture ball structures.
4. Slice a piece of material to fit air fryer container. Separate batter into two areas and press each out into a 8" round.
5. On portion of every mixture round, place half of the fried eggs and disintegrated bacon. Overlap the opposite side of the mixture over and press to seal the edges.
6. Spot calzones on ungreased material and into air fryer bushel. Change the temperature to 350°F and set the clock for 12 minutes, turning calzones partially through cooking. Outside layer will be brilliant and firm when done.
7. Let calzones cool on a cooking rack 5 minutes prior to serving.

Per serving Calories: 477
Protein: 28g Fiber: 3g Net starches: 7g
Fat: 35g Sodium: 665mg
Sugar: 3g

Eggs are an extraordinary wellspring of protein, and probably the least demanding base for a good keto breakfast. No compelling reason to start up the skillet for this formula, however—the entirety of the scrumptious flavors meet up in minutes in your air fryer.

Pantry Staples: Salt, ground dark pepper
Hands On schedule: 5 minutes
Cook Time: 15 minutes
Serves: 2
Fixings
- 3 enormous eggs
- 1 tablespoon salted margarine, softened
- ¼ cup cultivated and slashed green chime pepper
- 2 tablespoons stripped and hacked yellow onion
- ¼ cup slashed cooked no-sugar-added ham
- ¼ teaspoon salt
- ¼ teaspoon ground dark pepper

1. Break eggs into an ungreased 6" round nonstick heating dish. Blend in spread, chime pepper, onion, ham, salt, and dark pepper.
2. Spot dish into air fryer container. Change the temperature to 320°F and set the clock for 15 minutes. The eggs will be completely cooked and firm in the center when done.
3. Cut fifty-fifty and serve warm on two medium plates.

Per serving Calories: 201 Protein: 13g Fiber: 1g Net sugars: 2g Fat: 14g Sodium: 650mg

C I N N A M O N   R O L L S

Try not to be scared by the mozzarella—the cinnamon flavor will assume control over the gentle taste of the cheddar. In the event that you appreciate a coating, you can blend 1 tablespoon confectioners' erythritol with 3 tablespoons unsweetened almond milk or hefty whipping cream and sprinkle it over the rolls when they have cooled.

Pantry Staples: Vanilla concentrate
Hands On schedule: 10 minutes
Cook Time: 20 minutes
Yields 12 rolls
Fixings
- 2½ cups destroyed mozzarella cheddar
- 2 ounces cream cheddar, mellowed
- 1 cup whitened finely ground almond flour
- ½ teaspoon vanilla concentrate
- ½ cup confectioners' erythritol
- 1 tablespoon ground cinnamon

1. In a huge microwave-safe bowl, join mozzarella cheddar, cream cheddar, and flour. Microwave the combination on high 90 seconds until cheddar is liquefied.
2. Add vanilla concentrate and erythritol, and blend 2 minutes until a batter structures.
3. Once the batter is sufficiently cool to work with your hands, around 2 minutes, spread it out into a 12" × 4" square shape on ungreased material paper. Equitably sprinkle mixture with cinnamon.
4. Beginning at the long side of the mixture, move longwise to shape a log. Cut the sign into twelve even pieces.
5. Split moves between two ungreased 6" round nonstick preparing dishes. Spot one dish into air fryer crate. Change the temperature to 375°F and set the clock for 10 minutes.
6. Cinnamon rolls will be done when brilliant around the edges and generally firm. Rehash with second dish. Permit moves to cool in dishes 10 minutes prior to serving.

Per serving (1 roll) Calories: 145
Protein: 8g Fiber: 1g Net sugars: 3g
Sugar liquor: 6g Fat: 10g
Sodium: 177mg Sugars: 10g Sugar: 1g

M E S S Y   R I N G E R   P E P P E R   E G G S

This breakfast meets up rapidly however isn't lacking in flavor. The eggs absorb the juices of the peppers, making for a heavenly and crisp tasting dinner. Go ahead and get inventive and utilize your decision of cooked meat, for example, disintegrated without sugar bacon.

Pantry Staples: Salt, coconut oil
Hands On schedule: 10 minutes
Cook Time: 15 minutes
Serves: 4
Fixings
- 4 medium green chime peppers, tops eliminated, cultivated
- 1 tablespoon coconut oil
- 3 ounces hacked cooked no-sugar-added ham
- ¼ cup stripped and hacked white onion
- 4 huge eggs
- ½ teaspoon salt
- 1 cup destroyed gentle cheddar

1. Spot peppers upstanding into ungreased air fryer crate. Sprinkle each pepper with coconut oil. Gap ham and onion uniformly among peppers.

2. In a medium bowl, whisk eggs, at that point sprinkle with salt. Empty blend equally into each pepper. Top each with ¼ cup Cheddar.
3. Change the temperature to 320°F and set the clock for 15 minutes. Peppers will be delicate and eggs will be firm when done.
4. Serve warm on four medium plates.

Per serving Calories: 281
Protein: 18g Fiber: 2g Net starches: 6g Fat: 18g
Sodium: 767mg Starches: 8g Sugar: 4g

EGG WHITE CUPS

This formula is ideal for when you're in the state of mind for something light. Egg whites assume the kind of whatever you blend in with them. Go ahead and make these cups your own by adding mushrooms, ham, or a most loved flavoring mix.

Pantry Staples: Salt
Hands On schedule: 10 minutes
Cook Time: 15 minutes
Serves: 4
*   2 cups 100% fluid egg whites
*   3 tablespoons salted margarine, dissolved
*   ¼ teaspoon salt
*   ¼ teaspoon onion powder
*   ½ medium Roma tomato, cored and diced
*   ½ cup slashed new spinach leaves

1. In an enormous bowl, whisk egg whites with spread, salt, and onion powder. Mix in tomato and spinach, at that point empty uniformly into four 4" ramekins lubed with cooking shower.
2. Spot ramekins into air fryer crate. Change the temperature to 300°F and set the clock for 15 minutes. Eggs will be completely cooked and firm in the middle when done. Serve warm.

Per serving Calories: 146
Protein: 14g Fiber: 0g Net sugars: 1g
Fat: 8g Sodium: 416mg Sugars: 1g

SPINACH OMELET

Verdant green vegetables like spinach are an incredible piece of a low-carb diet, as they are brimming with nutrients and fiber. This formula is delectable and messy, and it will keep you going the entire morning.
Pantry Staples: Salt
Hands On schedule: 5 minutes
Cook Time: 12 minutes
Serves: 2

Fixings
*   4 enormous eggs
*   1½ cups slashed new spinach leaves
*   2 tablespoons stripped and slashed yellow onion
*   2 tablespoons salted margarine, dissolved
*   ½ cup destroyed gentle cheddar
*   ¼ teaspoon salt

1. In an ungreased 6" round nonstick heating dish, whisk eggs. Mix in spinach, onion, margarine, Cheddar, and salt.
2. Spot dish into air fryer bin. Change the temperature to 320°F and set the clock for 12 minutes. Omelet will be done when carmelized on the top and firm in the center.
3. Cut into equal parts and serve warm on two medium plates.

Per serving Calories: 368
Protein: 20g Fiber: 1g Net starches: 2g
Fat: 28g Sodium: 722mg
Starches: 3g Sugar: 1g

CHEDDAR SOUFFLÉS

If you've at any point been threatened by soufflés, this formula is for you. In under 30 minutes you can appreciate this scrumptious breakfast. The light, messy taste matches well a few cuts of sans sugar bacon or some new strawberries.

Hands On schedule: 15 minutes
Cook Time: 12 minutes
Serves: 4
Fixings
*   3 huge eggs, whites and yolks isolated
*   ¼ teaspoon cream of tartar
*   ½ cup destroyed sharp cheddar
*   3 ounces cream cheddar, mellowed

1. In a huge bowl, beat egg whites along with cream of tartar until delicate pinnacles structure, around 2 minutes.
2. In a different medium bowl, beat egg yolks, Cheddar, and cream cheddar together until foamy, around 1 moment. Add egg yolk blend to whites, delicately collapsing until joined.
3. Empty blend equitably into four 4" ramekins lubed with cooking shower. Spot ramekins into air fryer bushel. Change the temperature to 350°F and set the clock for 12 minutes. Eggs will be seared on the top and firm in the middle when done. Serve warm.

Per serving Calories: 183
Protein: 9g Fiber: 0g Net starches: 1g
Fat: 14g Sodium: 221mg Starches: 1g

BACON AND CHEDDAR QUICHE

This supper returns to essentials with exemplary breakfast top picks: bacon and eggs. Each nibble is so loaded with cushioned eggs, softened cheddar, and fresh bacon that it will make you wish you'd multiplied the formula. In any case, don't stress; they cook in under 15 minutes, so you can rapidly prepare another bunch any time!

Pantry Staples: Salt
Hands On schedule: 5 minutes
Cook Time: 12 minutes
Serves: 2

- 3 huge eggs
- 2 tablespoons substantial whipping cream
- ¼ teaspoon salt
- 4 cuts cooked without sugar bacon, disintegrated
- ½ cup destroyed gentle cheddar
1. In a huge bowl, whisk eggs, cream, and salt together until consolidated. Blend in bacon and Cheddar.
2. Empty blend equally into two ungreased 4" ramekins. Spot into air fryer container.
3. Change the temperature to 320°F and set the clock for 12 minutes. Quiche will be feathery and set in the center when done.
Let quiche cool in ramekins 5 minutes. Serve warm.

Per serving Calories: 380
Protein: 24g Fiber: 0g Net starches: 2g
Fat: 28g Sodium: 971mg Starches: 2g Sugar: 1g

BREAKFAST MEATBALLS

These meatballs are ideal for breakfast in a hurry. You can undoubtedly twofold the formula and keep them shrouded in the cooler for as long as multi week. Trade out the pork for turkey wiener if you like.

Fixings
- Salt, ground dark pepper
- **Hands On schedule**: 10 minutes
- **Cook Time**: 15 minutes
- **Yields** 18 meatballs
- 1 pound ground pork breakfast wiener
- ½ teaspoon salt
- ¼ teaspoon ground dark pepper
- ½ cup destroyed sharp cheddar

- 1 ounce cream cheddar, mellowed
- 1 huge egg, whisked

1. Consolidate all **Fixings** in a huge bowl. Structure combination into eighteen 1" meatballs.

2. Spot meatballs into ungreased air fryer crate. Change the temperature to 400°F and set the clock for 15 minutes, shaking container multiple times during cooking. Meatballs will be seared outwardly and have an inside temperature of at any rate 145°F when totally cooked. Serve warm.

Per serving (3 meatballs) Calories: 288
Protein: 11g Fiber: 0g Net carbs: 1g
Fat: 24g Sodium: 742mg Carbs: 1g Sugar: 1g

BUNLESS BREAKFAST TURKEY BURGERS

This light breakfast will get you up and abandoning burdening you. The delicious turkey patty gets a decent earthy colored covering that seals in its flavors. Go ahead and top with a seared egg or a sprinkle of sriracha for a little warmth.

Pantry Staples: Salt, ground dark pepper
Hands On schedule: 5 minutes
Cook Time: 15 minutes
Serves: 4
- 1 pound ground turkey breakfast wiener
- ½ teaspoon salt
- ¼ teaspoon ground dark pepper
- ¼ cup cultivated and cleaved green ringer pepper
- 2 tablespoons mayonnaise
- 1 medium avocado, stripped, pitted, and cut

1. In an enormous bowl, blend wiener in with salt, dark pepper, ringer pepper, and mayonnaise. Structure meat into four patties.
2. Spot patties into ungreased air fryer bin. Change the temperature to 370°F and set the clock for 15 minutes, turning patties part of the way through cooking. Burgers will be done when dim earthy colored and they have an inside temperature of in any event 165°F.
3. Serve burgers finished off with avocado cuts on four medium plates.

Per serving Calories: 276 Protein: 22g Fiber: 3g Net starches: 1g Fat: 17g Sodium: 917mg Starches: 4g Sugar: 0g

WIENER CRUSTED EGG CUPS

Who doesn't cherish frankfurter and eggs for breakfast? This is an incredible formula for a gathering that needs different add-ins. Everybody gets their own and can add their number one hacked vegetables and flavors. Have a go at dunking in salsa and acrid cream!

Pantry Staples: Salt, ground dark pepper
Hands On schedule: 10 minutes
Cook Time: 15 minutes
Serves: 6

* 12 ounces ground pork breakfast frankfurter
* 6 huge eggs
* ½ teaspoon salt
* ¼ teaspoon ground dark pepper
* ½ teaspoon squashed red pepper pieces

1. Spot frankfurter in six 4" ramekins (around 2 ounces for every ramekin) lubed with cooking oil. Press wiener down to cover base and about ½" up the sides of ramekins. Break one egg into every ramekin and sprinkle equitably with salt, dark pepper, and red pepper drops.
2. Spot ramekins into air fryer crate. Change the temperature to 350°F and set the clock for 15 minutes. Egg cups will be done when hotdog is completely cooked to in any event 145°F and the egg is firm. Serve warm.

Per serving Calories: 267 Protein: 14g
Fiber: 0g Net starches: 1g
Fat: 21g Sodium: 679mg Starches: 1g
Sugar: 0g

SMALLER THAN EXPECTED BAGELS

Bagels are an exemplary fast and simple breakfast, yet the carb check of the customary bagel is excessively high for a keto diet. These Smaller than normal Bagels will give you what you've been missing—without bargaining your keto objectives. Present with cream cheddar and all that bagel preparing to balance the flavor!

Pantry Staples: Preparing powder
Hands On schedule: 5 minutes
Cook Time: 10 minutes
Yields 6 smaller than normal bagels
Fixings

* 2 cups whitened finely ground almond flour
* 2 cups destroyed mozzarella cheddar
* 3 tablespoons salted spread, partitioned
* 1½ teaspoons preparing powder

* 1 teaspoon apple juice vinegar
* 2 huge eggs, partitioned

1. In a huge microwave-safe bowl, join flour, mozzarella, and 1 tablespoon spread. Microwave on high 90 seconds, at that point structure into a delicate wad of mixture.
2. Add preparing powder, vinegar, and 1 egg to mixture, mixing until completely joined.
3. When batter is adequately cool to work with your hands, around 2 minutes, partition equally into six balls. Punch a hole in each chunk of mixture with your finger and delicately stretch each ball out to be 2" in breadth.
4. In a little microwave-safe bowl, dissolve remaining spread in microwave on high 30 seconds, at that point let cool 1 moment. Race with residual egg, at that point brush blend over every bagel.
5. Line air fryer bin with material paper and spot bagels onto ungreased material, working in clusters if required.
6. Change the temperature to 350°F and set the clock for 10 minutes. Part of the way through, use utensils to flip bagels for cooking.
7. Permit bagels to set and cool totally, around 15 minutes, prior to serving. Store extras in a fixed pack in the fridge as long as 4 days.

Per serving (1 little bagel) calories: 415
Protein: 19g fiber: 4g net sugars: 6g
Fat: 33g sodium: 447mg Sugar: 2g

JALAPEÑO AND BACON BREAKFAST PIZZA

If you love jalapeño poppers, you'll be a tremendous devotee of this jalapeño-and bacon covered breakfast. The cheddar and egg make a rich hull that sets consummately with zesty peppers for a delectable supper. It's a liberal formula that actually keeps you on target.

Pantry Staples: Salt
Hands On schedule: 5 minutes
Cook Time: 10 minutes
Serves: 2
Fixings

* 1 cup destroyed mozzarella cheddar
* 1 ounce cream cheddar, broken into little pieces
* 4 cuts cooked without sugar bacon, slashed
* ¼ cup hacked salted jalapeños
* 1 huge egg, whisked
* ¼ teaspoon salt

1. Spot mozzarella in a solitary layer on the lower part of an ungreased 6" round nonstick preparing dish. Dissipate cream cheddar pieces, bacon, and jalapeños over mozzarella, at that point pour egg equally around heating dish.
2. Sprinkle with salt and spot into air fryer bin. Change the temperature to 330°F and set the clock for 10 minutes. At the point when cheddar is earthy colored and egg is set, pizza will be finished.
3. Let cool on a huge plate 5 minutes prior to serving.

Per serving Calories: 361
Protein: 26g Fiber: 0g Net carbs: 5g Fat: 24g Sodium: 1,324mg Carbs: 5g Sugar: 2g

PIZZA EGGS

Appetizing spices and filling protein make this an incredible informal breakfast alternative. To make this supper significantly seriously filling, add your #1 hacked vegetables, like mushrooms or spinach, or 2 tablespoons low-carb marinara to make it taste much more like pizza.

Pantry Staples: Salt, garlic powder
Hands On schedule: 5 minutes
Cook Time: 10 minutes
Serves: 2
Fixings
- 1 cup destroyed mozzarella cheddar
- 7 cuts pepperoni, hacked
- 1 huge egg, whisked
- ¼ teaspoon dried oregano
- ¼ teaspoon dried parsley
- ¼ teaspoon garlic powder
- ¼ teaspoon salt

1. Spot mozzarella in a solitary layer on the lower part of an ungreased 6" round nonstick preparing dish. Disperse pepperoni over cheddar, at that point pour egg equitably around preparing dish.
2. Sprinkle with outstanding **Fixings** and spot into air fryer bushel. Change the temperature to 330°F and set the clock for 10 minutes. At the point when cheddar is earthy colored and egg is set, dish will be finished.
3. Give cool access dish 5 minutes prior to serving.

Per serving Calories: 241
Protein: 19g Fiber: 0g
Net starches: 4g Fat: 15g Sodium: 834mg
Starches: 4g Sugar: 1g

MESSY CAULIFLOWER "HASH TANS"

Cauliflower has an incredible surface and impartial flavor that permits it to recreate your #1 potato dishes. This formula utilizes ground cheddar crisps, which can regularly be found close to the shop part of your supermarket. Brands like Whisps and Parm Crisps are amazing alternatives that contain just cheddar and no flour fillers.

Pantry Staples: Salt
Hands On schedule: 30 minutes
Cook Time: 24 minutes
Yields 6 hash tans
Fixings
- 2 ounces 100% cheddar crisps
- 1 (12-ounce) liner sack cauliflower, cooked concurring to bundle directions
- 1 huge egg
- ½ cup destroyed sharp cheddar
- ½ teaspoon salt

1. Let cooked cauliflower cool 10 minutes.
2. Spot cheddar crisps into food processor and heartbeat on low 30 seconds until crisps are finely ground.
3. Utilizing a kitchen towel, wring out abundance dampness from cauliflower and spot into food processor.
4. Add egg to food processor and sprinkle with Cheddar and salt. Heartbeat multiple times until combination is for the most part smooth.
5. Slice two bits of material to fit air fryer bin. Separate blend into six even scoops and spot three on each piece of ungreased material, keeping at any rate 2" of space between each scoop. Press each into a hash earthy colored shape, about ¼" thick.
6. Spot one clump on material into air fryer crate. Change the temperature to 375°F and set the clock for 12 minutes, turning hash browns partially through cooking. Hash browns will be brilliant earthy colored when done. Rehash with second bunch.
7. Permit 5 minutes to cool. Serve warm.

Per serving (1 hash earthy colored)
Calories: 120 Protein: 8g Fiber: 1g
Net carbs: 2g Fat: 8g Sodium: 390mg
Carbs: 3g Sugar: 1g

FLAPJACK FOR TWO

This formula is a simple twist on a breakfast exemplary. You get all the soft flapjack goodness that you love in minutes (and less carbs!). Utilize this formula as a base and get imaginative with your #1 flavor concentrates and add-ins. Hacked nuts, blackberries, and low-carb maple syrup cause incredible Fixings and will to handily take this formula to a higher level.

Pantry Staples: Vanilla concentrate
Hands On schedule: 5 minutes
Cook Time: 30 minutes
Serves: 2

- 1 cup whitened finely ground almond flour
- 2 tablespoons granular erythritol
- 1 tablespoon salted spread, dissolved
- 1 huge egg
- ⅓ cup unsweetened almond milk
- ½ teaspoon vanilla concentrate

1. In a huge bowl, combine all Fixings as one, at that point empty a large portion of the player into an ungreased 6" round nonstick preparing dish.
2. Spot dish into air fryer container. Change the temperature to 320°F and set the clock for 15 minutes. The flapjack will be brilliant earthy colored on top and firm, and a toothpick embedded in the middle will confess all when done. Rehash with outstanding hitter.
3. Cut down the middle in dish and serve warm.

Per serving Calories: 434
Protein: 15g Fiber: 6g Net starches: 5g
Sugar liquor: 12g Fat: 38g Sodium: 111mg
Starches: 23g Sugar: 2g

SCOTCH EGGS

A group of hard-bubbled eggs can be incredible for feast prep, however this formula takes things to a higher level. The eggs are enveloped by tasty frankfurter for a more complete dinner. The additional fat from the frankfurter will keep you full and give you the energy expected to get past the day.

Pantry Staples: Salt, ground dark pepper
Hands On schedule: 10 minutes
Cook Time: 12 minutes
Yields 8 eggs

- 1 enormous egg, whisked
- 1 pound ground pork breakfast frankfurter
- ½ cup whitened finely ground almond flour
- ½ teaspoon salt
- ¼ teaspoon ground dark pepper

- 8 huge hard-bubbled eggs, shells eliminated

1. In a huge bowl, blend crude egg in with hotdog, flour, salt, and pepper.
2. Structure ¼ cup of the combination around 1 hard-bubbled egg, totally covering the egg. Rehash with residual combination and hard-bubbled eggs.
3. Spot eggs into ungreased air fryer bin. Change the temperature to 400°F and set the clock for 12 minutes, turning partially through cooking.
4. Eggs will be done when carmelized. Allow eggs to cool 5 minutes prior to serving.

Per serving (1 egg) Calories: 325
Protein: 17g Fiber: 1g Net sugars: 1g
Fat: 25g Sodium: 630mg
Sugars: 2g

CINNAMON GRANOLA

If you've been feeling the loss of that cereal crunch while on a keto diet, this formula is for you! You can appreciate it with unsweetened almond milk or sprinkled over low-carb yogurt. Go ahead and add your #1 nuts and seeds, or even low-carb chocolate chips.

Hands On schedule: 10 minutes
Cook Time: 7 minutes
Yields 4 cups
Fixings

- 2 cups shelled walnuts, hacked
- 1 cup unsweetened coconut chips
- 1 cup fragmented almonds
- 2 tablespoons granular erythritol
- 1 teaspoon ground cinnamon

1. In a huge bowl, blend all **Fixings** . Spot blend into an ungreased 6" round nonstick preparing dish.
2. Spot dish into air fryer bushel. Change the temperature to 320°F and set the clock for 7 minutes, mixing part of the way through cooking.
3. Give cool access dish 10 minutes prior to serving. Store in impermeable compartment at room temperature as long as 5 days.

Per serving (⅔ cup) Calories: 445
Protein: 8g Fiber: 9g Net starches: 4g
Sugar liquor: 4g Fat: 42g
Sodium: 0mg Starches: 17g Sugar: 3g

Jalapeño Egg Cups

The exquisite decency of an exemplary tidbit has at last gone to the breakfast table! Zest up your morning with eggs that sneak up all of a sudden. Make certain to make enough for second helpings—you'll be happy you did.

Pantry Staples: Salt, ground dark pepper, garlic powder

Hands On schedule: 10 minutes
Cook Time: 14 minutes
Serves: 4
Fixings
- 4 huge eggs
- ½ teaspoon salt
- ¼ teaspoon ground dark pepper
- ¼ cup hacked cured jalapeños
- 2 ounces cream cheddar, mollified
- ¼ teaspoon garlic powder
- ½ cup destroyed sharp cheddar

1. In a medium bowl, beat eggs along with salt and pepper, at that point empty equally into four 4" ramekins lubed with cooking splash.
2. In a different huge bowl, blend jalapeños, cream cheddar, garlic powder, and Cheddar. Spoon ¼ of the blend into the focal point of one ramekin. Rehash with residual combination and ramekins.
3. Spot ramekins in air fryer crate. Change the temperature to 320°F and set the clock for 14 minutes. Eggs will be set when done. Serve warm.

Per serving
Calories: 177 Protein: 11g
Fiber: 0g Net sugars: 1g Fat: 13g
Sodium: 591mg Carbs: 1g
Sugar: 1g

Sometimes appetizers can be more exciting than meals, and all of us have eaten a tray of delicious small bites in place of a meal at least a time or two! That fun cocktail party tradition doesn't have to end just because you're sticking to a low-carb lifestyle. Whether you're hosting an event or just looking for a keto version of your restaurant favorites, the recipes in this chapter like Bacon-Wrapped Jalapeno Poppers and Garlic Cheese Bread will keep you and your guests satisfied without sabotaging your diet!

PROSCIUTTO-WRAPPED PARMESAN ASPARAGUS

Prosciutto is a thinly sliced Italian ham reminiscent of a less salty bacon. In this recipe it is used to offset the bitterness of asparagus for a more complete and satisfying vegetable appetizer.

HandsOn Time: 10 minutes
Cook Time: 10 minutes
Serves 4

- 1 pound asparagus
- 12 (0.5-ounce) slices prosciutto
- 1 tablespoon coconut oil, melted
- 2 teaspoons lemon juice
- 1/8 teaspoon red pepper flakes
- 1/3 cup grated Parmesan cheese
- 2 tablespoons salted butter, melted

Directions
- ✓ On a clean work surface, place an asparagus spear onto a slice of prosciutto.
- ✓ Drizzle with coconut oil and lemon juice. Sprinkle red pepper flakes and Parmesan across asparagus. Roll prosciutto around asparagus spear. Place into the air fryer basket.
- ✓ Adjust the temperature to 375°F and set the timer for 10 minutes.
- ✓ Drizzle the asparagus roll with butter before serving.

Per serving
Calories: 263
Protein: 13.9 G Fiber: 2.4 G
Net Carbohydrates: 4.3 G Fat: 20.2 G
Sodium: 368 Mg Carbohydrates: 6.7 G Sugar: 2.2 G

BACON-WRAPPED ONION RINGS

These perfectly crispy onion rings can elevate your game day or take your juicy bunless burger to the next level. A medium onion has around 10 grams of carbs, which can seem high when you're limiting yourself to 20-50 grams of carbs per day. The zero-carb breading increases the fat and protein content for this appetizer, making it an even better keto option, as long as you enjoy in moderation.

HandsOn Time: 5 minutes
Cook Time: 10 minutes

Serves 4

- 1 large onion, peeled
- 1 tablespoon sriracha
- 8 slices sugar-free bacon

Directions
- ✓ Slice onion into 1/4"-thick slices. Brush sriracha over the onion slices. Take two slices of onion and wrap bacon around the rings. Repeat with remaining onion and bacon. Place into the air fryer basket.
- ✓ Adjust the temperature to 350°F and set the timer for 10 minutes.
- ✓ Use tongs to flip the onion rings halfway through the cooking time. When fully cooked, bacon will be crispy. Serve warm.

Per serving
Calories: 105
Protein: 7.5 G Fiber: 0.6 G Net Carbohydrates: 3.7 G
Fat: 5.9 G
Sodium: 401 Mg Carbohydrates: 4.3 G Sugar: 2.3 G

MINI SWEET PEPPER POPPERS

These crunchy bites are perfectly portioned, poppable peppers to please your palate. This bright and colorful twist on jalapeno poppers comes in bite-sized fun with bold flavor!

HandsOn Time: 15 minutes
Cook Time: 8 minutes
Yields 16 halves (4 per serving)

- 8 mini sweet peppers
- 4 ounces full-fat cream cheese, softened
- 4 slices sugar-free bacon, cooked and crumbled
- 1/4 cup shredded pepper jack cheese

Directions
- ✓ Remove the tops from the peppers and slice each one in half lengthwise. Use a small knife to remove seeds and membranes.
- ✓ In a small bowl, mix cream cheese, bacon, and pepper jack.
- ✓ Place 3 teaspoons of the mixture into each sweet pepper and press down smooth. Place into the fryer basket.
- ✓ Adjust the temperature to 400°F and set the timer for 8 minutes.

✓ Serve warm.

Per serving

Calories: 176 Protein: 7.4 G
Fiber: 0.9 G
Net Carbohydrates: 2.7 G Fat: 13.4 G Sodium: 309
Mg Carbohydrates: 3.6 G Sugar: 2.2 G

<u>SPICY SPINACH ARTICHOKE DIP</u>

This spicy twist on a classic appetizer pairs cool and creamy with jalapenos for the heavenly appetizer that every party needs! It's right at home on a platter of pork rinds or your favorite low-carb veggies, such as sliced cucumbers or celery sticks.

HandsOn Time: 10 minutes

Cook Time: 10 minutes

Serves 6

- 10 ounces frozen spinach, drained and thawed
- 1 (14-ounce) can artichoke hearts, drained and chopped
- 1/4 cup chopped pickled jalapenos
- 8 ounces full-fat cream cheese, softened
- 1/4 cup full-fat mayonnaise
- 1/4 cup full-fat sour cream
- 1/2 teaspoon garlic powder
- 1/4 cup grated Parmesan cheese
- 1 cup shredded pepper jack cheese

Directions

✓ Mix all ingredients in a 4-cup baking bowl. Place into the air fryer basket.

✓ Adjust the temperature to 320°F and set the timer for 10 minutes.

✓ Remove when brown and bubbling. Serve warm.

Per serving

Calories: 226 Protein: 10.0 G Fiber: 3.7 G
Net Carbohydrates: 6.5 G Fat: 15.9 G Sodium: 776 Mg
Carbohydrates: 10.2 G Sugar: 3.4 G

<u>PERSONAL MOZZARELLA PIZZA CRUST</u>

This pizza crust is nothing short of bread-like magic! Its applications are endless, and your air fryer can cook it and crisp it faster than your oven ever could! Top this crust with your favorite pizza toppings such as pepperoni, low-carb pizza sauce, and a sprinkle of cheese.

HandsOn Time: 5 minutes

Cook Time: 10 minutes

Serves 1

- 1/2 cup shredded whole-milk mozzarella cheese

- 2 tablespoons blanched finely ground almond flour
- 1 tablespoon full-fat cream cheese
- 1 large egg white

Directions

✓ Place mozzarella, almond flour, and cream cheese in a medium microwave-safe bowl. Microwave for 30 seconds. Stir until smooth ball of dough forms. Add egg white and stir until soft round dough forms.

✓ Press into a 6" round pizza crust.

✓ Cut a piece of parchment to fit your air fryer basket and place crust on parchment. Place into the air fryer basket.

✓ Adjust the temperature to 350°F and set the timer for 10 minutes.

✓ Flip after 5 minutes and at this time place any desired toppings on the crust. Continue cooking until golden. Serve immediately.

Per serving

Calories: 314
Protein: 19.9 G Fiber: 1.5 G
Net Carbohydrates: 3.6 G Fat: 22.7 G
Sodium: 457 Mg Carbohydrates: 5.1 G Sugar: 1.8 G

<u>GARLIC CHEESE BREAD</u>

Who would've ever thought it would be so easy to satisfy your Garlic Cheese Bread cravings without an ounce of flour? Here's a keto-friendly appetizer that tastes just like delivery! Take it to the next level by dipping these strips in a low-carb marinara sauce!

HandsOn Time: 10 minutes

Cook Time: 10 minutes

Serves 2

- 1 cup shredded mozzarella cheese
- 1/4 cup grated Parmesan cheese
- 1 large egg
- 1/2 teaspoon garlic powder

Directions

✓ Mix all ingredients in a large bowl. Cut a piece of parchment to fit your air fryer basket. Press the mixture into a circle on the parchment and place into the air fryer basket.

✓ Adjust the temperature to 350°F and set the timer for 10 minutes.

✓ Serve warm.

Per serving

Calories: 258
Protein: 19.2 G Fiber: 0.1 G Net Carbohydrates: 3.6 G Fat: 16.6 G Sodium: 612 Mg Carbohydrates: 3.7 G Sugar: 0.7 G Hidden Carbs

Note

Don't forget that cheese and eggs have carbs. Many nutrition labels round down if the amount is less than 1. An egg, for example, has 0.06 grams of carbs, even though it's often assumed to be carb-free.

AIR FRYER COCONUT PIE

Planning Time: 15 minutes
Cook Time: 12 minutes
Serves:: 8 **Servings**

Fixings
- 1/2 cups coconut milk
- 2 eggs
- 1/2 teaspoons vanilla concentrate
- 1/4 cup spread
- 1/2 cup Priest natural product
- 1 cup coconut, destroyed
- 1/2 cup coconut flour

Strategy
1. Splash a 6" pie plate with nonstick shower and let sit until required.
2. Add each fixing into a major bowl and mix until very much consolidated, utilizing a wooden spatula.
3. Move player into the nonstick pie plate and spot into the air fryer.
4. Cook for 10-12 minutes at 350º.

Note: Halfway through cooking, check for doneness by embeddings a toothpick and check to guarantee pie isn't consuming.
Serve and appreciate.
Data/Serving
Calories 255 kcal, Carbs 17g, Fat 22g, Protein 8g

PB FROSTED DOUGHNUTS

Planning Time: 10 minutes
Cook Time: 11 minutes
Serves:: 6 **Servings**

Fixings
- 1/3 cup stevia powder
- 1/4 cups almond flour
- 1/2 tsp heating pop
- 1/2 tsp heating powder
- 1 egg
- 3/4 tsp salt
- 1 tsp vanilla
- 1/2 cup buttermilk
- 2 tbsps (liquefied and cooled) unsalted margarine + 1 tbsp extra for garnish

Coating
- 2 tbsps milk
- 1/2 cup powdered stevia
- 1 squeeze salt
- 2 tbsps peanut butter

Filling
- 1/2 cup blueberry jam

Technique
1. Add salt, heating pop, preparing powder, stevia powder and almond flour into a major bowl and speed until consolidated.
2. Add vanilla, heating pop, preparing powder and egg into another bowl and beat to consolidate.
3. Make an opening in the flour blend and add the vanilla combination.
4. Blend combination exhaustive until all around joined.
5. Add flour onto a ledge to keep mixture from staying.
6. Ply and pat batter until a 3/4in thickness is reached on the pre-arranged ledge.
7. Remove 3 1/2in rounds of mixture from the straightened batter and coat with cooled margarine.
8. Cut a material paper round and place in a fryer bin.
9. Add mixture into the pre-arranged fryer crate and cook for 11 minutes at 350º.
10. Add blueberry jam into a crush bottle.
11. Fill doughnuts with blueberry as wanted.
12. Add each frosting fixing into a bowl, speed to consolidate and spill over doughnuts until covered.

Nourishing Data/Serving
Calories 250 kcal, Carbs 11g, Fat 21g, Protein 8g

AIR FRYER CHOCOLATE CAKE

Planning Time: 10 minutes
Cook Time: 20 minutes
Serves:: 6 **Servings**
Fixings
- 1/3 cup truvia
- 3 eggs
- 1/2 cup substantial whipping cream
- 4 tbsps spread
- 1/4 cup Coconut Flour
- 1 tsp Vanilla concentrate
- 2 tbsp Cocoa powder, unsweetened
- 1 tsp preparing powder
- 1/4 tsp Salt

Icing

- 4 tbsps mollified Margarine, unsalted
- 4 tbsps (mollified) cream cheddar
- 1 tsp vanilla concentrate
- 1 tbsp truvia

Strategy

1. Warmth up air fryer to 350º.
2. Set up a lubed 6 cup biscuit tin and let sit until required.
3. Add spread into a major broiler secure bowl, place in a microwave and warmth for 30-60 seconds.
4. Add truvia into the spread and mix until completely joined.
5. Add vanilla concentrate, whipping cream and eggs into the combination and beat until completely consolidated utilizing a blender.
6. Add each dry fixing into the margarine bowl and blend until player arrives at a smooth and fine consistency.

Tip: if player shows up excessively thick, add all the more hefty whipping cream to disperse.

7. Empty cake hitter into the pre-arranged biscuit cups.
8. Spot in the pre-arranged fryer bushel and cook until an embedded toothpick comes out clean, for 10-12 minutes. Tip: check for doneness at 10 minutes to forestall over preparing.
9. Let sit to cool.
10. Add each icing fixing into a bowl and beat until entirely consolidated.
11. Spread icing blend over the cakes.

Dietary Data/Serving
Calories 296 kcal, Protein 4g, Dietary Fiber 2g, Carbs 5g, Complete Fat 28g

KETO KALE CHIPS

Planning Time: 5 minutes
Cook Time: 7 minutes
Serves:: 2 **Servings**

Fixings
Additional virgin olive oil, as fundamental
1 major pack (hard spines eliminated and tore into little pieces) pre-hacked kale
Pepper, as fundamental
Salt, as fundamental
Stew powder, as essential

Strategy
1. Add kale pieces into the fryer bushel.
2. Splash evoo over kale pieces until covered as wanted, close the air fryer and shake to cover kale chips uniformly.
3. Sprinkle pepper, salt and stew powder over kale chips until entirely covered.
4. Cook kale until wanted doneness is reached, for 6-7 minutes at 375º. Note; Shake kale occasionally while cooking.
5. Serve and appreciate kale chips.

Data/Serving
Calories 217 kcal, Carbs 5g, Fat 22g, Protein 2g

AIR SEARED DOUGHNUTS

Planning Time: 15 minutes
Cook Time: 10 minutes
Serves:: 10 **Servings**

Fixings (doughnut)
- 1/4 cup hefty whipping cream
- 1/2 cup acrid cream
- 1 teaspoon vanilla concentrate
- 4 major eggs
- 1/4 teaspoon nutmeg
- 1/2 cup coconut flour
- 1/4 cup erythritol
- 1/4 teaspoon preparing pop
- 1 squeeze salt
- ¼ cup avocado oil

Doughnut Covering
- 1 teaspoon cinnamon
- 1/4 cup erythritol

Strategy
1. Warmth up air fryer to 355º.
2. Add vanilla concentrate, eggs, stirring cream and harsh cream into a major bowl and beat to consolidate.
3. Continuously add the dry **Fixings** into the vanilla concentrate blend and blend until very much consolidated.
4. Empty hitter into a doughnut dish, around 3/4 of the skillet filled.
5. Move doughnut dish into the fryer crate and cook until all around cooked, for around 10-15 minutes.
6. Move doughnuts from air fryer and let sit until cooled.
7. Add avocado oil into a skillet over drug heat.
8. Add doughnuts into the hot oil and cook until brilliant earthy colored, for around 2 minutes for every side.
9. Sprinkle cinnamon over doughnuts and serve.

Nourishing Data/Serving
Calories 141 kcal, Protein 4g, Absolute Carbs 2g, All out Fat 12g

FRESH ZUCCHINI WASTES

Planning Time: 5 minutes
Cook Time: 30 minutes
Serves:: 8 (2 waste) **Servings**

Fixings (wastes)
- 2 tablespoon (partitioned) avocado oil
- 3 cups (crush out dampness) stuffed ground zucchini
- 6 tablespoons minced cilantro
- 2/3 cup diced onion
- 1 cup almond flour
- 3/4-1 teaspoon ocean salt
- 1 egg white
- Newly ground dark pepper
- 2 teaspoons coconut flour
- Avocado oil

Lime Mayo Sauce
- 5 teaspoons new lime juice
- 1/2 cup mayo
- Ocean Salt, as important
- 4 teaspoons new slashed dill, firmly stuffed
- Newly ground dark pepper

Technique
1. Add crushed zucchini into a major bowl.
2. Add 2 teaspoons avocado oil into a major skillet over medications heat.
3. Add onions into the hot oil and cook until brilliant earthy colored and delicate.
4. Add zucchini to the cooked onions.
5. Add coconut flour, almond flour, salt, cilantro and ground dark pepper into the skillet and mix to consolidate.
6. Add egg white into the zucchini combination and consolidate until zucchini is completely covered.
7. Warmth up air fryer to 400º.
8. Shower fryer bin with avocado oil.
9. Scoop a few modest bunches of the zucchini combination
10. Working in clumps, add around 4-5 zucchini waste balls into the air fryer bushel per time and splash top with avocado oil.
11. Cook wastes for around 10-15 minutes, until top is crisped and edges are brilliant earthy colored.
12. Flip wastes with a spatula and air fry for 5-7 additional minutes.

Nourishing Data/Serving

Calories 222 kcal, Protein 3.8g, Dietary Fiber 2.8g, Absolute Carbs 6.9g, All out fat 21.8g

CHOCOLATE BROWNIES

Planning Time: 10 minutes
Cook Time: 35 minutes
Serves:: 6 **Servings**

Fixings
- 1/2 cup margarine
- 1/2 cup chocolate chips, no-sugar added
- 1/4 cup erythritol
- 3 eggs
- 1 teaspoon vanilla concentrate

Strategy
1. Add chocolate and spread into a stove secure bowl and dissolve in a microwave briefly. Note: don't overcook the chocolate
2. Mix the dissolved blend altogether until joined.
3. Add vanilla, erythritol and eggs into a bowl and beat until foamy and light.
4. Continuously add the chocolate blend into the egg bowl and beat until combination is consolidated and completely joined.
5. Empty hitter into a pre-arranged cake container until an embedded toothpick tells the truth, for 20-30 minutes.
6. Serve and appreciate.

Healthful Data/Serving
Calories 224 kcal, Protein 4g, Dietary Fiber 1g, Carbs 3g, Fat 23g

LEMON DOUGHNUTS

Planning Time: 10 minutes
Cook Time: 10 minutes
Serves:: 8 **Servings**

Fixings
- 4 tablespoons liquefied coconut oil
- 4 huge eggs
- 2/3 cup lemon juice
- 3 tablespoons fluid stevia
- 1 teaspoon cinnamon
- 1 cup coconut flour
- 1 squeeze salt
- 1 teaspoon preparing pop

Strategy
1. Warmth up air fryer to 350º.
2. Oil a doughnut dish with avocado oil.

3. Add dissolved coconut oil, lemon juice, stevia, salt and eggs into a little bowl and speed to consolidate.
4. Add coconut flour, heating pop and cinnamon into a subsequent bowl and sift to consolidate.
5. Add flour blend into the lemon juice combination until completely consolidated and a player like consistency is reached.
6. Empty player into the pre-arranged skillet and spread similarly.
7. Spot container in the pre-arranged fryer and cook for 10 minutes until doughnut edges become brilliant, at 350º.
8. Let sit to cool for 5-10 minutes prior to moving to a wire rack.
9. Spill with wanted keto coat.

Nourishing Data/Serving
Calories 179 kcal, Protein 5g, Dietary Fiber 0.2g, Carbs 9g, Absolute Fat 11.2

CHOCOLATE MAGMA CAKE

Planning Time: 10 minutes
Cook Time: 10 minutes
Serves:: 2 **Servings**

Fixings
- 2 tbsps cocoa powder
- 1 egg
- 2 tbsps water
- 1 tbsp brilliant flaxmeal
- 1/8 tsp stevia
- 1/2 tsp heating powder
- 1 tbsp softened coconut oil
- 1 squeeze salt
- 1 scramble vanilla

Technique
1. Add each fixing into 2-cup ramekin and race to consolidate.
2. For 1 moment, heat up air fryer to 350º.
3. Spot ramekin into the air fryer and cook for 8-9 minutes until wanted doneness is reached, at 350º.
4. Allow cake to sit until cooled, serve and appreciate.

Dietary Data/Serving
Calories 299 kcal, Carbs 16g, Fat 24g, Protein 15g

PARMESAN ZUCCHINI

Planning Time: 10 minutes
Cook Time: 16 minutes
Serves:: 6 **Servings**

Fixings
- 1 huge egg
- 2 (cut into 1/4in cuts) medium zucchini
- 1/4 almond flour
- 1/2 cup parmesan cheddar, ground
- 1 tsp Italian flavoring
- 1/2 tsp garlic powder
- Olive oil

Strategy
1. Add egg into a bowl and beat well.
2. Add Italian flavoring, garlic powder, almond flour and ground parmesan cheddar into a different bowl and consolidate.
3. Submerge zucchini cuts in egg wash and drench in the Italian flavoring blend.
4. Move covered zucchini cuts onto an air fryer plate fixed with material paper.
5. Rehash measure until plate is filled.
6. Shower a modest quantity of olive oil over cuts of zucchini.
7. Cook zucchini cuts for 8 minutes at 370º.
Tip: Cook zucchini cuts in 2 clusters.
8. Flip zucchini cuts, shower with additional olive oil and cook for 8 additional minutes.
9. Air fry second zucchini clump, serve and appreciate.

Nourishing Data/Serving
Calories 92 kcal, Protein 6.1g, Dietary Fiber 1.8g, Carbs 4.9g, All out Fat 5.7g

SINGED MOZZARELLA STICKS

Planning Time: 10 minutes
Cook Time: 10 minutes
Serves:: 6 **Servings**

Fixings
- 2 (beaten) huge eggs
- 12 (cut down the middle) Mozzarella sticks
- 1/2 cup powdered parmesan cheddar
- 1/2 cup almond flour
- 1/2 tsp salt
- 1 tsp Italian flavoring

Strategy

1. Add salt, Italian flavoring, parmesan cheddar and almond flour into a bowl and consolidate.
2. Add eggs into a subsequent bowl and whisk together.
3. Dunk mozzarella stick in egg wash and plunge in the parmesan blend until mozzarella sticks are completely covered.
4. Move covered mozzarella sticks into a bowl in a solitary layer, cover and freeze for 30 minutes.
5. Move mozzarella sticks into the fryer bushel.
6. Cook for 5 minutes at 400º.
7. Open fryer, let mozzarella sticks sit briefly prior to moving to a serving platter.

Wholesome Data/Serving

Calories 188 kcal, Carbs 11g, Fat 14g, Protein 7g

A IR S INGED P ICKLES WITH M AYO

Planning Time: 15 minutes
Cook Time: 20 minutes
Serves:: **7 Servings**
Fixings

- 3/4 cup weighty cream
- 1 enormous egg
- 4 cups pork skins
- 1/4 teaspoon cayenne pepper
- 2 tablespoons freeze dried dill
- 1/2 cup almond flour
- 2 teaspoons dark pepper
- 2 teaspoons paprika
- 35 dill pickle cuts

Present with
- Farm dressing
- Mayo

Strategy

1. Add cayenne, hefty cream and egg into a little bowl and beat until consolidated.
2. Add pork skins into fast electric blender or food processor and cycle until a scrap like consistency is reached.
3. Add 1/2 cup pork skin morsels into a little bowl.
4. Add dark pepper, paprika, dill, almond flour and the leftover pork skin pieces into a different bowl and blend until consolidated.
5. Orchestrate bowls as follows: unadulterated pork skin bowl, egg wash bowl and the almond flour/pork skin bowl.
6. Inundate each pickle cut into every one of the dishes above in a similar request until entirely covered. Tip: first plunge in the unadulterated pork skin bowl, at that point move to the egg wash lastly submerge in the almond flour combination.
7. Rehash measure until no pickle cut remaining parts.
8. Add covered pickle cuts into the fryer crate in one layer, working in clumps.
9. Cook pickles until brilliant earthy colored, for 8-10 minutes, at 390º.
10. Serve pickles with farm dressing and mayo as wanted.

Nourishing Data/Serving

Calories 210 kcal, Protein 7.5g, Dietary Fiber 1.7g, Absolute Carbs 8g, Complete Fat 17.9g

S INGED A VOCADO C HIPS

Planning Time: 10 minutes
Cook Time: 10 minutes
Serves:: **2 Servings**
Fixings

- 1 egg
- 1 (split, hollowed and cut into wedges) avocado
- 1/2 tsp salt
- 1/2 cup pork skin pieces

Strategy

1. Gather salt and egg into a bowl and beat into a single unit.
2. Add pork skin pieces into a different low bowl.
3. Dunk avocado wedges into egg wash, at that point pork skin pieces until completely covered.
4. Move covered wedges into fryer bin in one layer.
5. Cook avocado wedges until sautéed softly, for 8-10 minutes at 400º.
6. Shake air fryer halfway while cooking.

Dietary Data/Serving

Calories 516 kcal, Carbs 5g, Fat 37g, Protein 41g

S INGED A VOCADO C HIPS

Planning Time: 10 minutes
Cook Time: 10 minutes
Serves:: **2 Servings**
Fixings

- 1 egg
- 1 (split, hollowed and cut into wedges) avocado
- 1/2 tsp salt
- 1/2 cup pork skin scraps

Technique
1. Gather salt and egg into a bowl and beat into a single unit.
2. Add pork skin pieces into a different low bowl.
3. Plunge avocado wedges into egg wash, at that point pork skin scraps until completely covered.
4. Move covered wedges into fryer bin in one layer.
5. Cook avocado wedges until carmelized gently, for 8-10 minutes at 400º.
6. Shake air fryer halfway while cooking.

Nourishing Data/Serving
Calories 516 kcal, Carbs 5g, Fat 37g, Protein 41g

COOKED ZUCCHINI ROUNDS

Planning Time: 5 minutes
Cook Time: 30 minutes
Serves:: 4 **Servings**

Fixings
- 2 tablespoons avocado oil
- 1 pound (cut into 1/4in thick circles) zucchini
- 1/2 teaspoon dark Pepper
- 1 teaspoon salt
- 1 teaspoon garlic powder

Strategy
1. Warmth up air fryer to 400º.
2. Add flavors and avocado oil into a little bowl and consolidate.
3. Add zucchini adjusts into the flavoring blend and join until completely covered.
4. Move covered zucchini adjusts into the pre-arranged fryer container and cook for 30 minutes.
5. Check zucchini like clockwork through cooking and cook until wanted doneness is reached.
6. Serve simmered zucchini adjusts and appreciate.

Wholesome Data/Serving
Calorics 142 kcal, Carbs 6g, Fat 14g, Protein 1g

KETO RAVIOLI

Planning Time: 5 minutes
Cook Time: 10 minutes
Serves:: 6 **Servings**

Fixings
- 1 (9 oz.) box cheddar ravioli
- 1 (14 oz.) container marinara sauce
- 2 cups pork skin scraps
- 1 tsp avocado oil
- 1/4 cup Parmesan cheddar
- 1 cup buttermilk

Technique
1. Add pork skin scraps and avocado oil into a bowl and join.
2. Submerge ravioli into the buttermilk, at that point the pork skin pieces.
3. Press to affix pork skin pieces onto the ravioli.
4. Add the pre-arranged ravioli on material paper and spot in the fryer container.
6. Cook for 5 minutes at 200ºF.
7. Fill in as wanted with most loved keto plunging sauce.

Dietary Data/Serving
Calories 611 kcal, Carbs 25g, Fat 32g, Protein 51g

FIRM PARMESAN EGGPLANT

Planning Time: 15 minutes
Cook Time: 25 minutes
Serves:: 4 **Servings**
Fixings
- 1/2 cup pork skin pieces
- 1 (cut into 1/2" cuts) huge eggplant
- Salt, as vital
- 3 tablespoons parmesan cheddar, finely ground
- 3 tablespoon almond flour
- 1 teaspoon Italian flavoring
- 1 tablespoon water
- 1 egg
- 1 cup marinara sauce
- Avocado oil
- 1/4 cup mozzarella cheddar, ground

Embellishment with
New slashed cilantro

Technique
1. Equitably season egg plants with salt on all sides and let sit for approx. 15 minutes.
2. Meanwhile, add almond flour, water and egg into a bowl and join until hitter is framed.
3. Add salt, Italian flavoring, parmesan cheddar and pork skin scraps into a different bowl and blend very until joined.
4. Indeed, even brush hitter over each cut of eggplant and dunk covered cuts into the pork skin blend until each side is covered uniformly.
5. Move breaded cuts of eggplant into a plate and splash with avocado oil.
6. Move eggplant cuts into a fryer crate and cook for 8 minutes at 360º.
7. Gently spread mozzarella cheddar and 1 tbsp marinara sauce on cooked eggplant cuts and cook until cheddar is softened, for 1-2 additional minutes.

8. Serve quickly with your ideal pasta.

Nourishing Data/Serving
Calories 336 kcal, Carbs 7g, Fat 24g, Protein 25g

SINGED BISON CAULIFLOWER

Planning Time: 5 minutes
Cook Time: 15 minutes
Serves:: 4 **Servings**

Fixings
- Avocado oil
- 1 (cut into reduced down pieces) cauliflower head
- 1 tbsp softened spread
- 1/2 cup bison sauce
- Salt and pepper, as vital

Technique
1. Shower fryer crate with avocado oil.
2. Add pepper, salt, bison sauce and softened spread into a bowl and mix until very much joined.
3. Add cauliflower lumps into the pre-arranged fryer bushel and splash with additional avocado oil.
4. Cook cauliflower pieces at 400º for 7 minutes.
5. Eliminate cooked cauliflower from the air fryer to a major blending bowl.
6. Spill the spread blend over cauliflower until entirely covered and mix to consolidate.
7. Return covered cauliflower into the fryer crate and cook until fresh, for 7-8 additional minutes.

Nourishing Data/Serving
Calories 101 kcal, Protein 3g, Net Carbs 4g, Fat 7g

AIR FRYER OKRA

Planning Time: 15 minutes
Cook Time: 17 minutes
Serves:: 4 **Servings**
Fixings
- 1 egg
- 7 oz. (remove stem closures and cut in 1/2" cuts) new okra
- 1 cup pork skin scraps
- 1 cup skim milk
- Avocado oil
- 1/2 tsp ocean salt

Technique
1. Add milk and egg into a genuinely enormous bowl and beat until consolidated.

2. Add cut okra into the milk blend and mix until completely covered.
3. Add salt and pork skin pieces into a zip-top pack and shake to consolidate.
4. Utilize opened spoon to move okra cuts from egg wash into the pork skin sack, shaking off the abundance egg.
5. Shake sack again until okra cuts are very much covered.
6. Add covered okra cuts in the fryer crate and shower with avocado oil.
7. Cook okra cuts for 5 minutes at 390º.
8. Shake air fryer with substance, at that point splash with avocado oil and cook for 5 additional minutes.
9. For crispier and brilliant earthy colored cuts, shake air fryer once more, splash with avocado oil and cook for 2-5 additional minutes.
10. Serve and appreciate.

Dietary Data/Serving
Calories 440 kcal, Carbs 7g, Fat 28g, Protein 40g

CRUNCHY ALMOND PICKLES

Planning Time: 10 minutes
Cook Time: 6 minutes
Serves:: 4 **Servings**
Fixings
- 3 tbsps Parmesan cheddar
- 1/2 cup pork skins, squashed
- 1/2 cup almond flour
- 16 dill pickles, cut
- 1 tsp avocado oil
- 1 (beaten) huge egg

Strategy
1. Add parmesan cheddar with pork skin scraps into a bowl and blend.
2. Add egg into a different bowl and beat.
3. Add almond flour into another bowl.
4. Dunk each cut of pickle into the flour bowl, at that point the egg wash and ultimately plunge into the parmesan bowl until completely covered.
5. Splash fryer container with avocado oil.
6. In a solitary layer, add the pickles into the pre-arranged air fryer container.
7. Shower pickles with avocado oil until covered.
8. Cook pickles at 360º for 6 minutes.
9. Serve and appreciate.

Wholesome Data/Serving
Calories 275 kcal, Protein 24g, All out Fat 19g, Net Carbs 3g, Dietary Fiber 2g

HOT MAYO COULIS WITH SINGED ASPARAGUS

Planning Time: 10 minutes
Cook Time: 5 minutes
Serves:: 2 **Servings**

Fixings
- Avocado oil
- 10 (intense woody closures cut off, flushed and dried) new asparagus lances
- 1 tbsp substantial whipping cream
- 1 major egg

Breading
- 1/3 cup parmesan cheddar, finely ground
- 1/3 cup almond flour, whitened
- 1/2 tsp paprika
- 1/2 tsp salt

Mayo Coulis
- 1 tsp dijon mustard
- 1/4 cup mayo
- 1/4 tsp dark pepper
- 1/4 tsp cayenne

Strategy
1. Add each mayo coulis fixing into a little bowl, consolidate well and spot in a fridge until required.
2. Add weighty cream and egg into a bowl, beat until joined and void into a major low bowl.
3. Add each breading fixing into a different low bowl and join well.
4. Dunk asparagus lances in egg wash, at that point in breading, place on a material paper lined plate.
5. Rehash measure until no asparagus stick remains.
6. Work in clusters if fundamental, add covered asparagus lances into the fryer container in one layer.
7. Shower lances with avocado oil.
8. Cook for 3-5 minutes at 350º, until brilliant.
9. Serve sticks promptly with hot coulis.

Healthful Data/Serving
Calories 420 kcal, Protein 9g, Dietary Fiber 3.5g, Absolute Carb 7g, Complete Fat 40g

ALMOND CHEDDAR STICKS

Planning Time: 10 minutes
Cook Time: 7 minutes
Serves:: 8 **Servings**
Fixings
- 1 enormous egg
- 8 cheddar sticks
- 1/2 cup parmesan cheddar, ground
- 1/4 cup almond flour
- 1/4 teaspoon dried thyme
- 1 teaspoon Italian Flavoring
- 1 teaspoon garlic powder

Strategy
1. Add egg into a little bowl and whisk altogether.
2. Add garlic powder, thyme, Italian flavoring, parmesan cheddar and almond flour into a different bowl and join well until a smooth consistency is reached.
3. Uniformly cover cheddar sticks with egg wash and dunk in the parmesan/flour combination until completely covered.
4. For careful covering, rehash stage 4 again.
5. Move cheddar sticks into a treat sheet fixed with material paper and spot in a cooler until entirely chilled.
6. Spot frozen cheddar sticks in the fryer bin in one layer.
7. Cook the cheddar sticks for 7-12 minutes at 370º.

Nourishing Data/Serving
Calories 62 kcal, Protein 4g, Absolute Carbs 2g, Complete Fat 4g

STUFFED JALAPENO POPPERS

Planning Time: 10 minutes
Cook Time: 5 minutes
Serves:: 5 **Servings**

Fixings
- 6 ounces low-fat cream cheddar
- 10 (split upward and eliminate seeds) new jalapenos
- 2 (cooked and disintegrated) bacon cuts
- 1/4 cup cheddar, destroyed
- Avocado oil cooking splash

Strategy
1. Add cream cheddar into a stove secure bowl and microwave until softened, for 15 seconds.
2. Add destroyed cheddar, disintegrated bacon and cream cheddar into a bowl and consolidate completely.
3. Add destroyed cheddar filling into every jalapeno half and move into the fryer container.
4. Splash avocado oil over jalapeno poppers.
5. Seal the cover and cook for 5 minutes at 370º.
6. Take out poppers from the fryer and let sit to cool before you serve.

Healthful Data/Serving
Calories 138 kcal, Carbs 8g, Fat 10g, Protein 5g

CHEDDAR STUFFED MUSHROOMS

Planning Time: 7 minutes
Cook Time: 8 minutes
Serves:: 5 **Servings**
Fixings

- 4 ounces cream cheddar
- 8 ounces (eliminate stems and make enormous round cut where stem remained) huge new mushrooms
- 1/8 cup destroyed sharp cheddar
- ¼ cup destroyed parmesan cheddar
- 1 tsp Worcestershire sauce
- 1/8 cup destroyed white cheddar
- Salt and pepper, as essential
- 2 cleaved garlic cloves

Strategy

1. Add cream cheddar into a stove secure bowl and microwave until delicate, for 15 seconds.
2. Add each cheddar and the cream cheddar into a genuinely large bowl and add Worcestershire sauce, pepper and salt and blend until very much joined.
3. Add cheddar filling into the mushrooms and move into the fryer container.
4. Seal fryer top and cook stuffed mushrooms at 370º for 8 minutes.
5. Allow stuffed mushrooms to sit to cool before you serve.

Nourishing Data/Serving
Calories 139 kcal, Carbs 4g, Fat 12g, Protein 7g

CRUNCHY AVOCADO FRIES

Planning Time: 10 minutes
Cook Time: 10 minutes
Serves:: 2 **Servings**

Fixings

- 1 egg
- 1 (divided, hollowed and cut into wedges) avocado, ready however firm
- 1/2 tsp salt
- 1/2 cup pork skin pieces

Strategy

1. Gather salt and egg into a bowl and beat into a single unit. Add pork skin pieces into a different bowl. Inundate avocado wedges in the egg wash and move into the bowl with pork skin. Warmth up air fryer to 400ºF.
2. Add the breaded avocados into the wire crate of the preheated air fryer in one layer. Cook until very much cooked, for 8-10 minutes. Shake air fryer crate halfway while cooking.

Healthful Data/Serving
Calories 196 kcal, Protein 9.5g, Absolute Carbs 6.2g, Fat 15.4g

CAULI-PIECES

Planning Time: 5 minutes
Cook Time: 10 minutes
Serves:: 4 **Servings**

Fixings

- 1 cup pork skin scraps
- 1 egg
- 1/2 tsp salt
- 1/2 head (cut into florets) cauliflower
- Newly ground dark pepper
- 1/2 tsp garlic powder
- 1/2 cup hot sauce
- 1 cup farm dressing

Strategy

1. Add pepper, garlic powder, salt, and egg into a bowl and blend until consolidated. Add pork skin morsels into a different bowl. Warmth up air fryer to 400ºF. Submerge cauliflower florets into the egg wash and move into the bowl with pork skin pieces.
2. Add the breaded cauliflower into the air fryer crate and cook for 4-5 minutes. Shake crate and cook until very much cooked, for 4-5 additional minutes. Meanwhile, add hot sauce and farm dressing into a bowl and consolidate.
3. Serve cauli-pieces with hot farm sauce.

Healthful Data/Serving
Calories 391 kcal, Protein 9.9g, Carbs 13.4g, Fat 32.1g

BACON-ASPARAGUS WRAPS

Planning Time: 5 minutes
Cook Time: 20 minutes
Serves:: 6 **Servings**

Fixings

- 1 lb. (trim off closes) asparagus
- 1 lb. (split) bacon
- Creole flavoring, to taste
- Salt and pepper, to taste
- 1 tablespoon avocado oil

Technique

1. Add managed asparagus into a bowl and coat with avocado oil. Sprinkle creole flavoring, pepper and salt over covered asparagus and throw until

completely covered. Wrap 2 asparagus lances in 1/2 bacon cut and move into the wire bin of the air fryer.
2. Cook until wanted freshness is reached, for 20 minutes. Flip bacon wrapped asparagus halfway during cooking. Serve immediately or move into well lidded compartments and store for as long as 7 days.

Nourishing Data/Serving
Calories 350 kcal, Fat 32g, Protein 11g, Carbs 3g

SINGED GARLIC

Planning Time: 5 minutes
Cook Time: 20 minutes
Serves:: 4 Servings
Fixings
- 2 tbsps avocado oil
- 1 (medium-sized) head garlic

Technique
1. Cut 1/4" off the highest point of the garlic head. Spill avocado oil over uncovered piece of the garlic cloves and wrap firmly in foil. Add the wrapped garlic into a wire bushel of an air fryer and cook for 20 minutes at 400ºF. Check for delicateness and doneness.
2. Cook for 5-10 additional minutes until all around cooked. Let sit to cool before you serve.

Nourishing Data/Serving
Calories 89 kcal, Protein 0.8g, Carbs 4.5g, Fat 8.2g

SCOTCH EGGS

Planning Time: 20 minutes
Cook Time: 25 minutes
Serves:: 4 Servings
Fixings
- 1 tbsp (cleave finely) sage
- 1 lb. pork wiener
- 1/8 tsp nutmeg, ground
- 2 tbsps new cleaved cilantro
- 1/8 tsp ground dark pepper
- 1/8 tsp salt
- 1 cup parmesan cheddar, destroyed
- 4 (stripped) eggs, hardboiled
- 2 tsps mustard, coarse-ground

Technique
1. Add dark pepper, salt, nutmeg, cilantro, sage, mustard and frankfurter into a major bowl and gently blend until joined. Structure combination into 4 even patties. Spot an egg on every patty and structure patty

around the egg. Rehash measure with the leftover patties and eggs.
2. Submerge each egg and patty in destroyed parmesan cheddar, delicately press and move until completely covered. Move eggs in the wire bin of an air fryer and coat daintily with avocado oil.
3. Cook scotch eggs for 15 minutes at 400ºF. Flip eggs halfway through air fryer and coat with avocado oil. Serve scotch eggs with mustard.

Wholesome Data/Serving
Calories 533 kcal, Fat 43g, Protein 33g, Carbs 2g

ROMANO ZUCCHINI FRIES

Planning Time: 5 minutes
Cook Time: 10 minutes
Serves:: 4 Servings
Fixings
- 1 (beaten) egg, huge
- 2 (cut into 1/2-by-3" sticks) zucchini, medium
- ½ cup (ground) pecorino romano cheddar
- ½ cup almond flour
- 1 squeeze pepper and salt
- 1 tsp Italian flavoring
- Avocado oil

Strategy
1. Add pepper, salt, preparing, ground pecorino romano cheddar and almond flour into a level lined bowl and mix until all around consolidated. Plunge zucchini stick into the bowl with the beaten egg until completely covered. Drench covered zucchini into the cheddar flour blend until completely covered.
2. Move the covered zucchini sticks onto a platter and rehash measure with the leftover zucchini sticks. Work in groups, cover the wired bin of the air fryer with avocado oil. Add zucchini sticks into the air fryer bushel in one layer.
3. Seal the cover and cook until crisped, at 400ºF for 10 minutes. Let sit to cool, serve and delve in.

Healthful Data/Serving
Calories 147 kcal, Fat 10g, Fat 9g, Carbs 6g

BISON CAULI-CHILDREN WITH TURKEY

Planning Time: 10 minutes
Cook Time: 5 minutes
Serves:: 4 Servings

Fixings
- 1/2 tsp garlic powder

- 2 cups cauliflower florets
- 1 egg
- 8 oz. prepared rotisserie turkey bosom
- 2 tbsps bison sauce
- 3/4 cup parmesan cheddar

Breading
- 4 tbsps parmesan cheddar
- 6 tbsps almond flour

Technique

1. Add wild ox sauce, 3/4 cup parmesan cheddar, egg, garlic powder, turkey bosom and cauliflower florets into a major bowl and join well. Structure combination into 1 tsp-sized balls.

2. Warmth up air fryer to 400ºF. Add 6 tbsps almond flour and 4 tbsps parmesan cheddar into a subsequent bowl and mix until joined. Fold cauli-balls into the parmesan combination until completely covered and shape into cauli-toddler shapes.

3. Coat the wire container of an air fryer with avocado oil until equitably covered. Work in clumps, add in the cauli-turkey children in a single layer, seal the cover and air fry for 6 minutes. Flip the toddlers and cook for 3 additional minutes, until very much cooked and seared.

4. Rehash measure until cauli-turkey children are very much cooked and carmelized.

Healthful Data/Serving
Calories 49 kcal, Protein 3g, Carbs 1g, Fat 3g

CREAM FILLED JALAPENO POPPERS

Planning Time: 10 minutes
Cook Time: 5 minutes
Serves:: 5 **Servings**

Fixings
- 6 ounces cream cheddar
- 10 (split upward and eliminate seeds) jalapenos
- 2 (cooked and disintegrated) bacon cuts
- 1/4 cup cheddar, destroyed
- Avocado oil cooking splash

Strategy

1. Add cream cheddar into a microwave-safe bowl and warmth until mollified, for 15 seconds in a microwave. Add destroyed cheddar, disintegrated bacon and cream cheddar into a bowl and blend until consolidated. Fill the poppers with the bacon blend.

2. Add the filled jalapeño into the wired bushel of the air fryer and cover uniformly with avocado oil. Seal the cover and cook until wanted delicacy is reached, for 5-7 minutes at 370ºF. Allow poppers to sit to cool before you serve.

Wholesome Data/Serving
Calories 62 kcal, Fat 4g, Protein 3g, Carbs 3g

AIR FRYER PICKLES WITH HERBED SAUCE

Planning Time: 10 minutes
Cook Time: 10 minutes
Serves:: 12 **Servings**

Fixings
- 1 cup coconut flour
- 12 (split lengthways and wipe off softly) pickle lances
- 2 eggs, huge
- 2 1/2 oz. pkg. pork skins, disintegrated

Tarragon Sauce
- 1/2 tbsp tarragon, dried
- 8 oz. acrid cream
- 1 tsps garlic powder
- 1 tsp vinegar
- 1/2 tsp salt
- 1/4 tsp pepper

Technique

1. Add pork skins into level lined bowl. Add eggs into a little bowl and race until beaten. Add coconut flour into a third bowl. Dunk pickle pieces in the coconut flour until covered. Inundate in the egg wash and move into the bowl with pork skin until completely covered.

2. Spot breaded pickles in the wire crate of the air fryer and cook at 400ºF for 7 minutes. Add each sauce fixing in a bowl and speed to join. Serve seared pickles with spice sauce.

Healthful Data/Serving
Calories 126 kcal, Fat 7g, Protein 6g, Carbs 7g

ASIAN KKWARI-GOCHU

Planning Time: 5 minutes
Cook Time: 10 minutes
Serves:: 4 **Servings**
Fixings

- Salt and pepper, as essential
- 1 (6 ounces) sack shishito peppers, wash and wipe off.
- 1/3 cup finely ground parmesan cheddar
- 1/2 tablespoons olive oil
- 1 Lemon, squeezed

Strategy

1. Add the cleaned shishito peppers into a bowl and throw with pepper, salt, and olive oil until completely covered. Move peppers into the wire container of an air fryer and cook until rankled for 10 minutes at 350ºF. Note: check sometimes to forestall consuming.
2. Serve peppers, finished off with ground parmesan cheddar and lemon juice.

Healthful Data/Serving
Calories 65 kcal, Protein 3.1g, Net Carb 1g, Fiber 1.5g, Fat 4g

YUMMY CHICKEN WINGS

Planning Time: 5 minutes
Cook Time: 30 minutes
Serves:: 3 **Servings**
Fixings

- 1/4 cup coconut oil
- 1/2 lbs. (cut at the joints with a major knife) chicken wings
- 1/4 cup hot sauce

Prcscnt with Farm plunge Celery sticks

Strategy

1. Add chicken wings in the wire bushel of an air fryer and cook for 15-20 minutes at 390ºF. Flip the chicken wings over and cook until crisped and brilliant earthy colored, for 10-15 additional minutes.
2. Add coconut oil into the skillet over drug warmth and liquefy. Add hot sauce into the coconut oil and mix until joined. Spill sauce over chicken wings and throw until covered.

Healthful Data/Serving
Calories 405 kcal, Fat 35g, Protein 23g, Carbs 1g

3-CHEDDAR FILLED MUSHROOMS

Planning Time: 5 minutes
Cook Time: 8 minutes
Serves:: 5 **Servings**

Fixings

- 4 ounces (decreased fat) cream cheddar
- 8 ounces (eliminate stems and cleave into little pieces) new mushrooms, huge
- 1/8 cup (destroyed) sharp cheddar
- ¼ cup (destroyed) parmesan cheddar
- 1 tsp Worcestershire sauce
- 1/8 cup (destroyed) white cheddar
- Salt and pepper, as fundamental
- 2 (hacked) garlic cloves

Strategy

1. Scoop out mushroom tissue from where stem remained until a huge depression is made. Add cream cheddar into a heatproof bowl, place in a microwave and warmth until softened, for 15 seconds.
2. Add Worcestershire sauce, pepper, salt, each destroyed cheddar and the softened cream cheddar into a normal bowl and blend until joined. Fill the mushroom openings with the cream cheddar filling.
3. Move the stuffed mushrooms into the wire bin of an air fryer and cook at 370ºF for 8 minutes. Allow the stuffed mushrooms to sit until cooled before you serve.

Healthful Data/Serving
Calories 196 kcal, Protein 5.4g, Carbs 5.9g, Fat 18.3g

BROILED PORK SCRATCHING

Planning Time: 5 minutes
Cook Time: 15 minutes
Serves:: 1 serving

Fixings
300g pork skin, entirety

Strategy

1. On a platter, add the pork skin with the skin side up and spread out. Spot platter with the spread pork skin into a cooler for 24 hours until dried out.
2. Move pork skin onto the wire crate of an air fryer and cook plaint, for 4 minutes at 446ºF. Cut pork skin into little pieces with a kitchen scissors, and return into the air fryer crate.
3. Cook until snapped, for 5 additional minutes. Leave uncrackled pork skins noticeable all around fryer container and move popped pork pieces onto a plate fixed with paper towel to deplete.

4. Cook for 2 additional minutes and rehash measure in sync 3 above, eliminating popped pork pieces to the plate and leaving the uncrackled ones noticeable all around fryer. Rehash measure until pork skins are completely snapped.

Dietary Data/Serving
Calories 1675 kcal, Fat 131.5g, Protein 107.5g, Carbs 0.6g

HOT BACON PIECES

Planning Time: 5 minutes
Cook Time: 10 minutes
Serves:: 4 **Servings**
Fixings
- 1/4 cup hot sauce
- 4 (cut into 6 equivalent pieces ea) bacon strips
- 1/2 cup pork skins, squashed

Strategy
1. Add bacon bits into a bowl and top with hot sauce until entirely covered. Empty pork skin pieces into a level lined bowl. Inundate bacon bits into skin until entirely covered. Move bacon bits into the wire bushel of an air fryer. Seal the cover and cook for 8-10 minutes at 350ºF. Note: Check once in a while to forestall consuming.

Dietary Data/Serving
Calories 121 kcal, Protein 7.3g Carbs 0g, Fat 8.7g

CRISPED ONION RINGS

Planning Time: 10 minutes
Cook Time: 20 minutes
Serves:: 6 (3 onion rings) **Servings**

Fixings
- 2 eggs
- 1 (stripped and cut into 1/2" thick rings) yellow onion, huge
- 1/4 cup ground flax seed
- 3/4 cup almond flour
- 1/4 teaspoon garlic powder
- 1/4 teaspoon paprika
- 1/4 teaspoon dark pepper, ground
- 1/2 teaspoon salt
- Avocado oil

Strategy
1. Coat an air fryer container with avocado oil and warmth up air fryer to 400ºF. Break and beat eggs into a bowl and let sit. Add the flavors, flax seed and almond flour into a subsequent bowl and race until very much blended. Submerge every onion ring into the bowl with the egg wash until entirely covered.
2. Shake off overabundance and dunk into the almond flour blend until completely covered. Move covered onion rings into a platter. Work in bunches, add onion rings into the air fryer bushel in one layer and coat daintily with avocado oil.
3. Cook for 5-7 minutes, turn and cook for 5 additional minutes. Check from time to time to forestall consuming. Rehash measure with the leftover groups. Serve onion rings immediately and appreciate.

Nourishing Data/Serving
Calories 77 kcal, Protein 3g, Carbs 4g, Fat 4g

DELICIOUS CHOCOLATE BROWNIES

Planning Time: 10 minutes
Cook Time: 35 minutes
Serves:: 6 **Servings**

Fixings
- 1/2 cup margarine
- 1/2 cup chocolate chips, no-sugar added
- 1/4 cup erythritol
- 3 eggs
- 1 teaspoon vanilla concentrate

Strategy
1. Add chocolate and spread into a broiler secure bowl and liquefy in a microwave briefly. Note: don't overcook the chocolate. Mix the softened combination altogether until joined.
2. Add vanilla, erythritol and eggs into a bowl and beat until foamy and light. Slowly add the chocolate blend into the egg bowl and beat until combination is consolidated and completely joined.
3. Empty hitter into a pre-arranged cake dish until an embedded toothpick confesses all, for 20-30 minutes. Serve and appreciate.

Healthful Data/Serving
Calories 224 kcal, Protein 4g, Dietary Fiber 1g, Carbs 3g, Fat 23g

RICH AIR SEARED DOUGHNUTS

Planning Time: 15 minutes
Cook Time: 10 minutes
Serves:: 10 **Servings**

Fixings (doughnut)
- 1/4 cup hefty whipping cream
- 1/2 cup acrid cream
- 1 teaspoon vanilla concentrate

- 4 major eggs
- 1/4 teaspoon nutmeg
- 1/2 cup coconut flour
- 1/4 cup erythritol
- 1/4 teaspoon heating pop
- 1 squeeze salt
- ¼ cup avocado oil
- Doughnut Covering
- 1 teaspoon cinnamon
- 1/4 cup erythritol

Technique

1. Warmth up air fryer to 355º. Add vanilla concentrate, eggs, stirring cream and harsh cream into a major bowl and beat to consolidate. Slowly add the dry **Fixings** into the vanilla concentrate blend and blend until very much joined.

2. Empty player into a doughnut dish, around 3/4 of the container filled. Move doughnut container into the fryer crate and cook until very much cooked, for around 10-15 minutes. Move doughnuts from air fryer and let sit until cooled.

3. Add avocado oil into a skillet over drug heat. Add doughnuts into the hot oil and cook until brilliant earthy colored, for around 2 minutes for every side. Sprinkle cinnamon over doughnuts and serve.

Nourishing Data/Serving

Calories 141 kcal, Protein 4g, Absolute Carbs 2g, Complete Fat 12g

DELIGHTFUL FRESH SINGED PICKLES

Planning Time: 15 minutes
Cook Time: 6 minutes
Serves:: 4 **Servings**

Fixings

- 3 tbsps (ground) parmesan cheddar
- 1/2 cup pork skins, squashed
- 1/2 cup almond flour
- 16 dill pickles, cut
- 1 tsp avocado oil
- 1 (beaten) egg, huge

Strategy

1. Add parmesan cheddar and pork skinpieces into a bowl and blend until consolidated. Add the beaten egg into another bowl. Add almond flour into a third bowl.

2. Inundate the pickle in the bow, with flour, move into the bowl with egg wash and ultimately, dunk into the morsel bowl. Coat the wire bushel of an air

fryer equally. Add the breaded pickles into the air fryer bushel in one layer.

3. Splash avocado oil over breaded pickles and cook at 370ºF for 6 minutes. Eliminate, let sit to cool, serve and dive in.

Healthful Data/Serving
Calories 155 kcal, Protein 17g, Fat 11g, Net Carbs 2g, Fiber 2g

KALE CHIPS

Planning Time: 10 minutes
Cook Time: 7 minutes
Serves:: 2 **Servings**

Fixings

- 2 tbsps avocado oil
- 1 pack (dispose of hard spines and tear leaves into little pieces) kale, enormous
- 1/2 tsp salt
- 1/2 tsp bean stew powder
- 1/2 tsp pepper

Technique

1. Add kale pieces into the wire bin of air fryer and coat with avocado oil and shake until entirely covered. Sprinkle pepper, salt and stew powder over kale to prepare. Cook until wanted doneness is reached, for 6-7 minutes at 360ºF.

Healthful Data/Serving
Calories 189 kcal, Protein 4.5g, Net Carbs 11.1g, Fat 14.4g

CRUNCHY SPINACH CHIPS

Planning Time: 5 minutes
Cook Time: 5 minutes
Serves:: 2 **Servings**
Fixings

- 1 teaspoon avocado oil
- 1 bundle (eliminate stem and cut into little pieces) spinach
- 1/2 teaspoon salt
- 1/2 teaspoon garlic powder

Technique

1. Warmth up air fryer to 370ºF. Add each fixing into a normal bowl and blend until joined. Add the prepared spinach into the bushel of the preheated air fryer. Cook spinach for 3 minutes. Shake and cook for 2 additional minutes. Serve and appreciate.

Healthful Data/Serving
Calories 37 kcal, Fat 1g, Protein 3g, Carbs 6g

YUMMY LEMON DOUGHNUTS

Planning Time: 10 minutes
Cook Time: 10 minutes
Serves:: 8 **Servings**

Fixings

- 4 tablespoons liquefied coconut oil
- 4 huge eggs
- 2/3 cup lemon juice
- 3 tablespoons fluid stevia
- 1 teaspoon cinnamon
- 1 cup coconut flour
- 1 squeeze salt
- 1 teaspoon preparing pop

Strategy

1. Warmth up air fryer to 350º and lube a doughnut container with avocado oil. Add liquefied coconut oil, lemon juice, stevia, salt and eggs into a little bowl and race to consolidate. Add coconut flour, preparing pop and cinnamon into a subsequent bowl and sift to join.

2. Add flour blend into the lemon juice combination until completely joined and a player like consistency is reached. Empty hitter into the pre-arranged skillet and spread similarly. Spot dish in the pre-arranged fryer and cook for 10 minutes until doughnut edges become brilliant, at 350º.

3. Let sit to cool for 5-10 minutes prior to moving to a wire rack. Spill with wanted keto coat.

Dietary Data/Serving

Calories 179 kcal, Protein 5g, Dietary Fiber 0.2g, Carbs 9g, Complete Fat 11.2

CRISPED ZUCCHINI SQUANDERS

Planning Time: 5 minutes
Cook Time: 30 minutes
Serves:: 8 (2 waste) **Servings**

Fixings

- 2 tablespoon (partitioned) avocado oil
- 3 cups (crush out dampness) pressed ground zucchini
- 6 tablespoons minced cilantro
- 2/3 cup diced onion
- 1 cup almond flour
- 3/4-1 teaspoon ocean salt
- 1 egg white
- Newly ground dark pepper
- 2 teaspoons coconut flour
- Avocado oil

Lime Mayo Sauce

- 5 teaspoons new lime juice
- 1/2 cup mayo
- Ocean Salt, as vital
- 4 teaspoons new cleaved dill, firmly stuffed
- Newly ground dark pepper

Strategy

1. Add crushed zucchini into a major bowl. Add 2 teaspoons avocado oil into a major dish over medications heat. Add onions into the hot oil and cook until brilliant earthy colored and delicate. Add zucchini to the cooked onions.

2. Add coconut flour, almond flour, salt, cilantro and ground dark pepper into the container and mix to join. Add egg white into the zucchini blend and join until zucchini is entirely covered. Warmth up air fryer to 400º.

3. Splash fryer crate with avocado oil. Scoop a few small bunches of the zucchini combination. Working in groups, add around 4-5 zucchini waste balls into the air fryer bushel per time and splash top with avocado oil.

4. Cook squanders for around 10-15 minutes, until top is crisped and edges are brilliant earthy colored. Flip squanders with a spatula and air fry for 5-7 additional minutes.

Wholesome Data/Serving

Calories 222 kcal, Protein 3.8g, Dietary Fiber 2.8g, All out Carbs 6.9g, Absolute fat 21.8g

NUT MARGARINE FROSTED DOUGHNUTS

Planning Time: 10 minutes
Cook Time: 11 minutes
Serves:: 6 **Servings**
Fixings

- 1/3 cup stevia powder
- 1/4 cups almond flour
- 1/2 tsp preparing pop
- 1/2 tsp preparing powder
- 1 egg
- 3/4 tsp salt
- 1 tsp vanilla
- 1/2 cup buttermilk
- 2 tbsps (liquefied and cooled) unsalted spread + 1 tbsp extra for garnish

Coating

- 2 tbsps milk
- 1/2 cup powdered stevia
- 1 squeeze salt
- 2 tbsps peanut butter

Filling

- 1/2 cup blueberry jam

Technique

1. Add salt, heating pop, preparing powder, stevia powder and almond flour into a major bowl and speed until consolidated. Add vanilla, heating pop, preparing powder and egg into another bowl and beat to join.
2. Make an opening in the flour blend and add the vanilla combination. Blend combination exhaustive until all around consolidated. Add flour onto a ledge to keep batter from staying.
3. Ply and pat batter until a 3/4in thickness is reached on the pre-arranged ledge. Remove 3 1/2in rounds of batter from the smoothed mixture and coat with cooled spread. Cut a material paper round and place in a fryer bushel.
4. Add mixture into the pre-arranged fryer container and cook for 11 minutes at 350º. Add blueberry jam into a press bottle. Fill doughnuts with blueberry as wanted. Add each frosting fixing into a bowl, rush to join and spill over doughnuts until covered.

Wholesome Data/Serving

Calories 250 kcal, Carbs 11g, Fat 21g, Protein 8g

F I R M C H E D D A R S T I C K S

Planning Time: 10 minutes
Cook Time: 10 minutes
Serves:: 6 **Servings**

Fixings

- 2 (beaten) eggs, huge
- 12 (string and cut down the middle) Mozzarella sticks
- 1/2 cup (powdered) parmesan cheddar
- 1/2 cup almond flour
- 1/2 tsp garlic salt
- 1 tsp Italian flavoring

Strategy

1. Add garlic salt, Italian flavoring, parmesan cheddar powder and almond flour into a bowl and blend until consolidated. Add eggs not a subsequent bowl and race until consolidated. Coat every 50% of your cheddar stick in the egg wash and move into the almond flour blend until entirely covered.
2. Move breaded cheddar stick into a well lidded holder. Rehash measure until each cheddar stick is covered. Spot the breaded cheddar stick in the resealable holder in a solitary layer. Spot a material paper sheet over layer and top with another layer of cheddar sticks.
3. Spot well lidded cheddar compartment into a cooler to chill for 30 minutes. Move chilled cheddar sticks into the wire crate of an air fryer. Cook for 5 minutes at 400ºF. In the wake of cooking, outside fryer crate and let cheddar sticks sit briefly.
4. Move cheddar adheres to a platter prior to serving.

Healthful Data/Serving
Calories 276 kcal, Fat 20g, Protein 18g, Carbs 4g

L I M E Y F I L L E D A R T I C H O K E S

Planning Time: 10 minutes
Cook Time: 30 minutes
Serves:: 4 **Servings**

Fixings

- 1 tbsp avocado oil
- 1 (enormous) artichoke, cut stem off and trim a little part off the top
- ½ cup (disintegrated) pork skins
- 2 tbsps lime juice
- ¼ cup parmesan cheddar, ground
- ½ cup (partitioned) mozzarella cheddar, destroyed
- 1 tsp minced garlic
- 2 tbsps new cleaved cilantro
- Salt and pepper, as vital

Strategy

1. Add 1" of water into the foundation of a pot over medications warmth, and bring to bubbling. Add 2 tablespoons lime juice into the bubbling water. Cut off the sharp and sharp finish of the artichoke leaves utilizing a kitchen scissors.
2. Move the artichokes into the bubbling water, looking up. Spot top over pot and stew until mollified, for 25 minutes. Remove artichoke from the water, channel and let sit to cool.
3. Put away not many tbsps mozzarella cheddar for sometime in the future. Meanwhile, add slashed cilantro, disintegrated pork skin, garlic, avocado oil, parmesan cheddar and mozzarella cheddar. Season with pepper and salt as essential and mix until consolidated.
4. Scoop cheddar combination and stuff into the artichokes until filled. Dissipate the held mozzarella cheddar over artichoke. Warmth up air fryer to 360ºF. Sprinkle avocado oil over stuffed artichokes.
5. Spot the stuffed artichokes in the wire bin of an air fryer and cook until wanted doneness is reached, for 20 minutes.

Nourishing Data/Serving
Calories 137 kcal, Fat 9g, Protein 8g, Carbs 4g

MESSY GARLIC BREAD

Fixings
- 5 round bread cuts
- 5 teaspoons sun-dried tomato pesto
- 3 slashed garlic cloves
- 4 Tbsp. softened spread
- 1 cup ground Mozzarella cheddar

Enhancement Alternatives:
- Chili drops
- Chopped basil leaves
- oregano

Guidelines
1) Preheat the Air Fryer to 356°F.
2) Cut the portion of bread into 5 thick cuts.
3) Add the margarine, pesto, and cheddar on the bread.
4) Put the cuts in the preheated cooker for six to eight minutes.
5) Enhancement with your selection of Fixings .

Note: Round or Roll bread was utilized for this formula. It is prescribed to add the finely cleaved garlic cloves to the liquefied margarine early for the best outcomes.

SHELLFISHES OREGANO

Fixings
- 2 dozen shucked shellfishes
- 1 cup unseasoned breadcrumbs
- 4 tablespoons liquefied margarine
- 3 clove minced garlic
- 1 teaspoon dried oregano
- ¼ cup cleaved parsley
- ¼ cup ground Parmesan cheddar

For the Container:
- 1 cup ocean salt

Guidelines
1) Preheat the AF to 400°F.
2) Blend the oregano, parsley, parmesan cheddar, breadcrumbs, and liquefied margarine in a medium compartment.
3) Utilizing a loading tablespoon of the morsel blend; add it to the uncovered shellfishes.

4) Fill the supplement with the salt, place the shellfishes inside and cook for three minutes.
5) Dress them up with a topping of lemon wedges and new parsley.
Yields: Four **Servings**

CORN TORTILLA CHIPS

Fixings
- 8 corn Tortillas
- 1 Tbsp. olive oil
- Salt if wanted

Guidelines
1) Preset the AF to 392°F.
2) Utilize a sharp knife to cut the tortillas.
3) Brush every tortilla with oil.
4) Air fry two clumps for three minutes each. Sprinkle with a spot of salt.

CRAB STICKS

Fixings
- 1 bundle 'DoDo' crab sticks
- Cooking shower

Guidelines
1) Remove every one of the sticks from the bundle; discover an edge, and unroll until level.
2) Tear the sheets into 1/3 widths.
3) Spot them on a plate and coat them with cooking splash.
4) Cook them in the AF for 10 minutes.
5) Note: If you shred the crab meat; you can slice the time down the middle, yet they will likewise effectively fall through the openings in the crate.

GARLIC BUNCHES

Fixings
- Marinara sauce
- 1 teaspoon ocean salt
- 1 Lb. frozen pizza outside batter

1 tablespoon each:
- Garlic powder
- Grated Parmesan cheddar
- Fresh hacked parsley

Directions
1) Preheat the Air Fryer to 360°F.
2) Carry out the batter until is around 1 ½ to 2-inches thick. Cut it roughly ¾-inches separated—longwise.
3) Fold the batter and make it into ties.
4) Add the cheddar, oil, and flavors in a bowl, and roll each bunch in the blend prior to setting it into the fry bin.

5) Set the clock for 12 minutes; flipping part of the way through the cooking interaction (six minutes).

MEATBALLS FOR THE GATHERING

Fixings
- 2 ½ Tablespoons Worcestershire sauce
- 1 pound ground hamburger
- 1 Tablespoon Tabasco
- ¾ cup ketchup
- 1 Tablespoon lemon juice
- ¼ cup vinegar
- ½ teaspoon dry mustard
- ½ cup earthy colored sugar
- 3 squashed gingersnaps

Guidelines
1) Join the entirety of the flavors in an enormous blending holder—mixing great.
2) Blend the hamburger and keep agitating the **Fixings** .
3) Make the balls and put them in the fryer. Cook on 375ºF for 15 minutes.
4) Spot them on the toothpicks prior to serving. Note: They are prepared when the middle is done, and they are firm.
Yields: 24 **Servings**

FETA TRIANGLES

Fixings
- 4 ounces feta cheddar
- 1 egg yolk
- 2 tablespoons finely slashed level leafed parsley
- 2 sheets frozen (thawed out) filo baked good
- 1 finely slashed scallion
- 2 tablespoons olive oil
- Ground dark pepper

1) Pre-set the warmth Noticeable all around Fryer to 390ºF.
2) Whisk the egg and mix in the scallion, feta, and parsley.
3) Cut the mixture into three strips.
4) Spot a loading teaspoon of the feta blend under the cake strip.
5) Overlap the tip to frame a triangle as you work your way around the strip.
6) Utilize a limited quantity of oil and brush every one of the triangles prior to putting them in the cooker container cooking them for three minutes.
7) Lower the warmth to 360ºF, and keep cooking for an extra two minutes.

Yields: Five **Servings**

MOZZARELLA STICKS

Fixings
- 2 eggs
- 1 pound or square Mozzarella cheddar
- 1 cup plain breadcrumbs
- ¼ cup white flour
- 3 tablespoons nonfat milk

Directions
1) Preheat the fryer to 400ºF.
2) Cut the cheddar into ½-inch x 3-inch sticks.
3) Whisk the milk and egg together in one bowl, with the oil and bread pieces in singular dishes also.
4) Dig the cut cheddar through the oil, egg, and breadcrumbs.
5) Spot the sticks on bread tin and put them in the cooler compartment for about a little while.
6) Spot them in little augmentations (don't stuff) into the AF crate.
7) Cook for 12 minutes.
Yields: Four **Servings**

LITTLE QUICHE WEDGES

Fixings
- 1 (3 ½ ounces or 100 g) Frozen or instant pizza outside
- 1 egg
- 1.4 ounces or 40 g of Ground cheddar
- ½ tablespoon oil
- 3 tablespoons whipping cream
- New ground pepper
- 2 little pie molds

1) Pre-set the warmth on the Air Fryer to 392ºF/200ºC.
2) Utilize a touch of cooking splash to lube the molds. Line them with the batter pushing down around the edges.
3) Whisk the cheddar, cream, and egg enhancing with some pepper and salt to taste. Void the combination into the molds.
4) Put the shape into the crate and set the clock for 12 minutes. Prepare the second one a similar way.
5) Take them from the molds and cut every one of the quiche into six wedges.
6) You can serve at room temperature or warm.

Y AM C HIPS

Fixings
- 2 Huge Yams
- 1 Tbsp. olive oil

1) Pre-set the warmth Noticeable all around Fryer to 350ºF.

2) Strip and cut the potatoes into chips. It is ideal to cut them into similar sizes so then will cook uniformly.

3) Spot the potatoes into a resealable baggie and add the oil. Shake the potatoes to cover them totally.

4) Empty the yams into the Air Fryer and cook for around fifteen minutes, contingent upon the thickness.

S CALED DOWN B LOSSOMING O NIONS

These little men are to some degree drawn-out in the prep, yet your visitors will flip over the charm factor! The award in acclaim merits your cautious knife abilities. Serve these warm with plunging sauce.

Active Time: 20 minutes
Cook Time: 14 minutes
Fixings | **Serves:** 5
- 10 ounces crude yellow pearl onions (around 20)
- 1/2 cup generally useful flour
- 1 teaspoon salt, in addition to additional for sprinkling
- 1/2 teaspoon ground dry mustard
- 1/2 teaspoon stew powder
- 1 huge egg
- 1/2 cup entire milk
- 1 cup panko bread pieces, squashed fine
- 1/2 cup cornmeal

1. Shallowly cut the root end off of every onion so it can sit level yet the areas stay appended. Strip and dispose of the skins. Utilizing a sharp knife, delicately cut around 3/4 of the route down through the onion into fifths, as though you were cutting a pie, uncovering a sum of ten areas, keeping the base flawless. Absorb the onions a bowl of ice water 30 minutes to help spread the areas. Move onions to a paper towel and eliminate abundance water.

2. Add flour, salt, mustard, and stew powder to a little bowl. In a different little bowl, whisk together egg and milk.

4. Consolidate bread pieces and cornmeal in a shallow dish.

5. Preheat air fryer at 375°F for 3 minutes.

6. Move onions in flour and flavor blend. Shake off overabundance flour. Dig onions in egg blend. Shake off abundance. Move in bread piece blend. Move to a plate. Rehash with residual onions.

7. Add half of onions to fryer container. Cook 7 minutes. Move to a plate and rehash with residual onions. Sprinkle with salt. Serve warm.

Per serving Calories: 192 | fat: 2.1 g | protein: 5.4 g | sodium: 416 mg | fiber: 1.7 g | carbs: 36.0 g | sugar: 4.5 g

L ITTLE S COTCH E GGS

Your partygoers will become hopelessly enamored with these Small Scotch Eggs. Quail eggs can be found at some claim to fame merchants just as Asian business sectors. These eggs have a comparable taste to chicken eggs yet are somewhat more extravagant because of the greater yolk-to-white proportion.

Active Time: 15 minutes
Cook Time: 10 minutes
Fixings | **Serves:** 4
- 12 quail eggs
- 1 cup ice
- 1 cup water
- 1/2 pound lean ground pork
- 1 teaspoon new thyme leaves
- 1/4 teaspoon salt
- 1/4 teaspoon newly ground dark pepper
- 1 enormous egg
- 1/2 cup panko bread pieces

1. Preheat air fryer at 250°F for 3 minutes.

2. Spot eggs in air fryer crate. Cook 4 minutes.

3. Add ice and water to a medium bowl. Move eggs to this water shower promptly to stop the cooking cycle. Following 5 minutes, strip eggs.

4. In a medium bowl, consolidate pork, thyme, salt, and pepper. Structure a slender layer of pork around each egg.

5. Preheat air fryer at 375°F for 3 minutes.

6. In a little bowl, whisk huge egg. In another bowl, add bread morsels.

7. Plunge shrouded eggs in whisked egg and afterward dig in bread scraps.

8. Spot eggs in air fryer bin. Cook 3 minutes. Turn. Cook an extra 3 minutes. Serve warm.

Per serving Calories: 168 | fat: 5.8 g | protein: 17.7 g | sodium: 250 mg | fiber: 0.1 g | carbs: 8.3 g |sugar: 0.5 g

PIMIENTO CHEDDAR STUFFED JALAPEÑOS

This gentle, smooth blend is extraordinary stuffed in hot jalapeño boats. Since the peppers are cultivated, a large portion of the warmth is eliminated. If you like things hot, blend the seeds in with the pimiento cheddar to warm things up.

Involved Time: 10 minutes
Cook Time: 16 minutes
Fixings | Serves: 4
- 6 medium jalapeño peppers
- ^{1}/2 cup pimiento cheddar

1. Cut jalapeño peppers the long way and dispose of seeds. (if you like the warmth, mix the seeds into the pimiento cheddar.)
2. Press equivalent sums pimiento cheddar into each jalapeño half.
3. Preheat air fryer at 350°F for 3 minutes.
4. Lay six stuffed peppers into air fryer bushel. Cook 8 minutes. Move cooked peppers to a serving plate. Rehash with outstanding peppers.
5. Move to a serving plate and serve warm.

Per serving Calories: 71 | fat: 5.2 g | protein: 4.1 g | sodium: 160 mg | fiber: 0.6 g | carbs: 1.7 g sugar: 1.0 g

JALAPEÑO POPPER BOMBS

Messy, hot, bready . . . yummy! These Jalapeño Popper Bombs have all the flavor southern style poppers have however without all the oil and with less cheddar. The mixture assists tone with bringing down the pepper heat, making these canapés charming for every one of your visitors.

Involved Time: 10 minutes
Cook Time: 12 minutes
Fixings | Serves: 3
- ^{1}/3 cup generally useful flour
- ^{1}/4 teaspoon salt
- ^{1}/4 teaspoon preparing powder
- 2 tablespoons diced jalapeño pepper, seeds eliminated
- 2 ounces cream cheddar, at room temperature
- 1 tablespoon destroyed Monterey jack cheddar
- 2 tablespoons destroyed cheddar
- 2 tablespoons entire milk
- ^{1}/2 teaspoon olive oil

1. In a medium bowl, consolidate flour, salt, and preparing powder.
2. In a little bowl, join remaining Fixings .
3. Empty combination from little bowl into dry Fixings in medium bowl.
4. Preheat air fryer at 325°F for 3 minutes.
5. Structure blend into nine (1") balls. Spot in delicately lubed pizza skillet (extra). It's okay if the poppers are contacting. Cook 12 minutes.
6. Move to a plate. Serve warm.

Per serving Calories: 155 | fat: 8.7 g | protein: 4.6 g | sodium: 350 mg | fiber: 0.5 g | starches: 12.3 g | sugar: 1.3 g

CHEDDAR ROLL BREADED GREEN OLIVES

You'll get fixated on this new disclosure. Cheddar batter folded over briny green olives? Indeed! Attempt this formula with dark olives as well!

Active Time: 15 minutes
Cook Time: 8 minutes
Fixings | Serves: 5
- ^{2}/3 cup generally useful flour
- ^{1}/2 teaspoon preparing powder
- ^{1}/2 cup finely ground sharp cheddar
- 4 tablespoons spread, liquefied
- 25 pimiento-stuffed standard Manzanilla green olives

1. In a food processor, beat flour, preparing powder, cheddar, and softened margarine until an uncooked ball structures.
2. Channel olives and wipe off with a paper towel.
3. Structure barely sufficient flour combination around an olive to cover it. Move between your hands to shape a smooth ball. Rehash with outstanding olives.
4. Preheat air fryer at 375°F for 3 minutes.
5. Spot olives in delicately lubed air fryer container. Cook 3 minutes. Delicately shake. Cook an extra 3 minutes. Tenderly shake. Cook an extra 2 minutes. Verify whether daintily seared. Give additional time if required; something else, move to a serving dish and let rest 5 minutes prior to serving warm.

SEARED FETA-DILL-BREADED KALAMATA OLIVES

The natural mix of feta, dill, and Kalamata olives is gathered in this one little nibble of delight. The firm outside mixture is consummated noticeable all around fryer. Serve these olives as a hors d'oeuvre, a bite, or even tossed into a new Greek plate of mixed greens!

Active Time: 15 minutes
CookTime: 8 minutes
Fixings | **Serves:**5
- ²/3 cup generally useful flour
- ¹/2 teaspoon preparing powder
- ¹/2 cup disintegrated feta cheddar
- ¹/2 teaspoon dried dill
- 4 tablespoons spread, liquefied
- 25 pitted standard Kalamata olives

1. In a food processor, beat flour, preparing powder, feta cheddar, dill, and softened margarine until a sticky ball structures.
2. Channel olives and wipe off with a paper towel.
3. Structure barely sufficient flour blend around an olive to cover it. Move between your hands to frame a smooth ball. Rehash with outstanding olives.
4. Preheat air fryer at 375°F for 3 minutes.
5. Spot olives in softly lubed air fryer bushel. Cook 3 minutes. Delicately shake. Cook an extra 3 minutes. Tenderly shake. Cook an extra 2 minutes. Verify whether softly cooked. Give additional time if required; something else, move to a serving dish and let rest 5 minutes prior to serving warm.

Per serving Calories: 225 | Fat: 16.7 g | Protein: 4.0 g | Sodium: 475 mg | Fiber: 0.5 g | Carbs: 13.5 g | Sugar: 0.7 g

BISON NECTAR CHICKEN WINGS

The pleasantness of the nectar helps temper the warmth from the bison sauce, making this a gentle mix ideal for the whole family. You might need to make a twofold bunch on the grounds that these wings vanish quickly.

Active Time: 15 minutes
CookTime: 44 minutes
Fixings | **Serves:**6
- 1 tablespoon water
- 2 pounds chicken wings, split at the joint, tips eliminated
- 1 tablespoon margarine
- ¹/2 cup wild ox sauce

- 2 tablespoons nectar

1. Spot 1 tablespoon water in the lower part of the air fryer to guarantee least smoke from fat drippings.
2. Preheat air fryer at 250°F for 3 minutes.
3. Spot half of wings in air fryer bin. Cook 6 minutes. Flip wings. Cook an extra 6 minutes.
4. While wings are cooking, join spread, wing sauce, and nectar in an enormous bowl. The chicken wings will dissolve the margarine, so don't stress over softening it previously.
5. Raise temperature on air fryer to 400°F. Flip wings and cook 5 minutes. Flip wings and cook an extra 5 minutes. Move to bowl with sauce and throw.
6. Rehash measure with residual wings and move all to a serving dish.

Per serving Calories: 368 | Fat: 22.9 g | Protein: 31.0 g | Sodium: 741 mg | Fiber: 0.0 g | Carbs: 5.8 g | Sugar: 5.8 g

PEANUT BUTTER AND STRAWBERRY JAM WINGS

This exemplary mix of peanut butter and jam is a characteristic supplement to the unassuming chicken wing. You could likewise attempt jalapeño jam decorated with new cilantro for a Mexican curve, or fig jam embellished with some goat cheddar disintegrates.

Involved Time: 15 minutes
CookTime: 44 minutes

Fixings | **Serves:**6
- 1 tablespoon water
- 2 pounds chicken wings, split at the joint, tips eliminated
- 2 teaspoons margarine
- ¹/4 cup velvety peanut butter
- ¹/2 cup strawberry jam
- 2 tablespoons apple juice vinegar
- 1 teaspoon hot sauce

1. Spot 1 tablespoon water in the lower part of the air fryer to guarantee least smoke from fat drippings.
2. Preheat air fryer at 250°F for 3 minutes.
3. Spot half of wings in air fryer bushel. Cook 6 minutes. Flip wings. Cook an extra 6 minutes.
4. While wings are cooking, consolidate margarine, peanut butter, jam, vinegar, and hot sauce in a huge bowl. The chicken wings will soften the spread, so don't stress over dissolving it in advance.
5. Raise temperature on air fryer to 400°F. Flip wings

and cook 5 minutes. Flip wings and cook an extra 5 minutes. Move to bowl with sauce and throw.
6. Rehash measure with outstanding wings and move all to a serving dish.

Per serving Calories: 480 | Fat: 27.6 g | Protein: 33.4 g | Sodium: 142 mg | Fiber: 0.8 g | Starches: 20.8 g | Sugar: 14.1 g

THAI SWEET BEAN STEW WINGS

The fresh skin on these wings from air singing is stunning with the tacky integrity of the sauce.

Involved Time: 15 minutes
CookTime: 44 minutes
Fixings | Serves:6
- 1 tablespoon water
- 2 pounds chicken wings, split at the joint, tips eliminated
- ¹/2 cup Sweet Bean stew Sauce (see Part 15)

1. Spot 1 tablespoon water in the lower part of the air fryer to guarantee least smoke from fat drippings.
2. Preheat air fryer at 250°F for 3 minutes.
3. Spot half of wings in air fryer container. Cook 6 minutes. Flip wings. Cook an extra 6 minutes.
4. While wings are cooking, add sauce to an enormous bowl.
5. Raise temperature on air fryer to 400°F. Flip wings and cook 5 minutes. Flip wings and cook an extra 5 minutes. Move to bowl with sauce and throw.
6. Rehash measure with outstanding wings and move all to a serving dish.

Per serving Calories: 472 | Fat: 21.1 g | Protein: 31.1 g | Sodium: 238 mg | Fiber: 0.0 g | Starches: 35.2 g | Sugar: 33.6 g

SALMON CROQUETTES

Generally, croquettes are a singed delicacy, as the word croquette comes from the French word croquer, which signifies "to crunch" or "to be crunchy." Notwithstanding, with the air fryer, you'll get all the freshness without the unfortunate cooking style. Serve these with your most loved plunging sauce.

Active Time: 15 minutes
CookTime: 24 minutes
Fixings | Serves:4
- 1 (14.75-ounce) can wild-got salmon, depleted
- ¹/3 cup mayonnaise
- 1 tablespoon minced celery
- 2 teaspoons dried dill, partitioned
- 1 teaspoon lime juice
- ¹/2 cup panko bread pieces, isolated
- 1 huge egg
- 1 teaspoon arranged horseradish
- ¹/4 cup cornmeal
- 1 teaspoon salt

1. In a medium bowl, join salmon, mayonnaise, celery, 1 teaspoon dill, lime juice, ¹/4 cup bread morsels, egg, and horseradish.
2. In a shallow dish, join ¹/4 cup bread pieces, cornmeal, remaining dill, and salt.
3. Preheat air fryer at 375°F for 3 minutes.
4. Structure 2 tablespoons salmon combination into sixteen children or egg shapes. Move in bread scrap combination. Proceed with rest of salmon.
5. Spot eight children in delicately lubed air fryer crate. Cook 4 minutes. Delicately turn toddlers 33% of the route around. Cook an extra 4 minutes. Tenderly turn children another third. Cook an extra 4 minutes. Move to a serving dish. Rehash with outstanding children. Let rest 5 minutes prior to serving warm.

Per serving Calories: 395 | Fat: 20.1 g | Protein: 31.6 g | Sodium: 1,154 mg | Fiber: 0.5 g | Carbs: 18.6 g | Sugar: 1.0 g

PEPPERONI PIZZA NIBBLES

Plunge these delightful little Pepperoni Pizza Chomps in a warm marinara sauce as an after-school nibble or as fast game-day food! The pungent pepperoni and melty mozzarella make a triumphant blend for anybody, and they are so natural to make.

Involved Time: 10 minutes
CookTime: 12 minutes
Fixings | Serves:2
- ¹/3 cup universally handy flour
- ¹/4 teaspoon salt
- ¹/4 teaspoon heating powder
- ¹/2 cup little diced pepperoni
- 2 ounces cream cheddar, at room temperature
- ¹/4 cup destroyed mozzarella cheddar
- ¹/2 teaspoon Italian flavoring
- 2 tablespoons entire milk
- 1 teaspoon olive oil

1. In a little bowl, consolidate flour, salt, and heating powder.
2. In a medium bowl, consolidate remaining **Fixings** until smooth. Add dry **Fixings** until all around joined.
3. Preheat air fryer at 325°F for 5 minutes.
4. Structure combination into nine (1") balls and add to pizza dish (frill). It's good if the pizza nibbles are contacting. Cook 12 minutes.
5. Move to a plate. Serve warm.

Per serving Calories: 366 | Fat: 22.8 g | Protein: 13.1 g | Sodium: 987 mg | Fiber: 0.6 g | Starches: 18.2 g | Sugar: 1.9 g

BROCCOLI SNACKERS

The marginally seared edges give this occasionally detested vegetable another taste and surface. Add a little plunging sauce for those difficult to-prevail upon people, and this may turn into another most loved bite!

Involved Time: 10 minutes
CookTime: 12 minutes

Fixings | **Serves:**4
- 1 enormous head of broccoli, slashed into florets
- 1 tablespoon olive oil
- ¹/2 teaspoon salt

1. Preheat air fryer at 350°F for 3 minutes.
2. In an enormous bowl, throw broccoli florets with olive oil.
3. Spot half of broccoli in fryer container. Cook 3 minutes. Shake. Cook an extra 3 minutes. Move to a serving bowl. Season with salt.
4. Rehash with outstanding broccoli and serve warm.

Per serving Calories: 81 | Fat: 3.4 g | Protein: 4.3 g | Sodium: 340 mg | Fiber: 4.0 g | Starches: 10.1 g | Sugar: 2.6 g

REDUCED DOWN PORK EGG ROLLS

These little men might be somewhat dreary to make, yet the final product is so worth the time. One approach to cut **Active Time** is by buying effectively destroyed cabbage and carrots. These are generally named "coleslaw blend" and can be found close to the bundled plates of mixed greens in the produce segment.

Involved Time: 30 minutes

CookTime: 24 minutes
Fixings | **Serves:**10
- ¹/2 pound lean ground pork
- 2 cups coleslaw blend (destroyed cabbage and carrots)
- 3 scallions, managed and minced
- 1 tablespoon hoisin sauce
- 1 tablespoon soy sauce
- ¹/4 teaspoon sriracha
- ¹/2 teaspoon lime juice
- 30 wonton coverings
- 2 teaspoons olive oil

1. In a huge skillet, heat ground pork over medium-high warmth. Sautéed food 5–6 minutes until not, at this point pink. Add coleslaw blend and mix into pork. Add scallions, hoisin sauce, soy sauce, sriracha, and lime juice. Sautéed food an extra 2 minutes. Eliminate from warmth and let rest 5 minutes off the burner.
2. Spot a wonton covering on a cutting board. Spot a little bowl of water close to the board. Spoon around 2 teaspoons combination in a line in the covering. Dunk your finger into the water and daintily run it around the edge of the wonton covering. Overlay ¹/4" of the edge of wonton toward the center. Move up the length to frame an egg roll. Rehash for every wonton covering.
3. Preheat air fryer at 325°F for 3 minutes.
4. Spot half of the egg abounds noticeable all around fryer container. Cook 3 minutes. Softly brush the highest points of egg moves with olive oil. Cook an extra 5 minutes. Rehash with second clump.
5. Move to a plate. Serve warm.

Per serving Calories: 106 | Fat: 1.2 g | Protein: 7.5 g | Sodium: 268 mg | Fiber: 0.9 g | Starches: 15.7 g | Sugar: 1.0 g

GREEN BEAN STEW FRESH WONTON SQUARES

Crunchy outwardly and smooth and gooey within, these squares burst with flavor in each nibble. Queso fresco, a rich and gentle Mexican cheddar, can be found in many merchants in squares and wedges.

Involved Time: 15 minutes
CookTime: 35 minutes
Fixings | **Serves:**6
- 30 wonton coverings
- 1 cup refried beans
- 2 (4-ounce) jars diced green chilies
- 1 cup ground queso fresco

1. Spot a wonton covering on a cutting board. Spot around 1¹/2 teaspoons beans in covering. Add roughly 1¹/2 teaspoons green chilies and around 1¹/2 teaspoons queso fresco.
2. Spot a little bowl of water close to the functioning region. Plunge your finger in the water bowl and run it around the border of the wonton. Carry all corners to the middle and press the straight edges together. Put away. Rehash with residual wontons.
3. Preheat air fryer at 325°F for 3 minutes.
4. Spot six wontons in air fryer container. Cook 7 minutes. Move to a plate and cook the excess clusters. Serve warm.

Per serving Calories: 220 | Fat: 4.8 g | Protein: 9.7 g | Sodium: 680 mg | Fiber: 3.9 g | Starches: 31.7 g | Sugar: 2.0 g

BRIE AND RED PEPPER JAM TRIANGLES

This is an overhaul on that square of cream cheddar finished off with red pepper jam that you see presented with wafers at many local gatherings. These triangles contain the entirety of the flavors in one flawless and pretty scrumptious chomp!

Involved Time: 10 minutes
CookTime: 16 minutes

Fixings | **Serves:**4
- 20 wonton coverings
- 10 teaspoons Brie cheddar
- 10 teaspoons red pepper jam
- 40 almond bits
- 1 tablespoon olive oil

1. Spot a wonton covering on a cutting board. Spot around ¹/2 teaspoon Brie and afterward ¹/2 teaspoon red pepper jam in covering. Spot 2 almond bits on top.
2. Spot a little bowl of water close to the functioning region. Plunge your finger in the water bowl and run it around the edge of the wonton. Overlap one corner to the contrary corner, framing a triangle. Press down edges to seal. Put away. Rehash with outstanding wontons.
3. Preheat air fryer at 325°F for 3 minutes.
4. Spot half of the triangles noticeable all around fryer bin. Cook 3 minutes. Delicately brush the highest points of triangles with olive oil. Cook an extra 5 minutes. Rehash with second clump.
5. Move to a plate. Serve warm.

Per serving Calories: 239 | Fat: 8.9 g | Protein: 6.9 g | Sodium: 292 mg | Fiber: 1.6 g | Starches: 32.2 g | Sugar: 7.8 g

REUBEN PIZZA FOR ONE

If you are a Reuben darling, at that point this is your pizza. With the entirety of the flavors from the exemplary Reuben sandwich, it guarantees that you never need your pizza some other way.

Involved Time: 10 minutes
CookTime: 17 minutes
Fixings | **Yields** 1 Individual Pizza

- ¹/4 pound new pizza batter, about the size of a tennis ball
- ¹/4 teaspoon caraway seeds
- 2 tablespoons Thousand Island dressing (or Russian dressing)
- ¹/4 cup slashed corned meat
- ¹/4 cup destroyed Swiss cheddar
- ¹/4 cup sauerkraut, depleted

1. Preheat air fryer at 200°F for 6 minutes.
2. Press out mixture to fit pizza container (extra). Sprinkle caraway seeds equally over batter. Cook 7 minutes.
3. Turn up the warmth to 275°F.
4. Eliminate container and spread dressing over batter, leaving ¹/4" external outside uncovered. Equally add corned meat. Sprinkle cheddar over meat. Cook an extra 10 minutes.
5. Tenderly exchange pizza to a cutting board. Uniformly add sauerkraut. Cut into six cuts and serve.

Per serving Calories: 848 | Fat: 42.5 g | Protein: 41.3 g | Sodium: 2,409 mg | Fiber: 3.1 g | Starches: 62.7 g | Sugar: 12.8 g

INDIVIDUAL PEPPERONI AND MUSHROOM PIZZA

This formula is for one, with the idea of adding pepperoni and mushrooms. In any case, you can twofold or fourfold this formula and get relatives engaged with adding their #1 **Fixings** to their individual pizzas.

Active Time: 10 minutes
CookTime: 17 minutes
Fixings | **YIELDS** 1 Individual PIZZA
- ¹/4 pound new pizza batter, about the size of a tennis ball

- 2 tablespoons marinara or pizza sauce
- 6 cuts pepperoni
- ¹/4 cup cut white mushrooms
- ¹/4 cup ground mozzarella cheddar

1. Preheat air fryer at 200°F for 6 minutes.
2. Press out mixture to fit pizza skillet (frill). Cook 7 minutes.
3. Turn up the warmth to 275°F. Eliminate bin and spread sauce over mixture, leaving ¹/4" external outside layer uncovered. Add pepperoni cuts and mushrooms. Sprinkle cheddar over both. Cook an extra 10 minutes.
4. Delicately move pizza to a cutting board. Cut into six cuts and serve.

Per serving Calories: 554 | Fat: 16.3 g | Protein: 21.9 g | Sodium: 2,154 mg | Fiber: 6.7 g | Carbs: 75.1 g | Sugar: 22.1 g

EVERYTHING BAGEL-SINGED CHICKPEAS

This formula seasons chickpeas with the famous all that bagel zest blend. Fresh and crunchy once cooked, these chickpeas make an incredible tidbit!

Involved Time: 5 minutes
CookTime: 16 minutes
Fixings | Serves:4
- 1 (15-ounce) can chickpeas/garbanzo beans, depleted and flushed
- 2 teaspoons olive oil
- 1 tablespoon all that bagel preparing blend (see sidebar)

1. Preheat air fryer at 350°F for 3 minutes.
2. In a little bowl, throw chickpeas in olive oil. Add to fryer container.
3. Spot in air fryer bin and cook 5 minutes. Shake. Cook an extra 5 minutes. Shake. Cook an extra 6 minutes.
4. Move to a little bowl and throw with preparing blend. Let cool and serve.

Per serving Calories: 122 | Fat: 3.2 g | Protein: 4.5 g | Sodium: 374 mg | Fiber: 4.0 g | Starches: 14.5 g | Sugar: 2.5 g

FIVE ZEST CRUNCHY EDAMAME

The sweet kind of the edamame matches pleasantly with the flavors in Chinese five zest. Firm outwardly and somewhat delicate within, these snackable chomps convey a sound portion of fiber, nutrients, and minerals.

Active Time: 5 minutes
CookTime: 16 minutes
Fixings | Serves:4
- 1 cup prepared to-eat edamame, shelled
- 1 tablespoon sesame oil
- 1 teaspoon five flavor powder
- ¹/2 teaspoon salt

1. Preheat air fryer at 350°F for 3 minutes.
2. In a little bowl, throw edamame in sesame oil. Add to fryer bushel.
3. Spot in air fryer crate and cook 5 minutes. Shake. Cook an extra 5 minutes. Shake. Cook an extra 6 minutes.
4. Move to a little bowl and throw with five flavor powder and salt. Let cool and serve.

Per serving Calories: 77 | Fat: 4.8 g | Protein: 4.2 g | Sodium: 292 mg | Fiber: 2.0 g | Starches: 3.9 g | Sugar: 0.8 g

BAR-B-QUE CAULIFLOWER NIBBLES

The kind of this dish can change contingent upon which grill sauce you pick—zesty or sweet, Korean or St. Louis style. The cauliflower assumes the kind of whatever you pair it with, meanwhile conveying your body a solid punch of nutrient C!

Active Time: 10 minutes
CookTime: 12 minutes
Fixings | Serves:4
- 1 huge head cauliflower, slashed into florets, center eliminated
- 2 teaspoons olive oil
- ¹/4 cup grill sauce of your decision

1. Preheat air fryer at 350°F for 3 minutes.
2. In a huge bowl, throw cauliflower florets with olive oil.
3. Spot half of cauliflower in fryer crate. Cook 3 minutes. Shake. Cook an extra 3 minutes.
4. Move to a medium bowl and throw with a large portion of the grill sauce. Rehash with outstanding cauliflower.
5. Move to a serving bowl and serve warm.

Per serving **Calories**: 102 | Fat: 2.6 g | Protein: 4.2 g | Sodium: 246 mg | Fiber: 4.4 g | Carbs: 17.7 g | Sugar: 10.0 g

MOZZARELLA STICKLETS

This is a small scale adaptation of those rotisserie delights found on numerous tidbit menus—less the oil. Serve these smaller than normal sticks with toothpicks and a warm marinara sauce.

Involved Time: 15 minutes
CookTime: 10 minutes
Fixings | **Serves:**6

- 2 tablespoons generally useful flour
- 1 huge egg
- 1 tablespoon entire milk
- $^1/2$ cup plain bread scraps
- $^1/4$ teaspoon salt
- $^1/4$ teaspoon Italian flavoring
- 10 mozzarella sticks, each cut into thirds
- 2 teaspoons olive oil

1. In a little bowl, add flour.
2. In another little bowl, whisk together egg and milk.
3. Consolidate bread morsels, salt, and Italian flavoring in a shallow dish.
4. Roll a mozzarella sticklet in flour, at that point dig in egg blend, and afterward move in bread morsel combination. Shake off overabundance between each progression. Put away on a plate and rehash with outstanding mozzarella. Spot in cooler 10 minutes.
5. Preheat air fryer at 400°F for 3 minutes.
6. Spot half of mozzarella sticklets in fryer crate. Cook 2 minutes. Shake. Delicately brush with olive oil. Cook an extra 2 minutes. Shake. Cook an extra 1 moment. Move to a serving dish.
7. Rehash with remaining sticklets and serve warm.

Per serving **Calories**: 181 | Fat: 9.5 g | Protein: 13.6 g | Sodium: 451 mg | Fiber: 0.4 g | Starches: 8.6 g | Sugar: 1.1 g

GOAT CHEDDAR AND PROSCIUTTO-STUFFED MUSHROOMS

Your taste buds will acclaim once they taste the smooth goat cheddar blended in with the pungency of the prosciutto, all stuffed in hearty mushrooms. The mix is hazardous, and the readiness is so straightforward.

Involved Time: 10 minutes
CookTime: 20 minutes
Fixings | **Serves:**4

- $^1/4$ cup disintegrated goat cheddar
- 1 tablespoon minced onion
- 1 teaspoon lemon juice
- $^1/2$ teaspoon salt
- $^1/2$ teaspoon newly ground dark pepper
- 16 ounces child bella (cremini) mushrooms, stems eliminated
- 2 tablespoons panko bread scraps
- 2 tablespoons margarine, liquefied
- 2 ounces prosciutto, attacked little pieces
- $^1/4$ cup julienned new basil

1. In a medium bowl, join goat cheddar, onion, lemon squeeze, salt, and pepper.
2. Preheat air fryer at 350°F for 3 minutes.
3. Equally stuff goat cheddar blend into mushroom covers. Disseminate bread pieces over stuffed mushrooms. Gradually pour softened spread over bread pieces.
4. Spot half of mushrooms in fryer bushel. Cook 10 minutes. Move to serving plate. Rehash with residual mushrooms.
5. Sprinkle with prosciutto and basil. Serve warm.

Per serving **Calories**: 155 | Fat: 10.7 g | Protein: 7.7 g | Sodium: 390 mg | Fiber: 0.8 g | Starches: 8.0 g | Sugar: 2.1 g

BROCCOLI AND CARROT CHOMPS

This formula is the ideal nibble since it's vegetable-based and low in calories while as yet being flavorful and fulfilling. It's a shrewd alternative to keep you on target.

Pantry Staples: Salt, ground dark pepper
Hands On schedule: 15 minutes
Cook Time: 12 minutes

Yields 20 nibbles
1 (10-ounce) liner sack broccoli, cooked by bundle
Guidelines

- $^1/2$ cup destroyed sharp cheddar
- 2 tablespoons stripped and ground carrot
- $^1/2$ cup whitened finely ground almond flour
- 1 enormous egg, whisked
- $^1/4$ teaspoon salt
- $^1/4$ teaspoon ground dark pepper

1. Let cooked broccoli cool 5 minutes, at that point wring out abundance dampness with a kitchen towel. In an enormous bowl, blend broccoli in with Cheddar, carrot, flour, egg, salt, and pepper. Scoop 2 tablespoons of the blend into a ball, at that point fold into a scaled down piece. Rehash with outstanding combination to frame twenty chomps.

2. Slice a piece of material to find a way into the lower part of air fryer bin. Spot nibbles into a solitary layer on ungreased material. Change the temperature to 320°F and set the clock for 12 minutes, turning chomps partially through cooking. Chomps will be brilliant earthy colored when done. Serve warm.

Per serving (5 Nibbles)
Calories: 191 Protein: 10g Fiber: 5g Net sugars: 4g
Fat: 13g Sodium: 291mg Starches: 9g Sugar: 3g

BACON-WRAPPED JALAPEÑO POPPERS

These poppers are a definitive flavorful treat, crisped flawlessly noticeable all around fryer. With a mix of smooth, messy, and hot flavors, they're ideal for your game day spread. They additionally warm well, so feel allowed to twofold the formula and store in the fridge as long as 5 days.

Pantry Staples: Garlic powder
Hands On schedule: 10 minutes
Cook Time: 12 minutes
Yields 12 poppers

- 3 ounces cream cheddar, mellowed
- ⅓ cup destroyed gentle cheddar
- ¼ teaspoon garlic powder
- 6 jalapeños (around 4" long), tops eliminated, cut into equal parts longwise and cultivated
- 12 cuts sans sugar bacon

1. Spot cream cheddar, Cheddar, and garlic powder in an enormous microwave safe bowl. Microwave 30 seconds on high, at that point mix. Spoon cheddar combination equitably into emptied jalapeños.

2. Fold 1 cut bacon over each jalapeño half, totally covering jalapeño, and secure with a toothpick. Spot jalapeños into ungreased air fryer container. Change the temperature to 400°F and set the clock for 12 minutes, turning jalapeños partially through cooking. Bacon will be firm when done. Serve warm.

Per serving (3 poppers)
Calories: 278 Protein: 15g
Fiber: 1g Net sugars: 2g Fat: 21g Sodium: 719mg
Sugar: 2g

FIERY CHEDDAR STUFFED MUSHROOMS

This tidbit is extraordinary on a careful spending plan and loads enormous flavor with only a couple **fixings** . The mushrooms get a firm outside while cooking that is supplemented by the delicate, messy stuffing. If you favor things milder, trade the pepper jack cheddar for monterey jack cheddar.

Pantry staples: salt, ground dark pepper
Hands on schedule: 10 minutes
Cook time: 8 minutes
Yields 20 mushrooms

- 4 ounces cream cheddar, mollified
- 6 tablespoons destroyed pepper jack cheddar
- 2 tablespoons hacked salted jalapeños
- 20 medium catch mushrooms, stems eliminated
- 2 tablespoons olive oil
- ¼ teaspoon salt
- ⅛ teaspoon ground dark pepper

1. In a huge bowl, blend cream cheddar, pepper jack, and jalapeños together.

2. Shower mushrooms with olive oil, at that point sprinkle with salt and pepper. Spoon 2 tablespoons cheddar blend into each mushroom and spot in a solitary layer into ungreased air fryer crate. Change the temperature to 370°f and set the clock for 8 minutes, checking part of the way through cooking to guarantee in any event, cooking, revamping if some are more obscure than others. At the point when they're brilliant and cheddar is percolating, mushrooms will be finished. Serve warm.

Per serving (2 mushrooms)
Calories: 87 Protein: 3g Fiber: 0g Net sugars: 2g
Fat: 7g sodium: 144mg Sugars: 2g

PEPPERONI CHIPS

Exemplary potato chips, even the heated assortment, can have upwards of 23 grams of carbs Per serving. Luckily, you don't need to sacrifice that fresh, exquisite flavor when on a keto diet—simply prepare a speedy clump of these scrumptious, protein-rich Pepperoni Chips.

Pantry Staples: None
Hands On schedule: 5 minutes
Cook Time: 8 minutes
Serves: 2

1. 14 cuts pepperoni
2. Spot pepperoni cuts into ungreased air fryer container.
3. Change the temperature to 350°F and set the clock for 8 minutes.
4. Pepperoni will be sautéed and fresh when done. Let cool 5 minutes prior to serving. Store in hermetically sealed holder at room temperature as long as 3 days.

Per serving
Calories: 69 Protein: 3g Fiber: 0g Net sugars: 0g
Fat: 5g Sodium: 246mg Sugar: 0g

BACON-WRAPPED ONION RINGS

These onion rings are simpler to make than the customary southern style rendition! The exquisite taste of the onion is matched with pungent bacon to make a flavorful side you'll need to make consistently.

Pantry Staples: None
Hands On schedule: 5 minutes
Cook Time: 10 minutes
Serves: 8

- 1 huge white onion, stripped and cut into 16 (¼"- thick) cuts
- 8 cuts sans sugar bacon

1. Stack 2 cuts onion and wrap with 1 cut bacon. Secure with a toothpick. Rehash with outstanding onion cuts and bacon.
2. Spot onion rings into ungreased air fryer container. Change the temperature to 350°F and set the clock for 10 minutes, turning rings partially through cooking. Bacon will be firm when done. Serve warm.
3.

Per serving
Calories: 84 Protein: 5g Fiber: 2g
Fat: 4g Sodium: 197mg Carbs: 8g Sugar: 3g

THREE CHEDDAR PLUNGE

Regardless of whether you lean toward vegetables or pork skins and cheddar crisps for plunging, this ultracreamy formula makes certain to be a champ. Add your own pizazz by throwing in cooked chicken, hacked scallions, or hot sauce.

Pantry Staples: None
Hands On schedule: 5 minutes
Cook Time: 12 minutes
Serves: 8 (**Yields** 1 cup)

- 8 ounces cream cheddar, mollified
- ½ cup mayonnaise
- ¼ cup sharp cream
- ½ cup destroyed sharp cheddar
- ¼ cup destroyed Monterey jack cheddar

1. In a huge bowl, consolidate all **Fixings** . Scoop blend into an ungreased 4-cup nonstick preparing dish and spot into air fryer container.

2. Change the temperature to 375°F and set the clock for 12 minutes. Plunge will be carmelized on top and percolating when done. Serve warm.

Per serving (2 tablespoons) Calories: 245 Protein: 5g Fiber: 0g Fat: 23g Sodium: 260mg Sugar: 1g

WILD OX CHICKEN PLUNGE

Since you don't eat customary chips on a keto diet doesn't mean your long periods of delectable plunges are finished. This plunge is delicious combined with 100% cheddar crisps like Parm Crisps, or threw into your morning omelet.

Pantry Staples: None
Hands On schedule: 10 minutes
Cook Time: 12 minutes
Serves: 8 (**Yields** 4 cups)

- 8 ounces cream cheddar, mollified
- 2 cups hacked cooked chicken thighs
- ½ cup bison sauce
- 1 cup destroyed gentle cheddar, isolated

1. In an enormous bowl, join cream cheddar, chicken, wild ox sauce, and ½ cup Cheddar. Scoop plunge into an ungreased 4-cup nonstick heating dish and top with residual Cheddar.

2. Spot dish into air fryer bin. Change the temperature to 375°F and set the clock for 12 minutes. Plunge will be sautéed on top and foaming when done. Serve warm.

Per serving (½ CUP)
Calories: 222 Protein: 14g Fiber: 0g Fat: 15g
Sodium: 680mg Sugar: 1g

Side dishes can often be one of the most difficult foods to come up with to round out a keto-friendly meal. Traditional white rice or macaroni and cheese may be easy to throw together, but once you start your low-carb lifestyle, these dishes are no longer your friends. The carbs in many traditional side dishes can leave you feeling sluggish and will definitely prevent you from reaching ketosis. Thankfully, there are many delicious alternatives that your air fryer can help you prepare quickly and easily without ever needing to turn on your oven. This chapter will show you how to make recipes like Sausage-Stuffed Mushroom Caps and Cheesy Cauliflower Tots that will start a side dish revolution!

LOADED ROASTED BROCCOLI

If you've ever thought broccoli was boring, this recipe will change your mind forever. It's stuffed to the gills with savory flavor and delicious fats to help keep you full, not to mention the great protein boost that comes from the broccoli itself!

HandsOn Time: 10 minutes
Cook Time: 10 minutes
Serves 2

- 3 cups fresh broccoli florets
- 1 tablespoon coconut oil
- 1/2 cup shredded sharp Cheddar cheese
- 1/4 cup full-fat sour cream 4 slices sugar-free bacon, cooked and crumbled 1 scallion, sliced on the bias

Directions
- ✓ Place broccoli into the air fryer basket and drizzle it with coconut oil.
- ✓ Adjust the temperature to 350°F and set the timer for 10 minutes.
- ✓ Toss the basket two or three times during cooking to avoid burned spots.
- ✓ When broccoli begins to crisp at ends, remove from fryer. Top with shredded cheese, sour cream, and crumbled bacon and garnish with scallion slices.

Per serving
Calories: 361 Protein: 18.4 G
Fiber: 3.6 G Net Carbohydrates: 6.9 G Fat: 25.7 G
Sodium: 564 Mg Carbohydrates: 10.5 G Sugar: 3.3 G

GARLIC HERB BUTTER ROASTED RADISHES

When roasted, radishes make a surprisingly excellent red potato substitute. When roasted in an air fryer, the crisp you're able to achieve is incomparable. Full of health benefits like vitamin C and healthy fiber, this is one side dish you'll always feel good about eating!

HandsOn Time: 10 minutes
Cook Time: 10 minutes
Serves 4

- 1 pound radishes
- 2 tablespoons unsalted butter, melted
- 1/2 teaspoon garlic powder
- 1/2 teaspoon dried parsley
- 1/4 teaspoon dried oregano
- 1/4 teaspoon ground black pepper

Directions
- ✓ Remove roots from radishes and cut into quarters.
- ✓ In a small bowl, add butter and seasonings. Toss the radishes in the herb butter and place into the air fryer basket.
- ✓ Adjust the temperature to 350°F and set the timer for 10 minutes.
- ✓ Halfway through the cooking time, toss the radishes in the air fryer basket. Continue cooking until edges begin to turn brown.
- ✓ Serve warm.

Per serving
Calories: 63 Protein: 0.7 G Fiber: 1.3 G
Net Carbohydrates: 1.6 G Fat: 5.4 G
Sodium: 28 Mg Carbohydrates: 2.9 G Sugar: 1.4 G

SAUSAGE-STUFFED MUSHROOM CAPS

Mushrooms are very low-carb, are high in potassium, and have a fresh, earthy taste. Stuffing them with sausage boosts their protein and fat contents, and more importantly it elevates their flavor to something you won't be able to get enough of!

HandsOn Time: 10 minutes
Cook Time: 8 minutes
Serves 2

- 6 large portobello mushroom caps
- 1/2 pound Italian sausage
- 1/4 cup chopped onion
- 2 tablespoons blanched finely ground almond flour
- 1/4 cup grated Parmesan cheese

- 1 teaspoon minced fresh garlic

Directions

- ✓ Use a spoon to hollow out each mushroom cap, reserving scrapings.
- ✓ In a medium skillet over medium heat, brown the sausage about 10 minutes or until fully cooked and no pink remains. Drain and then add reserved mushroom scrapings, onion, almond flour, Parmesan, and garlic. Gently fold ingredients together and continue cooking an additional minute, then remove from heat.
- ✓ Evenly spoon the mixture into mushroom caps and place the caps into a 6" round pan. Place pan into the air fryer basket.
- ✓ Adjust the temperature to 375°F and set the timer for 8 minutes.
- ✓ When finished cooking, the tops will be browned and bubbling. Serve warm.

Per serving

Calories: 404
Protein: 24.3 G Fiber: 4.5 G
Net Carbohydrates: 13.7 G Fat: 25.8 G
Sodium: 1,106 Mg Carbohydrates: 18.2 G Sugar: 8.1 G

CHEESY CAULIFLOWER TOTS

With the carb count in potatoes being so high, tater tots would be very difficult to fit into your macros. Luckily, cauliflower is a great substitute to give you that same crispy texture for a wonderfully kid-friendly side dish. Serve these warm with low- carb ketchup or your favorite dipping sauce.

HandsOn Time: 15 minutes
Cook Time: 12 minutes
Yields 16 tots (4 per serving)

- 1 large head cauliflower
- 1 cup shredded mozzarella cheese
- 1/2 cup grated Parmesan cheese 1 large egg
- 1/4 teaspoon garlic powder
- 1/4 teaspoon dried parsley
- 1/8 teaspoon onion powder

Directions

- ✓ On the stovetop, fill a large pot with 2 cups water and place a steamer in the pan. Bring water to a boil. Cut the cauliflower into florets and place on steamer basket. Cover pot with lid.
- ✓ Allow cauliflower to steam 7 minutes until fork tender. Remove from steamer basket and place into cheesecloth or clean kitchen towel and let cool. Squeeze over sink to remove as much excess moisture as possible. The mixture will be too soft to form into tots if not all the moisture is removed. Mash with a fork to a smooth consistency.
- ✓ Put the cauliflower into a large mixing bowl and add mozzarella, Parmesan, egg, garlic powder, parsley, and onion powder. Stir until fully combined. The mixture should be wet but easy to mold.
- ✓ Take 2 tablespoons of the mixture and roll into tot shape. Repeat with remaining mixture. Place into the air fryer basket.
- ✓ Adjust the temperature to 320°F and set the timer for 12 minutes.
- ✓ Turn tots halfway through the cooking time. Cauliflower tots should be golden when fully cooked. Serve warm.

Per serving

Calories: 181 Protein: 13.5 G Fiber: 3.0 G
Net Carbohydrates: 6.6 G Fat: 9.5 G Sodium: 417 Mg
Carbohydrates: 9.6 G Sugar: 3.2 G

Kid Friendly!

These are great to make for kids because they look just like a classic tater tot, but they're much better for you. The cheese also helps to mask the cauliflower taste, making this the ultimate way to sneak veggies in!

CRISPY BRUSSELS SPROUTS

Get ready to cook some Brussels sprouts your kids will be excited about eating! They're rich in nutrients, including heart- healthy omega-3 fatty acids. This version is a complete reversal of the bland and boring Brussels sprouts you grew up eating!

HandsOn Time: 5 minutes
Cook Time: 10 minutes
Serves 4

- 1 pound Brussels sprouts
- 1 tablespoon coconut oil
- 1 tablespoon unsalted butter, melted

Directions

- ✓ Remove all loose leaves from Brussels sprouts and cut each in half.
- ✓ Drizzle sprouts with coconut oil and place into the air fryer basket.
- ✓ Adjust the temperature to 400°F and set the timer for 10 minutes. You may want to gently stir halfway through the cooking time, depending on how they are beginning to brown.
- ✓ When completely cooked, they should be tender with darker caramelized spots. Remove from fryer basket and drizzle with melted butter. Serve immediately.

Per serving

Calories: 90

Protein: 2.9 G Fiber: 3.2 G Net Carbohydrates: 4.3 G
Fat: 6.1 G Sodium: 21 Mg Carbohydrates: 7.5 G
Sugar: 1.9 G

ZUCCHINI PARMESAN CHIPS

It can be difficult to get that satisfying crunch that a
lot of carb- filled foods carry, but it's easier than ever
with your air fryer. These thinly sliced zucchini chips
are a nutrient-rich treat for mealtime or snack time!

HandsOn Time: 10 minutes
Cook Time: 10 minutes
Serves 4

- 2 medium zucchini
- 1 ounce pork rinds
- 1/2 cup grated Parmesan cheese
- 1 large egg

Directions

✓ Slice zucchini in 1/4"-thick slices. Place
between two layers of paper towels or a
clean kitchen nj towel for 30 minutes to
remove excess moisture.

✓ Place pork rinds into food processor and
pulse until finely ground. Pour into medium
bowl and mix with Parmesan.

✓ Beat egg in a small bowl.

✓ Dip zucchini slices in egg and then in pork
rind mixture, coating as completely as
possible. Carefully place each slice into the
air fryer basket in a single layer, working in
batches as necessary.

✓ Adjust temperature to 320°F and set the
timer for 10 minutes.

✓ Flip chips halfway through the cooking
time. Serve warm.

Per serving
Calories: 121
Protein: 9.9 G Fiber: 0.6 G Net Carbohydrates: 3.2 G
Fat: 6.7 G Sodium: 364 Mg Carbohydrates: 3.8 G
Sugar: 1.6 G

ROASTED GARLIC

Roasted garlic is one of the easiest ways to add a
boost of flavor to any dish, from chicken to mashed
cauliflower to the Roasted Garlic White Zucchini
Rolls in Chapter 8. Unlike traditional oven recipes,
which can take over an hour to get the roasted garlic
right, your air fryer can extract all the savory flavor
in just minutes!

HandsOn Time: 5 minutes
Cook Time: 20 minutes
Yields 12 cloves (1 per serving)

- 1 medium head garlic
- 2 teaspoons avocado oil

Directions

✓ Remove any hanging excess peel from the
garlic but leave the cloves covered. Cut off
V4 of the head of garlic, exposing the tips of
the cloves.

✓ Drizzle with avocado oil. Place the garlic
head into a small sheet of aluminum foil,
completely enclosing it. Place it into the air
fryer basket.

✓ Adjust the temperature to 400°F and set the
timer for 20 minutes. If your garlic head is a
bit smaller, check it after 15 minutes.

✓ When done, garlic should be golden brown
and very soft.

✓ To serve, cloves should pop out and easily
be spread or sliced. Store in an airtight
container in the refrigerator up to 5 days.
You may also freeze individual cloves on a
baking sheet, then store together in a
freezer-safe storage bag once frozen.

Per serving
Calories: 11 Protein: 0.2 G
Fiber: 0.1 G Net Carbohydrates: 0.9 G Fat: 0.7 G
Sodium: 0 Mg Carbohydrates: 1.0 G Sugar: 0.0 G

HOW TO USE ROASTED GARLIC
Roasted garlic has a milder, sweeter taste than raw
garlic, which complements many dishes. Make a
uick roasted garlic and herb butter for your steak or
pork chops. Simply mash a clove of roasted garlic
with 1/4 cup softened butter and add your favorite
herbs.

KALE CHIPS

With just the right seasoning and only a few minutes
in your air fryer, you'll have a crispy snack that's easy
to take on the go! Plus, kale is high in fiber, helping
to promote a regular and healthy digestive tract.

HandsOn Time: 5 minutes
Cook Time: 5 minutes
Serves 4

- 4 cups stemmed kale
- 2 teaspoons avocado oil
- 2 teaspoon salt

Directions

✓ In a large bowl, toss kale in avocado oil and
sprinkle with salt. Place into the air fryer
basket.

✓ Adjust the temperature to 400°F and set the
timer for 5 minutes.

✓ Kale will be crispy when done. Serve
immediately.

BUFFALO CAULIFLOWER

auliflower steaks are a great vegetarian option that have nutrients and flavor. Roasting them with buffalo sauce gives you a light and spicy dish that is totally guilt-free! Serve with crumbled blue cheese or ranch dressing if you need to tone down the spice!

HandsOn Time: 5 minutes

Cook Time: 5 minutes

Serves 4

- 4 cups cauliflower florets
- 2 tablespoons salted butter, melted
- 2 (1-ounce) dry ranch seasoning packet
- 1/4 cup buffalo sauce

Directions
- ✓ In a large bowl, toss cauliflower with butter and dry ranch. Place into the air fryer basket.
- ✓ Adjust the temperature to 400°F and set the timer for 5 minutes.
- ✓ Shake the basket two or three times during cooking. When tender, remove cauliflower from fryer basket and toss in buffalo sauce. Serve warm.

Per serving
Calories: 87
Protein: 2.1 G Fiber: 2.1 G Net Carbohydrates: 5.2 G Fat: 5.6 G Sodium: 803 Mg Carbohydrates: 7.3 G Sugar: 2.1 G

GREEN BEAN CASSEROLE

This low-carb spin on a potluck favorite will be the newest addition to your holiday menu. You'll notice the dish is missing the cream of mushroom soup you might be used to, but don't worry; you'll get all the traditional flavor without all the unnecessary carbs!

HandsOn Time: 10 minutes

Cook Time: 15 minutes

Serves 4

- 4 tablespoons unsalted butter
- 1/4 cup diced yellow onion
- 1/2 cup chopped white mushrooms
- 1/2 cup heavy whipping cream
- 1 ounce full-fat cream cheese
- 1/2 cup chicken broth
- 1/4 teaspoon xanthan gum
- 1 pound fresh green beans, edges trimmed
- 1/2 ounce pork rinds, finely ground

Directions
- ✓ In a medium skillet over medium heat, melt the butter. Saute the onion and mushrooms until they become soft and fragrant, about 3-5 minutes.
- ✓ Add the heavy whipping cream, cream cheese, and broth to the pan. Whisk until smooth. Bring to a boil and then reduce to a simmer. Sprinkle the xanthan gum into the pan and remove from heat.
- ✓ Chop the green beans into 2" pieces and place into a 4-cup round baking dish. Pour the sauce mixture over them and stir until coated. Top the dish with ground pork rinds. Place into the air fryer basket.
- ✓ Adjust the temperature to 320°F and set the timer for 15 minutes.
- ✓ Top will be golden and green beans fork tender when fully cooked. Serve warm.

Per serving
Calories: 267 Protein: 3.6 G Fiber: 3.2 G Net Carbohydrates: 6.5 G Fat: 23.4 G Sodium: 161 Mg Carbohydrates: 9.7 G Sugar: 5.1 G

ARE GREEN BEANS KETO-FRIENDLY?

Green beans are legumes, but that doesn't mean you can't enjoy them on a ketogenic diet. Traditionally keto excluded legumes, including peanuts. Nowadays, a more rounded approach is taken and as long as the carbs are low and fit your macros, generally you can enjoy them. There are 3.6 grams net carbs in a 1-cup serving of green beans, which makes them a great choice!

Cilantro Lime Roasted Cauliflower

Although it's rich in nutrients, like vitamin C, cauliflower is usually a pretty bland-tasting vegetable. This gives you an excellent opportunity to flavor it just the way you like for an appetizing side. This cilantro lime flavoring will complement any steak dish perfectly!

HandsOn Time: 10 minutes

Cook Time: 7 minutes

Serves 4

- 2 cups chopped cauliflower florets
- 2 tablespoons coconut oil, melted
- 2 teaspoons chili powder
- 1/2 teaspoon garlic powder
- 1 medium lime
- 2 tablespoons chopped cilantro

Directions
- ✓ In a large bowl, toss cauliflower with coconut oil. Sprinkle with chili powder and garlic powder. Place seasoned cauliflower into the air fryer basket.

✓ Adjust the temperature to 350°F and set the timer for 7 minutes.
✓ Cauliflower will be tender and begin to turn golden at the edges. Place into serving bowl.
✓ Cut the lime into quarters and squeeze juice over cauliflower. Garnish with cilantro.

Per serving
Calories: 73
Protein: 1.1 G Fiber: 1.1 G
Net Carbohydrates: 2.2 G Fat: 6.5 G
Sodium: 16 Mg Carbohydrates: 3.3 G Sugar: 1.1 G

DINNER ROLLS

Do you miss bread on your keto diet? This low-carb substitute will satisfy any bread craving you may have and give you a great side dish to eat with your dinner. The dough can also be baked in a loaf pan or flattened out on a pizza pan to take care of you no matter which bread craving strikes!
HandsOn Time: 10 minutes
Cook Time: 12 minutes
Serves 6

- 1 cup shredded mozzarella cheese
- 1 ounce full-fat cream cheese
- 1 cup blanched finely ground almond flour
- 1/4 cup ground flaxseed
- 1/2 teaspoon baking powder
- 1 large egg

Directions
✓ Place mozzarella, cream cheese, and almond flour in a large microwave-safe bowl. Microwave for 1 minute. Mix until smooth.
✓ Add flaxseed, baking powder, and egg until fully combined and smooth. Microwave an additional 15 seconds if it becomes too firm.
✓ Separate the dough into six pieces and roll into balls. Place the balls into the air fryer basket.
✓ Adjust the temperature to 320°F and set the timer for 12 minutes.
✓ Allow rolls to cool completely before serving.

Per serving
Calories: 228 Protein: 10.8 G Fiber: 3.9 G
Net Carbohydrates: 2.9 G Fat: 18.1 G Sodium: 188 Mg
Carbohydrates: 6.8 G Sugar: 1.2 G

COCONUT FLOUR CHEESY GARLIC BISCUITS

Missing biscuits on a keto diet is completely understandable. There's practically no dish they don't side perfectly with. Try these fluffy and flavorful treats with shrimp scampi for a keto- friendly at-home restaurant experience!
HandsOn Time: 10 minutes
Cook Time: 12 minutes
Serves 4

- 1/3 cup coconut flour
- 1/2 teaspoon baking powder
- 1/2 teaspoon garlic powder
- 1 large egg
- 1/4 cup unsalted butter, melted and divided
- 1/2 cup shredded sharp Cheddar cheese
- 1 scallion, sliced

Directions
✓ In a large bowl, mix coconut flour, baking powder, and garlic powder.
✓ Stir in egg, half of the melted butter, Cheddar cheese, and scallions. Pour the mixture into a 6" round baking pan. Place into the air fryer basket.
✓ Adjust the temperature to 320°F and set the timer for 12 minutes.
✓ To serve, remove from pan and allow to fully cool. Slice into four pieces and pour remaining melted butter over each.

Per serving
Calories: 218
Protein: 7.2 G Fiber: 3.4 G
Net Carbohydrates: 3.4 G Fat: 16.9 G
Sodium: 177 Mg Carbohydrates: 6.8 G Sugar: 2.1 G

RADISH CHIPS

Radishes might not come to mind right away when thinking about healthy, low-carb vegetables, but this recipe might just change that forever. This quick and healthy snack packs plenty of flavor as well as dietary fiber to help you feel full and avoid overeating.
HandsOn Time: 10 minutes
Cook Time: 5 minutes
Serves 4

- 2 cups water
- 1 pound radishes
- 1/4 teaspoon onion powder
- 1/4 teaspoon paprika
- 1/2 teaspoon garlic powder
- 2 tablespoons coconut oil, melted

Directions

- ✓ Place water in a medium saucepan and bring to a boil on stovetop.
- ✓ Remove the top and bottom from each radish, then use a mandoline to slice each radish thin and uniformly. You may also use the slicing blade in the food processor for this step.
- ✓ Place the radish slices into the boiling water for 5 minutes or until translucent. Remove them from the water and place them into a clean kitchen towel to absorb excess moisture.
- ✓ Toss the radish chips in a large bowl with remaining ingredients until fully coated in oil and seasoning.
- ✓ Place radish chips into the air fryer basket.
- ✓ Adjust the temperature to 320°F and set the timer for 5 minutes.
- ✓ Shake the basket two or three times during the cooking time. Serve warm.

Per serving

Calories: 77 Protein: 0.8 G Fiber: 1.8 G
Net Carbohydrates: 2.2 G Fat: 6.5 G Sodium: 40 Mg
Carbohydrates: 4.0 G Sugar: 2.0 G

FLATBREAD

Flatbread is a great alternative for anything from a tortilla to a pizza crust. This easy recipe is flexible and versatile so you can make it any time of day to make your meal more filling.

HandsOn Time: 5 minutes
Cook Time: 7 minutes
Serves 2

- 1 cup shredded mozzarella cheese
- 4 cup blanched finely ground almond flour
- 1 ounce full-fat cream cheese, softened

Directions

- ✓ In a large microwave-safe bowl, melt mozzarella in the microwave for 30 seconds. Stir in almond flour until smooth and then add cream cheese. Continue mixing until dough forms, gently kneading it with wet hands if necessary.
- ✓ Divide the dough into two pieces and roll out to V4" thickness between two pieces of parchment. Cut another piece of parchment to fit your air fryer basket.
- ✓ Place a piece of flatbread onto your parchment and into the air fryer, working in two batches if needed.
- ✓ Adjust the temperature to 320°F and set the timer for 7 minutes.

- ✓ Halfway through the cooking time flip the flatbread. Serve warm.

Per serving

Calories: 296
Protein: 16.3 G Fiber: 1.5 G
Net Carbohydrates: 3.3 G Fat: 22.6 G
Sodium: 402 Mg Carbohydrates: 4.8 G Sugar: 1.5 G

AVOCADO FRIES

Avocados are an absolute staple on the keto diet. That's because they're low in carbs and very high in healthy fats that keep you full and focused. Some people like to eat avocados plain, but if you're not one of them, try these crispy Avocado Fries; they are a great, easy way to boost an avocado's flavor with little effort!

HandsOn Time: 15 minutes
Cook Time: 5 minutes
Serves 4

- 2 medium avocados
- 1 ounce pork rinds, finely ground

Directions

- ✓ Cut each avocado in half. Remove the pit. Carefully remove the peel and then slice the flesh into 4"-thick slices.
- ✓ Place the pork rinds into a medium bowl and press each piece of avocado into the pork rinds to coat completely. Place the avocado pieces into the air fryer basket.
- ✓ Adjust the temperature to 350°F and set the timer for 5 minutes.
- ✓ Serve immediately.

Per serving

Calories: 153
Protein: 5.4 G Fiber: 4.6 G
Net Carbohydrates: 1.3 G Fat: 11.9 G
Sodium: 121 Mg Carbohydrates: 5.9 G Sugar: 0.2 G

PITA-STYLE CHIPS

You'll never miss the real thing with these chips! They come out amazingly crunchy and perfect for dipping! Try them with the Bacon Cheeseburger Dip (Chapter 3) or add some Mexican-style toppings for yummy nachos!

HandsOn Time: 10 minutes
Cook Time: 5 minutes
Serves 4

- 1 cup shredded mozzarella cheese
- 1/2 ounce pork rinds, finely ground
- 1/4 cup blanched finely ground almond flour
- 1 large egg

Directions

- ✓ Place mozzarella in a large microwave-safe bowl and microwave for 30 seconds or until melted. Add remaining ingredients and stir until a mostly smooth dough forms into a ball easily. If dough is too hard, microwave for 15 seconds.
- ✓ Roll dough out between two pieces of parchment into a large rectangle and then use a knife to cut triangle shaped chips. Place the chips into the air fryer basket.
- ✓ Adjust the temperature to 350°F and set the timer for 5 minutes.
- ✓ Chips will be golden in color and firm when done. As they cool, they will become even more firm.
- ✓

Per serving
Calories: 161
Protein: 11.3 G Fiber: 0.8 G
Net Carbohydrates: 1.4 G Fat: 11.6 G
Sodium: 251 Mg Carbohydrates: 2.2 G Sugar: 0.6 G

ROASTED EGGPLANT

Eggplant is a very low-calorie vegetable that is high in fiber.
This combination can be great for promoting weight loss, and luckily eggplant is very easy to add to your diet. This simple roasting method makes for a tasty side that would go great with other veggies or a yummy chicken dish.

HandsOn Time: 15 minutes
Cook Time: 15 minutes
Serves 4

- 1 large eggplant
- 2 tablespoons olive oil
- 1/4 teaspoon salt
- 1/2 teaspoon garlic powder

Directions
Remove top and bottom from eggplant. Slice eggplant into 1/4"-thick round slices.

- ✓ 2 Brush slices with olive oil. Sprinkle with salt and garlic powder. Place eggplant slices into the air fryer basket.
- ✓ 3 Adjust the temperature to 390°F and set the timer for 15 minutes.
- ✓ 4 Serve immediately.

Per serving
Calories: 91 Protein: 1.3 G Fiber: 3.7 G
Net Carbohydrates: 3.8 G Fat: 6.7 G Sodium: 147 Mg
Carbohydrates: 7.5 G Sugar: 4.4 G

PARMESAN HERB FOCACCIA BREAD

This herb-baked focaccia substitute has only a fraction of carbs as the real thing, but it's the perfect sandwich bread to make sure you never feel left out while living your low-carb lifestyle.

HandsOn Time: 10 minutes
Cook Time: 10 minutes
Serves 6

- 1 cup shredded mozzarella cheese
- 1 ounce full-fat cream cheese
- 1 cup blanched finely ground almond flour
- 1/4 cup ground golden flaxseed
- 1/4 cup grated Parmesan cheese
- 1/2 teaspoon baking soda
- 2 large eggs
- 1/2 teaspoon garlic powder
- 1/4 teaspoon dried basil
- 1/4 teaspoon dried rosemary
- 2 tablespoons salted butter, melted and divided

Directions

- ✓ Place mozzarella, cream cheese, and almond flour into a large microwave-safe bowl and microwave for 1 minute. Add the flaxseed, Parmesan, and baking soda and stir until smooth ball forms. If the mixture cools too much, it will be hard to mix. Return to microwave for 10-15 seconds to rewarm if necessary.
- ✓ Stir in eggs. You may need to use your hands to get them fully incorporated. Just keep stirring and they will absorb into the dough.
- ✓ Sprinkle dough with garlic powder, basil, and rosemary and knead into dough. Grease a 6" round baking pan with 1 tablespoon melted butter. Press the dough evenly into the pan. Place pan into the air fryer basket.
- ✓ Adjust the temperature to 400°F and set the timer for 10 minutes.
- ✓ At 7 minutes, cover with foil if bread begins to get too dark.
- ✓ Remove and let cool at least 30 minutes. Drizzle with remaining butter and serve.

Per serving
Calories: 292 Protein: 13.1 G Fiber: 4.0 G
Net Carbohydrates: 3.6 G Fat: 23.4 G Sodium: 370 Mg Carbohydrates: 7.6 G Sugar: 1.2 G

SANDWICHES ARE BACK ON THE MENU!
For a filling meal, you can allow the bread to fully cool, then slice the entire round in half. Make it a club sandwich with turkey, bacon, lettuce, tomato,

and mayo, or whatever your favorite toppings may be. Replace the top and slice into six pieces to serve. It's an easy meal for the whole family!

QUICK AND EASY HOME FRIES

Jicama may seem like an intimidating vegetable from the outside but it's very easy to work with and well worth the extra effort. Peeling a jicama is a bit tricky but using a sharp knife to slice the peel off works easily. If you've never tasted it before, it's similar to a white potato in texture but with a hint of sweetness. It absorbs flavors easily, which makes jicama a good potato substitute. For a fraction of the carbs of the original, these home fries are the perfect smart swap for your keto diet.

HandsOn Time: 10 minutes
Cook Time: 10 minutes
Serves: 4

- 1 medium jicama, peeled
- 1 tablespoon coconut oil, melted
- 1/4 teaspoon ground black pepper
- 1/2 teaspoon pink Himalayan salt
- 1 medium green bell pepper, seeded and diced
- 1/2 medium white onion, peeled and diced

Directions

- ✓ Cut jicama into 1" cubes. Place into a large bowl and toss with coconut oil until coated. Sprinkle with pepper and salt. Place into the air fryer basket with peppers and onion.
- ✓ Adjust the temperature to 400°F and set the timer for 10 minutes.
- ✓ Shake two or three times during cooking. Jicama will be tender and dark around edges. Serve immediately.

Per serving
Calories: 97 protein: 1.5 g fiber: 8.0 g
Net carbohydrates: 7.8 g fat: 3.3 g sodium: 202 mg
Carbohydrates: 15.8 g sugar: 4.0 g

JICAMA FRIES

Jicama, also known as a Mexican potato, is a root vegetable native to Central and South America. A jicama is loaded with fiber, and it makes an excellent replacement for traditional French fries! One major selling point of air fryers is that they can get your French fries extremely crispy, with little to no oil. With this recipe you can take part in the fun, in a way that's much better for you!

HandsOn Time: 10 minutes
Cook Time: 20 minutes
Serves 4

- 1 small jicama, peeled
- 3/4 teaspoon chili powder
- 1/4 teaspoon garlic powder
- 1/4 teaspoon onion powder
- 1/4 teaspoon ground black pepper

Directions

- ✓ Cut jicama into matchstick-sized pieces.
- ✓ Place pieces into a small bowl and sprinkle with remaining ingredients. Place the fries into the air fryer basket.
- ✓ Adjust the temperature to 350°F and set the timer for 20 minutes.
- ✓ Toss the basket two or three times during cooking. Serve warm.

Per serving
Calories: 37
Protein: 0.8 G Fiber: 4.7 G
Net Carbohydrates: 4.0 G Fat: 0.1 G Sodium: 18 Mg
Carbohydrates: 8.7 G Sugar: 1.7 G

WHERE CAN YOU FIND JICAMA?
Jicama is more common to grocery stores than you might realize! Check your produce aisle near regular potatoes, but if your search is unsuccessful be sure to try an international market.

FRIED GREEN TOMATOES

Green tomatoes are tomatoes that haven't fully ripened. Because of this, they're tarter than a red tomato and firmer. Fried Green Tomatoes are a sweet and juicy side that taste like summer with every bite and come together easily in your air fryer, so you don't have to worry about frying them in oil!

HandsOn Time: 10 minutes • **Cook Time**: 7 minutes
Serves 4

- 2 medium green tomatoes
- 1 large egg
- 1/4 cup blanched finely ground almond flour
- 1/3 cup grated Parmesan cheese

Directions

- ✓ Slice tomatoes into V2"-thick slices. In a medium bowl, whisk the egg. In a large bowl, mix the almond flour and Parmesan.
- ✓ Dip each tomato slice into the egg, then dredge in the almond flour mixture. Place the slices into the air fryer basket.
- ✓ Adjust the temperature to 400°F and set the timer for 7 minutes.
- ✓ Flip the slices halfway through the cooking time. Serve immediately.

Per serving
Calories: 106
Protein: 6.2 g fiber: 1.4 g net carbohydrates: 4.5 g
fat: 6.7 g Sodium: 175 mg carbohydrates: 5.9 g sugar: 2.8 g

A favorite for many people in the Southern United States, Fried Pickles are a crispy and tart appetizer. They're traditionally battered with cornmeal and flour, but this keto-friendly alternative will give you all the flavor you need. Pair them with Southern "Fried" Chicken (Chapter 5) to keep the authentic Southern feel going!

HandsOn Time: 10 minutes
Cook Time: 5 minutes
Serves 4

- 1 tablespoon coconut flour
- 1/3 cup blanched finely ground almond flour
- 1 teaspoon chili powder
- 1/4 teaspoon garlic powder
- 1 large egg
- 1 cup sliced pickles

Directions

- ✓ Whisk coconut flour, almond flour, chili powder, and garlic powder together in a medium bowl.
- ✓ Whisk egg in a small bowl.
- ✓ Pat each pickle with a paper towel and dip into the egg. Then dredge in the flour mixture. Place pickles into the air fryer basket.
- ✓ Adjust the temperature to 400°F and set the timer for 5 minutes.
- ✓ Flip the pickles halfway through the cooking time.

Per serving
Calories: 85
Protein: 4.3 g fiber: 2.3 g
Net carbohydrates: 2.3 g fat: 6.1 g
Sodium: 351 mg carbohydrates: 4.6 g sugar: 1.2 g

B A S I C   A I R   F R Y E R   B R O C C O L I   C R I S P S

Planning Time: 5 minutes
Cook Time: 35 minutes
Servings: 2
Fixings

- 2 broccoli florets
- 2 tablespoons olive oil
- 2 tablespoon lime and Mexican chilies blend
- salt and vinegar, as wanted

Guidelines

1. Cleave the broccoli florets into scaled down pieces at that point cover with the flavors and olive oil.
2. Warmth the air fryer up to 200°F at that point place the broccoli florets inside the fryer bin.
3. Cook for 30-35 minutes at that point put away to cool for 20-30 minutes.
4. Serve and appreciate.

Sustenance Data
Calories: 200 | All out Fat: 19g | Absolute Carb: 8g | Protein: 2g

B A S I C   P L A T E   O F   M I X E D   G R E E N S   D R E S S I N G

Planning Time: 10 minutes
Cook Time: 0 moment
Servings: 10

Fixings

- 1/4 cup weighty whipping cream
- 1/2 cup mayo
- 1/2 cup harsh cream
- 1 teaspoon chives
- 1 teaspoon dried dill
- 1 teaspoon onion powder
- 1 teaspoon garlic powder
- 1-2 teaspoons squeezed lime
- salt and pepper, as wanted

Guidelines

1. Utilizing an enormous blending bowl, include every one of the Fixings and combine as one.

Refrigerate the blend for at any rate 2 hours.
Utilize chilled and appreciate.

Nourishment Data
Calories: 181 | Complete Fat: 18g | Absolute Starches: 2g | Protein: 1g

G A T H E R I N G   A I R   S E A R E D   M E A T B A L L S

Planning Time: 20 minutes
Cook Time: 15 minutes
Servings: 24

Fixings

- 1/4 cup vinegar
- 1/2 cup earthy colored sugar
- 1/2 teaspoon dry mustard
- 3/4 cup ketchup
- 1 pound mince hamburger
- 1 tablespoon tabasco
- 1 tablespoon squeezed lime
- 2 tablespoon Worcester sauce
- 3 squashed gingersnaps

Guidelines

1. Utilizing a medium measured blending bowl, include the flavoring at that point combine everything as one until very much covered.
2. Add the minced hamburger into the blending bowl and join.
3. Form the combination into smaller than expected meatballs at that point heat the air fryer up to 190°C.
4. When the air fryer is warmed up, place the meat balls into the fryer container at that point cook until firm for 15 minutes.
5. Put the cooked meatballs on sticks at that point serve and appreciate.

Nourishment Data
Calories: Absolute Fat: 3g | Complete Sugars: 8g | Protein: 3g

AIR SINGED MUSTARD AND NECTAR PORK BALLS

Planning Time: 5 minutes
Cook Time: 14 minutes
Servings: 4

Fixings

- 1 teaspoon nectar
- 1 teaspoon mustard
- 1 teaspoon garlic puree
- 1 tablespoon ground cheddar
- 50g stripped and diced onion
- 300g minced pork
- modest bunch cleaved new basil
- salt and pepper

Guidelines

1. Warmth the air fryer up to 200°C.
2. Add the minced pork, preparing and onion into a combining bowl at that point consolidate as one.
3. Structure the blend into smaller than normal balls at that point move into the air fryer crate.
4. Cook until all around accomplished for 14 minutes. Serve and appreciate.

Nourishment Data
Calories: 225 | Complete Fat: 17g | All out Sugars: 3g | Protein: 13g

AIR FRYER PIGS IN COVERS

Planning Time: 3 minutes
Cook Time: 15 minutes
Servings: 9

Fixings

- 3 major Brazilian sausages
- 9 bacon back
- salt and pepper, as wanted

Directions

1. Cut the sausages into 3 equivalent sizes at that point fold the bacon rashers over them.
2. Warmth the air fryer up to 180°C at that point cook the sausages for 15 minutes.
3. Once done, sprinkle the cooked sausages with salt and pepper at that point serve and appreciate.

Nourishment Data
Calories 206 | Complete Fat 18g | All out Starches 0g | Protein 8g 16%

SAGE AND ONION STUFFED AIR FRYER BALLS

Planning Time: 3 minutes
Cook Time: 15 minutes
Servings: 9
Fixings

- 1/2 teaspoon garlic puree
- 1/2 little stripped and diced onion
- 1 teaspoon sage
- 3 tablespoons breadcrumbs
- 100g sausage meat
- salt and pepper

Guidelines

1. Put every one of the Fixings in a medium estimated combining bowl and blend as one.
2. Warmth the air fryer up to 180°C.
3. Shape the blend into smaller than normal ball sizes and spot inside the fryer container.
4. Cook for 15 minutes at that point serve and appreciate.

Sustenance Data
Calories: 50 | All out Fat: 3g | Absolute Carbs: 3g | Protein: 2g

Planning Time: 10 minutes
Cook Time: 25 minutes
Servings: 4
Fixings

- 1 teaspoon parsley
- 1 tablespoon olive oil
- 1 teaspoon garlic puree
- 1 tablespoon breadcrumbs
- 6 little mushrooms
- 20g stripped and diced onion
- salt and pepper, to taste

Guidelines

1. Utilizing a medium measured blending bowl, include the garlic, olive oil, parsley, onion, salt and pepper and breadcrumbs at that point combine as one.
2. Wash the mushrooms at that point eliminate the stalks at the middle.
3. Top the middle off with the breadcrumbs combination.
4. Warmth the air fryer up to 180°C.
5. Once warmed, move the mushrooms into the fryer bushel and cook for 10 minutes.
6. Serve and appreciate once done.

Sustenance Data
Calories: 51 | Absolute Fat: 3g | All out Sugars: 3g | Protein: 1g

AIR SINGED CHICKEN SCOOPS

Planning Time: 1 hour 10 minutes
Cook Time: 20 minutes
Servings: 4
Fixings

- 1 major egg
- 1 teaspoon oregano
- 1 teaspoon mustard powder
- 2 chicken bosoms
- 2 teaspoons parsley
- 2 cuts bread breadcrumbs
- salt and pepper, to taste

Guidelines

1. Cleave the chicken up into lump measures at that point put away.
2. Utilizing a heating container, join the breadcrumbs and preparing together.
3. Break the egg into another blending bowl and beat.

4. Plunge every chicken piece into the beaten egg then into the breadcrumbs combination.
5. Move the chicken onto a serving platter and freeze for 60 minutes.
6. Preheat the stove to 180°C.
7. Spot in the cooler chicken pieces and cook for 25 minutes until done.
8. Serve and appreciate with any garnish of your decision.

Nourishment Data
Calories: 183 | Complete Fat: 4g | All out Sugars: 7g | Protein: 26g

AIR SEARED AIR POCKET AND SQUEAK

Planning Time: 3 minutes
Cook Time: 25 minutes
Servings: 4
Fixings

- 1 teaspoon tarragon
- 1 tablespoon blended spices
- 1 stripped and cut medium onion
- 2 beaten medium eggs
- 4 turkey bosom cuts
- 50g cheddar
- extra vegetables
- salt and pepper, as wanted

Directions

1. Put the vegetable extras inside a medium estimated blending bowl at that point pound them into little pieces.
2. Add the eggs, onion, preparing and cheddar into the vegetables.
3. Dice the turkey cuts and add them into the bowl of veggies at that point utilize your hands to fuse everything together.
4. Preheat the stove up to 180°C at that point cook in the bushel until the top is rising, for 25 minutes.
5. Serve and appreciate.

Nourishment Data
Calories: 113 | Complete Fat: 7g | All out Carbs: 3g | Protein: 7g

SOUTHERN LIKE CHICKEN AND WAFERS

Planning Time: 15 minutes
Cook Time: 20 minutes
Servings: 6

Fixings

- 1/4 teaspoon scoured sage
- 1/4 teaspoon ground cumin
- 1/2 teaspoon pepper
- 1 enormous egg
- 1 teaspoon paprika
- 1 teaspoon garlic salt
- 1 tablespoon new parsley, minced
- 2 cups (around 50) squashed saltines
- 3-4 pounds chicken, cut up

Guidelines

1. Utilizing a profound blending bowl, include the sage, cumin, pepper, paprika, salt, parsley and saltines at that point consolidate together.
2. Break the egg into a different bowl and beat. Dig the chicken in the egg blend then into the wafers combination until all around covered.
3. Warmth the air fryer up to 375°F at that point utilize the cooking splash to shower the fryer crate.
4. Organize the chicken pieces in a solitary layer inside the fryer crate at that point cook for 10 minutes.
5. Turn the chicken over then cook for an additional 10 minutes until brilliant earthy colored.
6. Rehash similar interaction with the excess chicken pieces at that point serve and appreciate.

Nourishment Data
Calories: 405 | Complete Fat: 22g | Absolute Starch: 13g | Protein: 36g

ITALIAN PREPARED MEATBALLS

Planning Time: 5 minutes
Cook Time: 12 minutes
Servings: 12

Fixings

- 1/3 cup ground parmesan cheddar
- 1/4 cup marinara sauce, no sugar
- 1 huge egg
- 1 pound ground meat
- 1 teaspoon minced onion
- 1 teaspoon powdered garlic
- 1 teaspoon Italian flavoring

Directions

1. Utilizing a medium estimated blending bowl, include every one of the Fixings at that point mix until appropriately fused.
2. Warmth the air fryer 350°F.
3. Shape the combination into 12 (1" estimated) roundabout balls at that point move the blend into the fryer crate.
4. Cook the meatballs for 10-12 minutes.
5. Once done, serve and appreciate.

Nourishment Data
Calories: 91 | Complete Fat: 5g | All out Starch: 1g | Protein: 9g

ASPARAGUS WRAPPED PROSCUITTO

Planning Time: 5 minutes
Cook Time: 4 minutes
Servings: 3

Fixings

- cut slim prosciutto
- stalks of asparagus

Directions

1. Utilize the cut prosciutto to wrap the asparagus follows around.
2. Warmth the air fryer up to 360°F at that point include the wrapped asparagus.
3. Cook the asparagus for 4 minutes at that point serve and appreciate.

Sustenance Data
Calories: 382 | Absolute Fat: 23g | All out Sugar: 1g | Protein: 42g

COOKED ASIAN AIR SINGED BROCCOLI

Planning Time: 10 minutes
Cook Time: 20 minutes
Servings: 4

Fixings

- 1/3 cup salted peanuts, cooked
- 1 teaspoon rice vinegar
- 1 pound broccoli florets
- 1 tablespoon minced garlic
- 1/2 tablespoon nut oil
- 2 teaspoon nectar
- 2 teaspoon sriracha
- 2 tablespoon low sodium soy sauce
- salt, to taste
- new squeezed lemon, if wanted

Guidelines

1. Utilizing an enormous blending bowl, include the nut oil, broccoli, ocean salt, garlic at that point join together.
2. Warmth the air fryer up to 400°F at that point spread the broccoli in the fryer container at that point cook for 15-20 minutes until fresh and brilliant.
3. Meanwhile, consolidate the soy sauce, nectar, rice vinegar, sriracha together in a microwave safe bowl.
4. Spot the bowl in a microwave and warmth until the nectar melts and everything is all around joined for 10-15 seconds.
5. Move the cooked broccoli to a serving platter at that point pour the soy sauce over and throw together.
6. Season with the salt and throw once more, at that point include the peanuts and squeezed lemon.
7. Serve and appreciate.

Sustenance Data
Calories: 154 | All out Fat: 10.8g | All out Sugars: 10.9g | Protein 6.4g

WILD OX SAUCED CAULIFLOWER

Planning Time: 5 minutes
Cook Time: 15 minutes
Servings: 4
Fixings

-   1/2 cup wild ox sauce
-   1 tablespoon softened margarine
-   1 cauliflower head, slashed into little nibbles
-   cooking oil splash
-   salt and pepper, to taste

Guidelines

1. Utilizing a blending bowl, include the wild ox sauce, liquefied margarine, salt and pepper at that point mix to join.
2. Shower the fryer container with the cooking splash at that point heat the air fryer up to 400°F.
3. Add the cauliflower nibbles into the fryer bushel at that point cook for 5 minutes.
4. Following 5 minutes, shower the cauliflower with the wild ox blend, dissolved spread at that point mix through.
5. Return the cauliflower back into the air fryer and cook until the cauliflower nibbles turn fresh for 7-8 additional minutes.
6. Once done, present with any keto cordial farm dressing and appreciate.

Sustenance Data
Calories: 118 | All out Fat: 10g | Absolute Sugars: 7g | Protein 3g

HERBED BRUSSELS FLEDGLINGS

Planning Time: 10 minutes
Cook Time: 8 minutes
Servings: 4
Fixings

-   1/4 teaspoon salt
-   1/2 teaspoon dried thyme
-   1 teaspoon dried parsley
-   1 teaspoon powdered garlic
-   1 pound washed and managed brussels sprouts
-   2 teaspoon oil

Guidelines

1. Utilizing an enormous blending bowl include every one of the Fixings at that point throw until the brussels is very much covered.
2. Warmth the air fryer up to 390°F at that point move the brussels sprouts into the fryer.
3. Cook the brussels sprouts for 8 minutes.
4. Once cooked, permit the brussels to chill at that point serve and appreciate.

Sustenance Data
Calories: 79 | All out Fat: 2g | Absolute Starches: 12g | Protein: 4g

LOW CARB MOZZARELLA STICKS

Planning Time: 10 minutes
Cook Time: 10 minutes
Servings: 6

Fixings

-   1/2 cup almond flour
-   1/2 cup parmesan cheddar
-   1/2 teaspoon garlic salt
-   1 teaspoon Italian flavoring
-   2 enormous eggs
-   12 sticks line of mozzarella cheddar, cut down the middle

Guidelines

1. Utilizing a medium measured blending bowl, add the parmesan cheddar in alongside the almond flour, garlic salt and Italian flavoring at that point join together.
2. Add the eggs into a different bowl at that point whisk together.

3. Dunk every mozzarella stick in the beaten egg and afterward dig it into the parmesan cheddar blend to cover.
4. Move the covered mozzarella into reseal capable holders. Note: on the off chance that you need to mastermind in layers, separate the layers with material paper.
5. Spot the holder into the freeze and chill for around 30 minutes.
6. Warmth the air fryer up to 400°F at that point add the mozzarella stick into the air fryer and cook for 5 minutes.

Once done, permit the mozzarella sticks to cool at that point serve and appreciate.

Sustenance Data
Calories: 304 | All out Fat: 19g | Absolute Sugars: 18g | Protein: 17g

MESSY JALAPEÑO POPPERS

Planning Time: 5 minutes
Cook Time: 10 minutes
Servings: 4

Fixings
- bacon
- jalapeno
- zest mix
- cream cheddar
- cheddar, destroyed

Guidelines
1. Join the cheddar and cream cheddar together.
2. Fill the jalapenos empty with the cheddar combination.
3. Warmth the air fryer up to 360°F at that point place the jalapeno in the fryer bin.
4. Cook for 10 minutes at that point serve and appreciate.

Sustenance Data
Calories: 214 | Absolute Fat: 15g | All out Carbs: 9g | Protein: 14g

AIR SINGED TOFU AND CAULIFLOWER RICE

Planning Time: 10 minutes
Cook Time: 20 minutes
Servings: 3
Fixings
for the tofu
- 1/2 square firm tofu
- 1/2 cup onion, diced
- 1 teaspoon turmeric
- 1 cup carrot, diced
- 2 tablespoons low salt soy sauce

for the cauliflower
- 1/2 cup frozen peas
- 1/2 cup broccoli, conveniently slashed
- 1 tablespoon rice vinegar
- 1 tablespoon ginger, minced
- 1/2 teaspoons toasted sesame oil, if wanted
- 2 minced garlic cloves
- 2 tablespoons low salt soy sauce
- 3 cups riced cauliflower

Guidelines
1. Utilizing an enormous blending bowl, squash the tofu at that point blend it in with the leftover tofu Fixings until very much joined.
2. Warmth the air fryer up to 370°F.
3. Spot the covered tofu in the fryer crate at that point cook for 10 minutes, shaking only a single time.
4. Meanwhile, add all the cauliflower Fixings into a medium measured combining bowl at that point consolidate as one.
5. When the 10 minutes for the tofu is finished, add the cauliflower blend into the air fryer, delicately shake the bin at that point cook for an additional 10 minutes, shaking partially through.
6. Cook for an additional 2-5 minutes if you feel the need at that point serve and appreciate.

BREAD WITH POTATO STUFFING

Fixings
- 8 cuts bread (white part as it were)
- 5 enormous potatoes
- 1 little pack finely slashed coriander
- 2 cultivated and finely cleaved green chilies
- ½ teaspoon turmeric
- 2 curry leaf branches
- ½ teaspoon mustard seeds
- 2 finely cleaved little onions
- 2 tablespoons oil (fricasseeing and brushing)
- Salt if wanted

Guidelines
1. Preheat the Air Fryer to 392ºF.
2. Remove the edges of the bread.
3. Strip the potatoes, and bubble. Utilize one teaspoon of salt, and crush the potatoes.

4. Meanwhile, on the burner utilize a skillet to consolidate the mustard seeds and one teaspoon of the oil. Add the onions when the seeds falter, keep singing until they become clear. Throw in the curry and turmeric.
5. Fry the blend a couple of moments, at that point add the salt, pureed potatoes; blend well, and let it cool.
6. Shape eight segments of the combination into an oval shape. Set aside.
7. Wet the bread with water, and press it into your palm to eliminate the overabundance water.
8. Spot the oval potato into the bread and roll the bread totally around the potato blend. Be certain they are totally fixed.
9. Brush the crate and the potato moves with oil, and set aside.
10. Set the Air Fryer clock for 12 to 13 minutes. Allow them to cook until firm and sautéed.

Yields: Four **Servings**

BROCCOLI

Fixings
- 2 Lbs. broccoli crowns
- 2 Tablespoons olive oil
- 1 teaspoon fit salt
- ½ teaspoon dark pepper
- 2 teaspoons ground lemon zing
- 1/3 cup Kalamata olives
- ¼ cup shaved Parmesan cheddar

Guidelines
1. Eliminate the stems from the broccoli and slice them into 1 to 1-1/2-inch florets. Pit and cut the olives down the middle.
2. Over high warmth, fill a medium skillet with six cups of water—carry it to bubbling. Throw in the florets and cook for three to four minutes. Eliminate and channel. Add the pepper, salt, and oil
3. Set the AF to 400ºF.
4. Spot the broccoli into the container, close the cabinet, and snap the clock for 15 minutes. Throw/flip at seven minutes for carmelizing. When done, place the broccoli in the bowl.
5. Embellishment with lemon zing, olives, and cheddar. Appreciate right away.

Yields: Two to Four **Servings**

Reality: The Kalamata olive is a local of southern Greece which is intermittently protected in olive oil or wine vinegar. It is an extra 'kick' for this treat!

WILD OX CAULIFLOWER

Fixings
- 1 cup breadcrumbs
- 4 cups cauliflower florets
- ¼cup wild ox sauce
- ¼ cup liquefied spread

For the Plunge: Your number one dressing

Guidelines
1. Spot the margarine in a microwaveable dish; eliminate and race in the bison sauce.
2. Dunk every one of the florets in the rich blend; the stem doesn't have to have sauce. Utilize the stem as a handle, hold it over a cup and let the overabundance trickle away.
3. Run the floret through the breadcrumbs as you would prefer. Drop them into the fryer. Cook for 14 to 17 minutes at 350ºF. (The unit won't have to preheat since it is determined in the time.)
4. You can shake the bushel a few times to be certain it is uniformly cooking. Appreciate with your #1 plunge, however make certain to consume it right in light of the fact that the crunchiness disappears rapidly.
5. Note: Warm in the stove. Try not to warm it in the microwave; it will be soft.

Yields: Four Servings

MESSY POTATOES

Fixings
- 7 medium potatoes
- ½ cup ground Gruyere (semi-develop) cheddar
- ½ cup cream
- ½cup milk
- 1 teaspoon dark pepper
- ½ teaspoon nutmeg

Directions
1. Strip and cut the potatoes skinny. Chestnut potatoes work extraordinary with this formula.
2. Preset the Air Fryer to 400ºF.
3. Mix the milk and cream; add the nutmeg pepper, and salt for preparing.
4. Liberally cover the potatoes with the blend.
5. Put the cuts in a 8 x 8 dish, pouring the remainder of the blend over the potatoes.
6. Spot the dish into Air Fryer and set the clock for 25 minutes.
7. Eliminate the dish and sprinkle the cheddar over the hot potatoes.

8. Keep cooking until the cheddar is dissolved and carmelized, typically an extra ten minutes.

Yields: **Serves:** Six

FRENCH SEARED POTATOES

Fixings
6 medium stripped potatoes
2 Tbsp. olive oil
Directions
- Preheat the Air Fryer to 360ºF.
- Strip and cut the potatoes into 3-inch strips x ¼-inch.
- Splash the cut potatoes for at least thirty minutes in water, and channel completely. Wipe them off with a towel.
- Coat the potatoes with the oil in an enormous blending holder.
- Drop the potatoes into the cooking bin for around thirty minutes or until they are the ideal doneness.
- Shake the bin a few times during the cooking stage.

- Note: The time may shift contingent upon the thickness of the potatoes.

POTATOES AU GRATIN

Fixings
- 7 Medium stripped chestnut potatoes

½ cup each:
- Cream
- Milk
- ½ teaspoon nutmeg
- 1 teaspoon dark pepper
- ½ cup semi-develop (Gruyere) ground cheddar

Guidelines
Preheat the Air Fryer to 390ºF.
1. Wash and cut the potatoes slender.
2. Mix together the cream and milk—enhancing with some pepper, salt, and nutmeg.
3. Utilize the milk blend to cover the potatoes.
4. Spot the cuts into an eight-inch heating container/dish and pour the rest of the milk/cream combination on top of the potatoes.
5. Spot the warmth safe dish onto the cooking bin—setting the clock for 25 minutes.
6. Take the bin out and sprinkle with the cheddar.
7. Heat ten additional minutes or until seared.
8. Note: You can utilize two eggs rather than milk.

Yields: Six Servings

CUSTOM MADE AF BREAD GARNISHES

Attempt these with a solid serving of mixed greens:
Fixings
- Lifeless Bread
- Margarine
- Discretionary: Olive oil

Guidelines
1. Preheat the Air Fryer for around a few minutes at 248ºF. (You can generally change the time however don't more blazing than 320ºF.)
2. Block a portion of the old bread to the sizes you need to use for your feast.
3. Pour in the olive oil and softened margarine.
4. Put the cubed bread into the container and cook for a few minutes.
5. Throw and cook for an extra a few minutes.
6. Totally cool and keep in an impermeable holder for close to two days.

PORTOBELLO MUSHROOMS

Fixings
- Oz. cubed ham (around two cuts)
- 4 Tbsp. additional virgin olive oil
- Oz. Portobello mushrooms
- 2 shiitake or catch mushrooms
- 1.8 Oz. Mozzarella cheddar (destroyed)
- 1 Tbsp. hacked garlic
- Discretionary: Ground dark pepper and salt

Directions
1. Preheat the AF cooker at 356ºF.
2. Clean, cap, and eliminate the stalks from the mushrooms; two or three paper towels to wipe them off.
3. Utilize 1/2 of the oil to brush the Portobello mushrooms tops and spot them cap side down on a heating plate fixed with aluminum foil or material paper.
4. Separation the mushrooms and top with cheddar, garlic, the other portion of mushrooms—diced, and the cubed ham.
5. Flavor with the pepper and salt. Sprinkle a touch of the oil over the mushrooms.
6. Cook for around 10 minutes. Topping with some dried or new parsley.

THE SPROUTING ONION

Fixings
- 4 little/medium onions
- 4 dabs of margarine
- 1 Tbsp. olive oil

Directions
1. Strip the skin from the onion and remove the top and base to uncover level finishes.
2. Absorb the onions salt water for four hours to remove the cruelty.
3. You'll have to chop the onion as far down as you can without cutting off the onion. Slice multiple times to make eight sections.
4. Preheat the fryer to 350ºF.
5. Put the onions in the fryer and shower with the oil—putting a touch of spread on every one.
6. Cook in the AF until the outside is dull, for the most part around thirty minutes.

Note: 4 spots is 4 loading tablespoons

Yields: Four Servings

ONION RINGS

Fixings
- For a side dish or fast bite; buy four ounces of frozen, battered onion rings.

Guidelines
1. Preheat the Air Fryer cooker to 360ºF.
2. Spot the frozen onion rings in the bin for ten minutes.
3. Take them from the cooker and give them a throw.
4. Reset the clock for an extra ten minutes or more if required.

SANS FAT FRIES

Fixings
- 1 to 2 yams
- 1 to 2 red potatoes
- Sprinkle of pepper and salt
- Cooking shower

Discretionary: Parsley

Guidelines
1. Preset the Air Fryer for 356ºF.
2. Strip and cut the potatoes; place in a holder of water until prepared for broiling.
3. Utilize two layers of paper towels to dry the wedges and shower them with the oil.

4. Spot a solitary layer of fries in the crate and set the clock for ten minutes.
5. After the time is up, give the fries a shake, get back to the AF for an extra eight to ten minutes.
6. Take them from the fryer and season as you wish.
7. Trimming with a touch of parsley.

POTATO CROQUETS

Fixings
- 7 little cubed red potatoes
- 1 egg yolk
- 2 Tablespoons universally handy flour
- ½ cup ground Parmesan cheddar

1 Squeeze Each:
- Cayenne
- Black pepper
- Salt

For the Breading:
- 1 cup universally handy flour
- 2 Tablespoons vegetable oil
- 2 beaten eggs
- ½ cup panko
- 1 Spot of nutmeg

Guidelines
1. Preset the temperature on the Air Fryer to 390ºF.
2. In salted water, heat up the potatoes for 15 minutes, channel, and squash. Cool totally.
3. Add the flour, cheddar, and egg yolk—enhancing with nutmeg, pepper, and salt,
4. Shape the filling into golf ball size.
5. Make a brittle combination of the breadcrumbs and oil. Put each ball into the flour combination, the eggs, and afterward the panko. Fold them into chamber shapes.
6. Put them in the cooking crate until sautéed—around seven to eight minutes.

Yields: It will most likely take 2 bunches relying upon how huge you made the balls.

Fixings
- 6 medium chestnut potatoes
- 1 ½ tsp. paprika
- ½ tsp. salt
- 2 Tbsp. canola oil
- ½ tsp. dark pepper

Guidelines
1. Altogether wash the potatoes under the tap. Heat up the potatoes in salted water around forty minutes.
2. Cool in the fridge for around thirty minutes. Quarter them when cooled.
3. Join the paprika, pepper, salt, and oil in a blending dish. Throw the potatoes in the blend.
4. Spot in the cooking container with the skin side down. Cook them until brilliant earthy colored; around 14 to 16 minutes.

Fixings
- 2 tomatoes
- Cooking shower
- Pepper
- Spices

Guidelines
1. Preheat the fryer to 320ºF.
2. Wash and cut the tomatoes into equal parts. Shower every one of them delicately with some cooking splash and spot them cut side confronting upwards. Sprinkle with your #1 flavors—new or dried—including the pepper, sage, rosemary, basil, oregano, and any others of your decision.
3. Put them into the crate for 20 minutes or until they are to the doneness you need to accomplish. If they are prepared to appreciate—if not—cook for a couple of more minutes.
4. This would be delicious breakfast or as a side dish.

Yields: Two Servings

Planning Time: 5 minutes
Cook Time: 20 minutes
Serves:: 3 Servings
Fixings
- 1/2 teaspoon avocado oil
- 8-10 (wash, cut and wipe off) radishes
- 1/2 tsp onion powder and garlic powder
- Salt and peppers, to taste

Technique
1. Add radish cuts to the wire bushel of an air fryer in one layer and coat equally with avocado oil. Sprinkle with onion powder, garlic powder, pepper, and salt. Seal air fryer.
2. Cook for 15-18 minutes at 390ºF. Check radish chips at 7 minutes, shake air fryer crate and cook until wanted doneness/freshness is reached.

Dietary Data/Serving
Calories 35 kcal, Protein 1g, Net Carbs 2g, Fat 3g

Planning Time: 15 minutes
Cook Time: 15 minutes
Serves:: 4 Servings
Fixings
- 1 egg
- 8 oz. (eliminate stems and cut into 1/2" cuts) new okra
- 1 cup pork skin morsels
- 1 cup coconut milk
- Avocado oil
- 1/2 tsp ocean salt

Technique
1. Add coconut milk and egg into a normal bowl and beat until consolidated. Add okra cuts into the milk combination and mix until covered. Add salt and pork skin morsels into a well lidded bowl and blend until joined.
2. Shake off abundance milk blend from the okra cuts and add into the pork skin bowl. Shake until okra is completely covered. Add okra cuts into the wire container of an air fryer and coat with avocado oil.
3. Cook for 5 minutes at 390ºF. Shake air fryer bin and coat with oil once more. Cook for 5 additional minutes, shake air fryer bin and coat with avocado oil. Cook until okra cuts are crisped and brilliant earthy colored, for 2-5 additional minutes.

Dietary Data/Serving
Calories 188 kcal, Protein 11.9g, Complete Carbs 2.3g, Fat 15g

Planning Time: 3 minutes
Cook Time: 7 minutes
Serves:: 2 **Servings**
Fixings

- 1/4 teaspoon avocado oil
- 1 pound (remove dry parts) asparagus
- Salt and pepper, to taste

Strategy

1. Brush asparagus daintily with avocado oil and season with pepper and salt.
2. Move the prepared asparagus into the wire bin of an air fryer and cook at 400ºF for 7 minutes. Shake air fryer bin halfway during cooking.
3. Serve and appreciate.
4.

Healthful Data/Serving
Calories 46 kcal, Dietary Fiber 4.8g, Protein 5g, Net Carbs 4.1g, Fat 0.8g

C RISPED   Z UCCHINI   G RATIN

Planning Time: 10 minutes
Cook Time: 15 minutes
Serves:: 4 **Servings**
Fixings

- 1 tbsp new hacked cilantro
- 2 (split lengthways and cut every half in two) zucchinis
- 4 tbsps pecorino romano cheddar, ground
- 2 tbsps disintegrated pork skins
- Salt and pepper, to taste
- 1 tbsp avocado oil

Strategy

1. Warmth up air fryer to 350ºF. Working in groups, add zucchini pieces into the wire bushel of the air fryer. Add dark pepper, avocado oil, pecorino romano cheddar, pork skin and cilantro into a bowl and blend until joined.
2. Sprinkle half of cilantro blend over first bunch of zucchini and cook until brilliant earthy colored, for 15 minutes. Rehash measure with the excess cluster of zucchini and the leftover cilantro blend. Serve and appreciate.

Healthful Data/Serving
Calories 75 kcal, Protein 3.8g, Carbs 2.6g, Fat 5.6g

C OOKED   O NIONS   AND   S WEET   P EPPERS

Planning Time: 15 minutes
Cook Time: 10 minutes
Serves:: 4 **Servings**
Fixings

- 1 cup red ringer pepper, cut
- 1 cup green ringer pepper, cut
- 1 tbsp avocado oil
- 1 cup red onion, cut
- 2 tbsps new cleaved parsley
- 1/2 tsp salt
- 1 tbsp new lemon juice

Strategy

1. Warmth up air fryer to 350ºF. Add salt, avocado oil, onion and peppers into a major bowl and throw until entirely covered. Empty combination into the wire container of an air fryer. Cook for 7-9 minutes, until onions are peppers are delicate. Mix halfway while cooking.
2. Empty air singed blend into a serving bowl, include lemon juice and parsley and throw until entirely covered. Serve and delve in.

Healthful Data/Serving
Calories 55 kcal, Protein 0.8g, Carbs 5.6g, Fat 3.5g

B ROILED   AND   C RISPED   B RUSSELS   F LEDGLINGS

Planning Time: 10 minutes
Cook Time: 20 minutes
Serves:: 4 **Servings**
Fixings

- 1 tablespoon avocado oil
- 2 cups (divided and quartered into huge pieces) brussels sprouts
- 1/4 teaspoon ocean salt

Strategy

1. For 5 minutes, heat up air fryer to 375ºF. Add sprout pieces into a major bowl and top with avocado oil. Throw blend until entirely covered, move into the wire container of the air fryer, and softly cover bin with additional avocado oil.
2. Cook until wanted firmness is reached, for 9 minutes. Sprinkle with salt and let sit to cool. Rehash measure with the leftover cluster of fledglings.

Wholesome Data/Serving
Calories 50 kcal, Protein 1g, Fiber 2g, Net Carbs 2g, Fat 4g

ASPARAGUS LANCES WITH MAYO SAUCE

Planning Time: 20 minutes
Cook Time: 5 minutes
Serves:: 2 **Servings**
Fixings

- Avocado oil
- 10 (trim off extreme woody closures, wash and wipe off) asparagus lances
- 1 tbsp substantial whipping cream
- 1 egg, huge
- 1/3 cup pecorino romano cheddar, finely ground
- 1/3 cup almond flour, whitened
- 1/2 tsp paprika
- 1/2 tsp salt

Sauce

- 1 tsp Dijon mustard
- 1/4 cup mayo
- 1/4 tsp dark pepper
- 1/4 tsp cayenne

Technique

1. Add cayenne, dark pepper, mayo and Dijon mustard into a little bowl, mix until consolidated and place in a fridge until required. Add substantial cream and egg into a bow and beat until joined. Move egg wash into a level lined bowl.
2. Add 1/2 tsp salt, 1/2 tsp paprika, 1/3 cup almond flour, and 1/3 cup pecorino romano cheddar into a different level lined bowl and mix until joined. Plunge asparagus lances into the egg wash bowl until covered. Drench asparagus lances into the almond flour blend until entirely covered.
3. Move breaded asparagus onto a material paper lined plate and rehash measure until no asparagus remains. Work in clusters, move breaded asparagus lances into the wire bushel of an air fryer. Splash avocado oil over lances and cook for around 5 minutes at 350ºF.
4. Let sit to cool somewhat. Serve without a moment's delay with mayo sauce.

Dietary Data/Serving
Calories 420 kcal, Protein 9g, Carbs 7g, Fat 40g

BROILED CAULIFLOWER

Planning Time: 10 minutes
Cook Time: 15 minutes
Serves:: 2 **Servings**
Fixings

- 1 tbsp avocado oil
- 3 (split and crushed) garlic cloves
- 1/2 tsp paprika, smoked
- 1/2 tsp salt
- 4 cups cauliflower florets

Strategy

1. Warmth up air fryer to 400ºF. Add paprika, salt, garlic and avocado oil into a bowl and consolidate. Add the cauliflower florets into the blend and throw until completely covered.
2. Move the covered cauli-florets into an air fryer bushel and cook for 15 minutes, until fresh. Shake air fryer crate once like clockwork.

Dietary Data/Serving
Calories 118 kcal, Protein 4.3g, Carbs 12.4g, Fat 7g

AIR SEARED BRUSSELS FLEDGLINGS WITH SPICES

Planning Time: 10 minutes
Cook Time: 8 minutes
Serves:: 4 **Servings**
Fixings

- 1/2 teaspoons oregano, dried
- 1 pound (perfect and managed) brussels sprouts
- 1 teaspoon garlic powder
- 1 teaspoon cilantro, dried
- 2 teaspoon avocado oil
- 1/4 teaspoon salt

Technique

1. Add each fixing into a major bowl and throw until sprouts is completely covered. Add combination into an air fryer bushel and seal the top.
2. Cook for 8 minutes at 390ºF. Let sit to cool prior to serving.

Nourishing Data/Serving
Calories 79 kcal, Protein 4g, Carbs 12g, Fat 2g

LEMON COOKED BROCCOLI WITH PISTACHIOS

Planning Time: 10 minutes
Cook Time: 20 minutes
Serves:: 4 **Servings**

Fixings

- 1/2 tablespoon avocado oil
- 1 pound (cut into florets) broccoli
- Salt
- 1 tablespoon minced garlic
- 2 teaspoons fluid stevia

- 2 tablespoons soy sauce, diminished sodium
- 1 teaspoon rice vinegar
- 2 teaspoons Sriracha
- 2 tbsp lemon juice
- 1/3 cup simmered salted pistachios

Technique
1. Add broccoli florets, salt, garlic, and avocado oil into a major bowl and throw until whisky covered. Add broccoli into an air fryer crate in one layer, and cook for 15-20 minutes, until crisped and brilliant earthy colored, at 400°F. Mix halfway through cooking.
2. Meanwhile, add rice vinegar, sriracha, soy sauce and stevia into a little warmth verification bowl and microwave until consolidated, for 10-15 seconds. Add the cooked broccoli into a bowl and top with the stevia blend. Throw broccoli blend until entirely covered.
3. Check for preparing and change salt as important. Top with lemon squeeze and broiled pistachios.

Healthful Data/Serving
Calories 156 kcal, Protein 4.3g, Carbs 6.2g, Fat 10.5g

SEARED BROCCOLI WITH SPICES

Planning Time: 10 minutes
Cook Time: 8 minutes
Serves:: 4 **Servings**

Fixings
- 1/2 teaspoon sage, dried
- 1 pound (clean and trim) broccoli
- 1 teaspoon garlic powder
- 1 teaspoon cilantro, dried
- 2 tbsp avocado oil
- 1/4 teaspoon salt

Strategy
1. Add each fixing into a major bowl and throw until broccoli is entirely covered. Empty combination into the air fryer bushel and seal the top.
2. Cook for 8 minutes at 400°F. Let sit to cool somewhat prior to serving.

Nourishing Data/Serving
Calories 102 kcal, Protein 3.4g, Carbs 8.4g, Fat 7.1g

AIR FRYER HARICOT VERTS

Planning Time: 15 minutes
Cook Time: 10 minutes
Serves:: 4 **Servings**
Fixings
- 3 (diced) bacon cuts
- 3 cups (cut) haricot verts, frozen
- 1 tsp salt
- 1/4 cup water
- 1 tsp ground dark pepper

Technique
1. Add water, bacon pieces, frozen haricot verts into heat-safe skillet and move dish into the wire container of an air fryer. Cook for 15 minutes for 375°F> Change the temperature of the air fryer from 375°F to 400°F and cook blend for 5 additional minutes.
2. Sprinkle pepper and salt haricot verts combination, and throw until consolidated. Remove dish from the air fryer bushel, let sit and cover with a top. Fill in as wanted and delve in.

Healthful Data/Serving
Calories 95 kcal, Dietary Fiber 2g, Fat 6g, Protein 3g, Net Carbs 4g

SESAME SHISHITO PEPPERS

Albeit these gentle peppers can be eaten crude, when you air-fry them to get a little roast, they are far better. Combined with only a tad of sesame oil, these make an incredible side dish or bite!

Active Time: 5 minutes
CookTime: 8 minutes
Fixings | **Serves:**2
- 6 ounces shishito peppers (about 3 1/2 cups)
- 1 teaspoon sesame oil
- 1 teaspoon salt, partitioned
- 1 teaspoon sesame seeds

1. In a medium bowl, throw peppers with sesame oil and 1/2 teaspoon salt.
2. Preheat air fryer at 375°F for 3 minutes.
3. Add peppers to fryer crate and cook 4 minutes. Shake peppers. Cook an extra 4 minutes until peppers are rankled.
4. Move peppers to a serving dish and embellishment with staying salt and sesame seeds.
   Per serving Calories: 21 | Fat: 2.2 g | Protein:

2.0 g | Sodium: 1,163 mg | Fiber: 2.8 g | Carbs: 6.1 g | Sugar: 2.8 g

COOKED CARROTS

The blend of cinnamon and nectar draws out the regular pleasantness of these cooked carrots. The air fryer adds a little singe to the outside, making another layer of flavor.

Active Time: 5 minutes
CookTime: 10 minutes
Fixings | Serves:4
- 3 huge carrots, stripped
- 1 teaspoon olive oil
- 1 tablespoon nectar
- $^1/_4$ teaspoon ground cinnamon
- $^1/_8$ teaspoon cayenne pepper
- $^1/_2$ teaspoon salt

1. Slice carrots down the middle longwise. At that point cut parts into 1" segments.
2. In a medium bowl, whisk together oil, nectar, cinnamon, cayenne pepper, and salt. Add carrots and throw.
3. Preheat air fryer at 375°F for 3 minutes.
4. Add carrots to fryer crate and cook 5 minutes. Throw. Cook an extra 5 minutes.
5. Move to a bowl and serve warm.

Per serving Calories: 47 | Fat: 1.2. g | Protein: 0.5 g | Sodium: 327 mg | Fiber: 1.6 g | Carbs: 9.7 g | Sugar: 6.7 g

SEARED OKRA

Okra gets unfavorable criticism for its disgusting nature when cooked. This ooze, or adhesive, is really eatable, yet the mouthfeel can dismiss a few group. Fortunately air searing makes these taste mind blowing and become an incredible side dish with chicken, steak, or fish!

Involved Time: 10 minutes
CookTime: 7 minutes
Fixings | Serves:2
- 2 enormous eggs
- $^1/_4$ cup entire milk
- $^1/_4$ cup plain bread scraps
- $^1/_4$ cup cornmeal
- 1 teaspoon salt
- $^1/_2$ pound new okra, cut into $^1/_2$" pieces
- 1 tablespoon margarine, dissolved

1. In a little bowl, whisk together eggs and milk. In a shallow dish, join bread morsels, cornmeal, and salt.
2. Preheat air fryer at 400°F for 3 minutes.
3. Plunge okra in egg combination. Dig in bread piece combination. Spot okra in air fryer bushel. Cook 4 minutes. Shake. Brush okra with dissolved spread. Cook an extra 3 minutes.
4. Move to a dish and serve warm.
   Per serving Calories: 187 | Fat: 8.4 g | Protein: 7.0 g | Sodium: 970 mg | Fiber: 3.6 g | Starches: 20.3 g | Sugar: 2.8 g

SINGED GREEN BEANS

These green beans are fast and fresh and ideal for nibbling on while appreciating a virus blend. Likewise, if you have some critical eaters, these might be the secret to get them to take a stab at something green!

Active Time: 10 minutes
CookTime: 14 minutes
Fixings | Serves:2
- 1 huge egg
- 1 tablespoon entire milk
- 1 tablespoon nectar
- 2 tablespoons cornmeal
- 2 tablespoons cornstarch
- 2 tablespoons finely ground Parmesan cheddar
- $^1/_2$ teaspoon salt, in addition to an additional squeeze for embellish
- 10 ounces green beans, managed (around 3 cups)

In a medium bowl, whisk together egg, milk, and nectar.
In a shallow dish, consolidate cornmeal, cornstarch, cheddar, and salt.
Preheat air fryer at 375°F for 3 minutes.
Coat green beans with egg blend and shake off any abundance. Dig in the cornmeal blend.
Spot green beans in air fryer crate. Cook 7 minutes. Tenderly throw green beans. Cook an extra 7 minutes.
Move green beans to a serving dish and embellishment with a touch of salt. Serve warm.

Per serving Calories: 171 | Fat: 2.9 g | Protein: 6.7 g | Sodium: 774 mg | Fiber: 4.5 g | Carbs: 31.0 g | Sugar: 9.8 g

ASIAN BRUSSELS FLEDGLINGS

The pungency of the soy sauce and the pleasantness of the maple syrup help counter the severe flavor that some may recognize in Brussels sprouts. Balanced significantly more with the little kick of warmth from the sriracha, this side dish will have your family requesting seconds!

Active Time: 5 minutes
CookTime: 14 minutes
Fixings | Serves:2

- ¹/4 cup newly pressed squeezed orange
- 1 tablespoon unadulterated maple syrup
- 1 tablespoon soy sauce
- ¹/4 teaspoon sriracha
- 1 tablespoon olive oil
- 1 pound Brussels sprouts, divided
- Squeeze salt

1. In an enormous bowl, whisk together squeezed orange, maple syrup, soy sauce, sriracha, and olive oil. Throw in Brussels sprouts. Refrigerate 30 minutes.
2. Preheat air fryer at 350°F for 3 minutes.
3. Add Brussels fledglings to air fryer. Cook 7 minutes. Throw. Cook an extra 7 minutes.
4. Move Brussels fledglings to a serving dish, season with salt, and serve warm.
   Per serving Calories: 123 | Fat: 3.7 g | Protein: 6.1 g | Sodium: 304 mg | Fiber: 6.4 g | Carbs: 20.2 g | Sugar: 8.1 g

CHILD BACON HASSELBACKS

If a prepared potato and home fries had a child, it'd be this dish. The cuts of potatoes permit the dissolved spread to cook down in the little hiding spots, making numerous fresh edges, and the bacon between cuts Yields a pungent pork flavor that no one but bacon can give.

Involved Time: 15 minutes
CookTime: 20 minutes
Fixings | Serves:3

- 6 child red potatoes, cleaned
- 1 cut uncooked bacon, diced
- 1 tablespoon olive oil
- 2 tablespoons margarine, liquefied
- Squeeze salt
- 6 teaspoons harsh cream
- ¹/4 cup slashed new parsley

1. Make cuts in the width of potatoes about ¹/4" separated without carving completely through.

Press a little dice of bacon between each cut. Brush potatoes with olive oil.
2. Preheat air fryer at 350°F for 3 minutes.
3. Add potatoes to air fryer container. Cook 10 minutes. Brush with dissolved spread, guaranteeing the margarine gets between cuts. Cook an extra 10 minutes.
4. Move potatoes to a serving dish. Season with salt. Add a bit of acrid cream to the highest point of every potato. Topping with cleaved parsley. Serve warm.
   Per serving Calories: 383 | Fat: 14.8 g | Protein: 8.2 g | Sodium: 181 mg | Fiber: 6.0 g | Starches: 54.7 g | Sugar: 4.7 g

HEATED GNOCCHI

Gnocchi are pillowy little potato dumplings that are generally presented with a rich sauce. In this formula, the cushions are as yet fleecy, however the air fryer gives them a fresh outside.

Involved Time: 5 minutes
CookTime: 27 minutes
Fixings | Serves:4

- 2 medium Chestnut potatoes, stripped and diced
- ¹/2 teaspoon onion powder
- ¹/2 teaspoon salt
- ¹/2 teaspoon newly ground dark pepper
- 1 enormous egg
- ¹/4 cup universally handy flour
- 1 tablespoon margarine, softened
- ¹/2 teaspoon garlic salt

1. Add potatoes to an enormous pot with sufficient water to cover potatoes. Bring to bubble. Decrease warmth and stew 4–5 minutes until potatoes are fork-delicate.
2. Channel potatoes and move to a medium bowl. Add onion powder, salt, and pepper to the bowl. Squash prepared potatoes until smooth. Add egg and blend until joined.
3. Sprinkle a portion of the flour on a level, clean surface. With floured hands, ply mixture to join a portion of the flour and lessen tenacity.
4. Sever a little wad of mixture. Work into a rope ¹/2" wide. Utilizing a knife cut into ¹/2" areas. If you'd like the exemplary lines on the gnocchi, roll every gnocchi under the prongs of a fork. Rehash with the remainder of the mixture.
5. Heat a pot of salted water to the point of boiling. Add gnocchi in two groups to water. Utilizing an

opened spoon, eliminate once they ascend to the top, after around 2 minutes.

6. Preheat air fryer at 350°F for 3 minutes.
7. Add gnocchi to air fryer bin. Cook 5 minutes. Tenderly throw. Cook an additional 5 minutes. Throw and brush gnocchi with margarine. Cook 4 minutes. Throw again and cook an extra 4 minutes.
8. Move gnocchi to a bowl and throw with garlic salt. Serve warm.

Per serving Calories: 116 | Fat: 3.8 g | Protein: 3.1 g | Sodium: 754 mg | Fiber: 1.8 g | Starches: 17.2 g | Sugar: 0.8 g

PECAN CRUSTED GOAT CHEDDAR BOMBS

Regardless of whether serving these alongside a succulent steak, adding a new turn to a late spring salad, or simply popping them in your mouth, these Pecan Crusted Goat Cheddar Bombs will add grins to the essences of each one of people around you.

Active Time: 10 minutes
CookTime: 16 minutes
Fixings | Serves:4

- 5 ounces goat cheddar, at room temperature
- 5 ounces mascarpone cheddar, at room temperature
- 1/4 teaspoon salt
- 1/4 teaspoon newly ground dark pepper
- 1 teaspoon new thyme leaves
- 1/4 cup generally useful flour
- 1 enormous egg, whisked
- 1/3 cup finely squashed pecans
- 1/3 cup panko bread morsels

1. In a medium bowl, consolidate goat cheddar, mascarpone cheddar, salt, pepper, and thyme. Structure into sixteen wads of equivalent size.
2. Add flour to a little bowl. Add whisked egg to another little bowl. Blend pecan pieces and bread scraps in a shallow dish.
3. Move cheddar bombs in flour. Shake off any abundance. Plunge cheddar bombs in egg. Shake off any overabundance. Dig cheddar bombs in bread scrap blend. Spot covered cheddar bombs in cooler 30 minutes.
4. Preheat air fryer at 375°F for 3 minutes.
5. Add eight cheddar bombs to daintily lubed air fryer crate. Cook 8 minutes. Rehash with residual cheddar bombs.
6. Move to a serving plate and serve warm.

Per serving Calories: 338 | Fat: 24.7 g | Protein: 13.5 g | Sodium: 338 mg | Fiber: 0.6 g | Carbs: 14.0 g | Sugar: 1.9 g

NUTTY BROILED OAK SEED SQUASH

The sweet orange tissue of this fall side dish is featured with a touch of margarine, sugar, cinnamon, and nutmeg. Adding the walnuts loans surface and heartiness, which helps make oak seed squash an occasional top choice!

Active Time: 10 minutes
CookTime: 35 minutes
Fixings | Serves:2

- 1/2 huge oak seed squash, seeds eliminated
- 1 teaspoon spread, liquefied
- 1 teaspoon earthy colored sugar
- 1 teaspoon nectar
- Squeeze ground cinnamon
- Squeeze ground nutmeg
- Squeeze salt
- 1 tablespoon walnut pieces

1. Turn the oak seed squash cut side up and cut off about 1/4" of the base so it can sit level.
2. In a little bowl, consolidate margarine, sugar, nectar, cinnamon, nutmeg, and salt. Brush over top of crush and pour any extra in the opening.
3. Preheat air fryer at 400°F for 3 minutes.
4. Add oak seed squash to air fryer. Cook 30 minutes. Add walnuts. Cook an extra 5 minutes.
5. Slice down the middle and move to two plates. Serve warm.

Per serving Calories: 102 | Fat: 4.2 g | Protein: 1.2 g | Sodium: 76 mg | Fiber: 2.0 g | Carbs: 17.0 g | Sugar: 5.3 g

PROSCIUTTO-WRAPPED ASPARAGUS

The air fryer realizes how to fresh up prosciutto, and wrapped asparagus is a such a reward. There is no requirement for preparing. The pungent idea of prosciutto loans barely sufficient flavor for these scrumptious lances. Appreciate as a side dish, tidbit, or canapé, either alone or with a custom made plunging sauce!

Involved Time: 10 minutes
CookTime: 12 minutes
Fixings | Serves:4

- 3 ounces prosciutto
- 18 thick lances of asparagus, managed of woody closures

1. Cut prosciutto the long way into eighteen even cuts. Twisting wrap the prosciutto takes from the lower part of the asparagus to the top, halting prior to covering the tip.
2. Preheat air fryer at 400°F for 3 minutes.
3. Spot enveloped asparagus by air fryer bin. Cook 6 minutes. Shake. Cook an extra 6 minutes until prosciutto is fresh.
4. Move to a plate and serve.
   Per serving Calories: 80 | Fat: 4.8 g | Protein: 6.5 g | Sodium: 86 mg | Fiber: 1.9 g | Starches: 4.0 g | Sugar: 1.7 g

SWEET BEAN STEW CHILD BOK CHOY

Air singing these child groups of bok choy **Yields** delicate cabbage with firm edges. The custom made Sweet Bean stew Sauce adjust the slight sharpness of the bok choy. Serve close by a piece of cod for a light and quality feast.

Involved Time: 10 minutes
CookTime: 12 minutes
Fixings | Serves:4

- 2 medium bunches child bok choy, quartered longwise
- ¹/4 cup Sweet Bean stew Sauce (see Section 15)
- Squeeze salt

1. Clean quartered child bok choy and let channel on paper towels. Wipe off.
2. Preheat air fryer at 350°F for 3 minutes.
3. Brush bok choy with Sweet Bean stew Sauce. Spot half in air fryer container and cook 3 minutes. Flip bok choy. Cook an extra 3 minutes. Rehash with remaining bok choy.
4. Move to a serving plate, season with a touch of salt, and serve warm.
   Per serving Calories: 134 | Fat: 0.3 g | Protein: 3.3 g | Sodium: 255 mg | Fiber: 2.1 g | Starches: 31.0 g | Sugar: 27.7 g

SQUASH WASTES

Essentially, these are singular chomps of a squash meal. The solitary difference? You get a smash with each chomp.
Involved Time: 10 minutes
CookTime: 22 minutes
Fixings

- 12 Wastes
- 2 cups ground summer squash (around 1 huge squash)
- ¹/2 cup destroyed cheddar
- 2 tablespoons minced yellow onion
- 1 tablespoon universally handy flour
- 1 tablespoon cornmeal
- 1 tablespoon unsalted margarine, dissolved
- 1 enormous egg
- ¹/4 teaspoon salt
- ¹/2 teaspoon newly ground dark pepper
- 1 cup plain bread morsels

1. Crush ground squash between paper towels to eliminate abundance dampness and move to a huge bowl. Add cheddar, onion, flour, cornmeal, margarine, egg, salt, and pepper and join.
2. Add bread morsels to a shallow dish.
3. Preheat air fryer at 350°F for 3 minutes.
4. Structure squash combination into twelve balls, roughly 2 tablespoons each. Roll each ball in bread morsels to cover all sides.
5. Spot half of the squanders on a pizza skillet (embellishment). Cook 6 minutes. Flip wastes and cook an extra 5 minutes. Move to a plate.
6. Rehash with outstanding wastes and serve warm.
   Per serving Calories: 60 | Fat: 2.9 g | Protein: 2.7 g | Sodium: 117 mg | Fiber: 0.5 g | Carbs: 5.3 g | Sugar: 0.8 g

SEARED OLD FASHIONED CORN

If you've at any point been to a state reasonable, at that point you realize that everything gets seared except if it's made sure about. This incorporates ideal cobs of sweet, brilliant corn.
Involved Time: 5 minutes
CookTime: 20 minutes
Fixings | Serves:4

- 1 enormous egg
- 1 cup buttermilk
- 1 cup universally handy flour
- 2 teaspoons salt
- ¹/2 teaspoon sugar

- 1 teaspoon dried thyme
- ¼ cup ground Parmesan cheddar
- 4 ears corn, shucked and divided, silk eliminated
- 3 tablespoons margarine, dissolved

1. In a medium bowl, whisk together egg and buttermilk.
2. In a shallow dish, join flour, salt, sugar, thyme, and Parmesan cheddar.
3. Preheat air fryer at 400°F for 3 minutes.
4. Move corn in egg combination and dig in flour blend. Shake off overabundance.
5. Add 4 half ears of corn to fryer bin and cook 7 minutes. Flip corn and brush with dissolved margarine. Cook an extra 3 minutes. Rehash with residual corn.
6. Move seared corn to a plate and serve warm.
   Per serving Calories: 260 | Fat: 11.3 g | Protein: 8.0 g | Sodium: 694 mg | Fiber: 2.5 g | Starches: 33.5 g | Sugar: 8.4 g

BROILED CORN SALAD

Via air fricasseeing the corn, you add a little roast, which thusly adds a ton of flavor. Refrigerate this plate of mixed greens covered for the time being to truly permit the flavors to wed together for a surprisingly better encounter.

Active Time: 5 minutes
CookTime: 7 minutes
Fixings | **Serves:**4
- 3 ears corn, shucked and split, silk eliminated
- 2 medium Roma tomatoes, cultivated and diced
- 1 cup canned dark beans, depleted and washed
- 1 medium avocado, stripped, pitted, and diced
- ½ cup hacked new cilantro
- ½ cup diced red onion
- ¼ cup balsamic vinegar
- 2 tablespoons olive oil
- ½ teaspoon salt
- ¼ teaspoon newly ground dark pepper

1. Preheat air fryer at 400°F for 3 minutes.
2. Add corn to fryer bin and cook 5 minutes. Shake bin. Cook an extra 2 minutes.
3. Move corn to a plate and permit to cool until simple to deal with. Cut bits from cob and add to a medium bowl.
4. Add remaining Fixings , join, and serve.

Per serving Calories: 264 | Fat: 12.4 g | Protein: 7.4 g | Sodium: 450 mg | Fiber: 8.8 g | Carbs: 33.1 g | Sugar: 9.1 g

RANKLED GRAPE TOMATOES

Adding warmth to tomatoes draws out their common sugars. Thrown with tart balsamic vinegar, this side dish is a brilliant backup to a steak new off the barbecue.

Active Time: 5 minutes
CookTime: 15 minutes
Fixings | **Serves:**4
- 8 ounces (roughly 30) grape tomatoes
- 2 teaspoons olive oil
- ¼ teaspoon salt
- 1 tablespoon balsamic vinegar
- 1 tablespoon cleaved new basil

1. Preheat air fryer at 350°F for 3 minutes.
2. In a little bowl, throw tomatoes, olive oil, and salt.
3. Move tomatoes to air fryer bin and cook 5 minutes. Shake bushel. Cook 5 minutes. Shake crate. Cook 5 minutes.
4. Move tomatoes to a bowl. Throw with balsamic vinegar and enhancement with slashed basil.
   Per serving Calories: 33 | Fat: 2.3 g | Protein: 0.5 g | Sodium: 148 mg | Fiber: 0.7 g | Carbs: 2.9 g | Sugar: 2.1 g

SINGED SPICED EGGS

Singed Spiced Eggs have every one of the customary kinds of the firsts with the additional surface of breading and air broiling the white of the egg. At that point spoon or line on the smooth yolk combination for something special that your visitors will discuss for some time.

Involved Time: 15 minutes
CookTime: 10 minutes
Fixings | **Serves:**5
- 5 hard-bubbled enormous eggs
- 1 enormous egg
- ¼ cup entire milk
- 1 cup panko bread scraps
- ¼ cup universally handy flour
- 1 teaspoon salt
- ¼ cup mayonnaise
- 1 teaspoon yellow mustard
- ½ teaspoon dill pickle juice
- 1 tablespoon finely diced dill pickles

- $^1/8$ teaspoon salt
- $^1/8$ teaspoon newly ground dark pepper
- $^1/8$ teaspoon smoked paprika

1. Strip eggs and dispose of shells. Cut each egg into equal parts longwise. Spot yolks in a little bowl.
2. In a different little bowl, whisk together egg and milk.
3. In a shallow dish, consolidate bread pieces, flour, and salt.
4. Preheat air fryer at 400°F for 3 minutes.
5. Coat egg white parts in egg blend and afterward dig in bread piece combination. Shake off abundance.
6. Add half of egg white parts to fryer bushel and cook 5 minutes. Rehash with outstanding egg whites.
7. While eggs are cooking, consolidate egg yolks with mayonnaise, mustard, pickle juice, pickles, salt, and pepper.
8. Move seared egg parts to a plate. Spoon the yolk filling into the egg white parts. Delicately sprinkle with paprika. Keep refrigerated and covered until prepared to serve.
   Per serving Calories: 230 | Fat: 13.7 g | Protein: 9.3 g | Sodium: 488 mg | Fiber: 0.3 g | Starches: 14.2 g | Sugar: 1.7 g

PREPARED POTATOES

The air fryer can cook the potatoes a lot quicker than your stove. Albeit a microwave can accomplish this cook in a considerably more limited time, the air fryer crisps up the external skin while cooking the middle flawlessly!

Involved Time: 5 minutes
CookTime: 45 minutes
Fixings | **Serves:**2
- 2 enormous Reddish brown potatoes (around 1 pound), scoured
- 2 teaspoons olive oil
- 2 tablespoons margarine, cut into 2 taps
- $^1/2$ teaspoon salt
- $^1/4$ teaspoon newly ground dark pepper

1. Preheat air fryer at 400°F for 3 minutes.
2. Rub olive oil over the two potatoes. Spot in air fryer bin.
3. Cook 30 minutes. Flip potatoes. Cook an extra 15 minutes.
4. Once cooled, cut every potato longwise about $^1/2$" profound. Squeeze closures to open up cut.

Add a pat of spread and season with salt and pepper. Serve warm.

Per serving Calories: 419 | Fat: 15.3 g | Protein: 7.6 g | Sodium: 1,606 mg | Fiber: 6.7 g | Starches: 63.4 g | Sugar: 3.5 g

SPREAD THYME CHILD REDS

Normally rich and firm, child red potatoes are improved with a touch of added margarine, thyme, garlic salt, and dark pepper. Cook these while the chicken or steak is on the outside barbecue or whenever you need a delicious side!

Active Time: 5 minutes
CookTime: 19 minutes
Fixings | **Serves:**6
- 1 pound child red potatoes, scoured and divided
- 2 tablespoons unsalted spread, softened
- $^1/2$ teaspoon dried thyme
- $^1/4$ teaspoon garlic salt
- $^1/8$ teaspoon newly ground dark pepper

1. Preheat air fryer at 350°F for 3 minutes.
2. In a huge bowl, join potatoes, spread, thyme, garlic salt, and pepper.
3. Spot potatoes in air fryer crate. Cook 10 minutes. Throw potatoes. Cook an extra 9 minutes.
4. Move to a serving bowl.
   Per serving Calories: 82 | Fat: 3.6 g | Protein: 1.4 g | Sodium: 94 mg | Fiber: 1.2 g | Carbs: 11.0 g | Sugar: 0.9 g

TWICE-PREPARED POTATOES

You might not have any desire to make these for your family, on the grounds that once you do, you should make this formula again and again!

Active Time: 10 minutes
CookTime: 47 minutes
Fixings | **Serves:**4
- 2 teaspoons olive oil
- 2 huge Reddish brown potatoes (around 1 pound), cleaned
- $^1/2$ teaspoon garlic salt
- $^1/4$ teaspoon newly ground dark pepper
- 1 tablespoon unsalted spread
- $^1/2$ cup destroyed cheddar
- $^1/4$ cup acrid cream
- 3 cuts bacon, cooked and disintegrated
- $^1/4$ cup cleaved new parsley

1. Preheat air fryer at 400°F for 3 minutes.
2. Rub olive oil over the two potatoes. Spot in air fryer crate.
3. Cook 30 minutes. Flip potatoes. Cook an extra 15 minutes.
4. Once cooled, cut every potato the long way. Scoop out potato to frame four boats with the skins, leaving a ¹/4" layer of potato tissue in each. Spot scooped-out potato in a medium bowl.
5. To scooped-out potato, crush in garlic salt, pepper, spread, cheddar, sharp cream, and bacon. Spoon combination into potato boats.
6. Spot boats once more into air fryer bin and cook an extra 2 minutes. Topping with parsley and serve warm.

Per serving Calories: 310 | Fat: 14.5 g | Protein: 10.5 g | Sodium: 504 mg | Fiber: 3.5 g | Carbs: 32.7 g | Sugar: 2.3 g

FARM PURPLE POTATOES

Throw these beautiful spuds with some farm dressing for velvety flavor. If you don't incline toward cilantro, just trade it out for some slashed new parsley!

Involved Time: 5 minutes
CookTime: 19 minutes
Fixings | Serves:6
- 1 pound little purple potatoes, scoured and divided
- 2 tablespoons margarine, liquefied
- ¹/4 teaspoon salt
- ¹/8 teaspoon newly ground dark pepper
- ¹/4 cup farm dressing
- ¹/4 cup slashed new cilantro

1. Preheat air fryer at 350°F for 3 minutes.
2. In an enormous bowl, join potatoes, spread, salt, and pepper.
3. Spot potatoes in air fryer container. Cook 10 minutes. Throw potatoes. Cook an extra 9 minutes.
4. Move to a serving bowl and throw with farm dressing. Trimming with cilantro and serve warm.
   Per serving Calories: 84 | Fat: 3.9 g | Protein: 1.4 g | Sodium: 115 mg | Fiber: 1.2 g | Starches: 11.0 g | Sugar: 0.9 g

BROILED GARLIC PUREED POTATOES

The skins of the potatoes add nourishment to your pureed potatoes, yet additionally add to the surface and natural kind of the dish.

Active Time: 10 minutes
CookTime: 14 minutes
Fixings | Serves:4
- 1 pound Yukon Gold potatoes (2 medium), scoured and diced into 1" 3D shapes
- 3 cloves garlic, split
- 2 tablespoons spread, liquefied
- ¹/2 teaspoon salt
- ¹/2 teaspoon newly ground dark pepper
- ¹/4 cup substantial cream
- 1 tablespoon spread (not liquefied)
- ¹/4 cup hacked new parsley

1. Preheat air fryer at 350°F for 3 minutes.
2. In a huge bowl, consolidate potatoes, garlic, and dissolved margarine.
3. Spot potato blend in air fryer crate. Cook 7 minutes. Throw. Cook an extra 7 minutes. Move to a huge bowl.
4. Add salt, pepper, a large portion of the cream, and 1 tablespoon spread and squash. Gradually add remaining cream until wanted consistency.
5. Trimming with parsley and serve warm.
   Per serving Calories: 203 | Fat: 13.4 g | Protein: 2.4 g | Sodium: 315 mg | Fiber: 2.7 g | Carbs: 17.8 g | Sugar: 1.7 g

PREPARED JALAPEÑO AND CHEDDAR CAULIFLOWER POUND

This dish is the ideal side when you're in a rush and Fixings . You probably have a large portion of the Fixings in your fridge as of now. The cream cheddar is utilized as a thickener to give the dish a smooth and velvety surface.

Pantry Staples: Salt, ground dark pepper
Hands On schedule: 10 minutes
Cook Time: 15 minutes
Serves: 6
- 1 (12-ounce) liner sack cauliflower florets, cooked by bundle Guidelines
- 2 tablespoons salted margarine, mellowed
- 2 ounces cream cheddar, mellowed
- ½ cup destroyed sharp cheddar
- ¼ cup salted jalapeños
- ½ teaspoon salt

- ¼ teaspoon ground dark pepper

1. Spot prepared cauliflower into a food processor with outstanding Fixings . Heartbeat multiple times until cauliflower is smooth and all Fixings are joined.
2. Spoon squash into an ungreased 6" round nonstick heating dish. Spot dish into air fryer crate. Change the temperature to 380°F and set the clock for 15 minutes. The top will be brilliant earthy colored when done. Serve warm.

Per serving
Calories: 117 Protein: 4g Fiber: 1g Net carbs: 2g
Fat: 9g Sodium: 390mg Carbs: 3g Sugar: 2g

BURGER BUN FOR ONE

This bun is the ideal speedy and simple bread substitute for everything from burgers to barbecued cheddar to breakfast sandwiches. Flavorful and prepared in minutes, this formula will hold you back from going after customary carb-filled bread!

Pantry Staples: Preparing powder
Hands On schedule: 2 minutes
Cook Time: 5 minutes
Serves: 1
- 2 tablespoons salted spread, softened
- ¼ cup whitened finely ground almond flour
- ¼ teaspoon preparing powder
- ⅛ teaspoon apple juice vinegar
- 1 huge egg, whisked

1. Empty spread into an ungreased 4" ramekin. Add flour, preparing powder, and vinegar to ramekin and mix until consolidated. Add egg and mix until player is for the most part smooth.
2. Spot ramekin into air fryer crate. Change the temperature to 350°F and set the clock for 5 minutes. At the point when done, the middle will be firm and the top marginally seared. Let cool, around 5 minutes, at that point eliminate from ramekin and cut into equal parts. Serve.

Per serving calories: 444 protein: 13g fiber: 3g net sugars: 3g fat: 41g
Sodium: 374mg starches: 6g sugar: 1g

BACON-BALSAMIC BRUSSELS FLEDGLINGS

The sweet balsamic and smoky bacon seasons in this formula make for a dish that can supplement pretty much any entrée. Regardless of whether you're getting a charge out of chicken or steak, these Brussels fledglings will amaze you with how delectable they are.

Pantry Staples: Salt, ground dark pepper
Hands On schedule: 5 minutes
Cook Time: 12 minutes
Serves: 4
- 2 cups managed and divided new Brussels sprouts
- 2 tablespoons olive oil
- ¼ teaspoon salt
- ¼ teaspoon ground dark pepper
- 2 tablespoons balsamic vinegar
- 2 cuts cooked sans sugar bacon, disintegrated

1. In an enormous bowl, throw Brussels sprouts in olive oil, at that point sprinkle with salt and pepper. Spot into ungreased air fryer container. Change the temperature to 375°F and set the clock for 12 minutes, shaking the bushel part of the way through cooking. Brussels fledglings will be delicate and sautéed when done.
2. Spot sprouts in a huge serving dish and shower with balsamic vinegar. Sprinkle bacon up and over. Serve warm.

Per serving calories: 112 protein: 3g
Fiber: 2g net carbs: 3g fat: 9g sodium: 254mg
carbs: 5g sugar: 2g

BROILED ASPARAGUS

You needn't bother with much flavoring to give this formula flavor, as the brilliant earthy colored finishes add a decent common pleasantness. This dish can be multiplied and utilized for feast prep close by Margarine and Bacon Chicken or Italian Meatballs for a balanced and flavorful spread.

Pantry Staples: Salt, ground dark pepper
Hands On schedule: 5 minutes
Cook Time: 12 minutes
Serves: 4
- 1 tablespoon olive oil
- 1 pound asparagus lances, closes managed
- ¼ teaspoon salt
- ¼ teaspoon ground dark pepper

- 1 tablespoon salted spread, dissolved

1. In a huge bowl, shower olive oil over asparagus lances and sprinkle with salt and pepper.
2. Spot lances into ungreased air fryer bin. Change the temperature to 375°F and set the clock for 12 minutes, shaking the bushel part of the way through cooking. Asparagus will be gently cooked and delicate when done.
3. Move to a huge dish and shower with spread. Serve warm.

Per serving calories: 73 protein: 2g
Fiber: 2g net carbs: 2g fat: 6g sodium: 169mg
carbs: 4g sugar: 2g

MESSY PREPARED ASPARAGUS

This formula puts a messy twist on straightforward asparagus. The delicate vegetable cooks in a smooth sauce and absorbs all the delicious flavor. Go ahead and add ½ teaspoon of your #1 Italian flavoring to truly make it pop.

Pantry Staples: Salt, ground dark pepper
Hands On schedule: 10 minutes
Cook Time: 18 minutes
Serves: 4

- ½ cup substantial whipping cream
- ½ cup ground Parmesan cheddar
- 2 ounces cream cheddar, mollified
- 1 pound asparagus, closes managed, hacked into 1" pieces
- ¼ teaspoon salt
- ¼ teaspoon ground dark pepper

1. In a medium bowl, whisk together substantial cream, Parmesan, and cream cheddar until joined.
2. Spot asparagus into an ungreased 6" round nonstick heating dish. Pour cheddar combination up and over and sprinkle with salt and pepper.
3. Spot dish into air fryer bushel. Change the temperature to 350°F and set the clock for 18 minutes. Asparagus will be delicate when done. Serve warm.

Per serving calories: 221 protein: 7g
Fiber: 2g net starches: 5g fat: 18g
Sodium: 435mg starches: 7g sugar: 3g

DIJON BROIL CABBAGE

If you like nectar mustard, you'll love the sweet sauce that is showered over the fresh cabbage in this dish. It's not difficult to make, and you may as of now have a large portion of the **Fixings** in your storeroom. It's an incredible side to imps or a rich chicken thigh.

Pantry Staples: Salt
Hands On schedule: 10 minutes
Cook Time: 10 minutes
Serves: 4

- 1 little head cabbage, cored and cut into 1"-thick cuts
- 2 tablespoons olive oil, partitioned
- ½ teaspoon salt
- 1 tablespoon Dijon mustard
- 1 teaspoon apple juice vinegar
- 1 teaspoon granular erythritol

1. Shower each cabbage cut with 1 tablespoon olive oil, at that point sprinkle with salt. Spot cuts into ungreased air fryer bushel, working in bunches if required. Change the temperature to 350°F and set the clock for 10 minutes. Cabbage will be delicate and edges will start to brown when done.
2. In a little bowl, whisk staying olive oil with mustard, vinegar, and erythritol. Sprinkle over cabbage in a huge serving dish. Serve warm.

Per serving calories: 111 protein: 3g
Fiber: 4g net starches: 7g sugar liquor: 1g
Fat: 7g sodium: 416mg starches: 12g
Sugar: 6g

GARLIC PARMESAN–BROILED CAULIFLOWER

As is valid for potatoes, there are such countless approaches to spruce up cauliflower. And keeping in mind that a great deal of plans require depleting and cooking it twice, this basic formula returns to fundamentals through simmering. Made generally with Fixings you'll have close by, this simple side goes with pretty much anything.

Pantry Staples: Salt
Hands On schedule: 5 minutes
Cook Time: 15 minutes
Serves: 6

- 1 medium head cauliflower, leaves and center eliminated, cut into florets
- 2 tablespoons salted margarine, dissolved
- ½ tablespoon salt

- 2 cloves garlic, stripped and finely minced
- ½ cup ground Parmesan cheddar, separated

1. Throw cauliflower in a huge bowl with margarine. Sprinkle with salt, garlic, and ¼ cup Parmesan.
2. Spot florets into ungreased air fryer bushel. Change the temperature to 350°F and set the clock for 15 minutes, shaking bin partially through cooking. Cauliflower will be cooked at the edges and delicate when done.
3. Move florets to an enormous serving dish and sprinkle with residual Parmesan. Serve warm.

Per serving Calories: 94
Protein: 4g fiber: 2g net starches: 4g fat: 6g
Sodium: 791mg starches: 6g sugar: 2g

CAULIFLOWER RICE BALLS

This dish is so scrumptious it may very well capture everyone's attention! The rice balls are crunchy outwardly and brimming with gooey cheddar inside—yet at the same time stacked with supplements. Fill in as a side or with warmed low-carb marinara and embellished with Parmesan.

Pantry Staples: Salt
Hands On schedule: 10 minutes
Cook Time: 8 minutes
Serves: 4
- 1 (10-ounce) liner sack cauliflower rice, cooked by bundle Guidelines
- ½ cup destroyed mozzarella cheddar
- 1 enormous egg
- 2 ounces plain pork skins, finely squashed
- ¼ teaspoon salt
- ½ teaspoon Italian flavoring

1. Spot cauliflower into an enormous bowl and blend in with mozzarella.
2. Whisk egg in a different medium bowl. Spot pork skins into another huge bowl with salt and Italian flavoring.
3. Separate cauliflower combination into four equivalent segments and structure each into a ball. Cautiously plunge a ball into whisked egg, at that point move in pork skins. Rehash with residual balls.
4. Spot cauliflower balls into ungreased air fryer crate. Change the temperature to 400°F and set the clock for 8 minutes. Rice balls will be brilliant when done.
5. Utilize a spatula to painstakingly move cauliflower balls to a huge dish for serving. Serve warm.

Per serving Calories: 158
Protein: 15g fiber: 2g net starches: 2g
Fat: 9g sodium: 509mg
Starches: 4g sugar: 2g

MESSY STACKED BROCCOLI

This dish is a top pick of children and grown-ups the same. It tastes like the fixing of a stacked prepared potato; with the very most awesome things—like cheddar and bacon—nobody will even miss the potato!

Pantry Staples: Salt, coconut oil
Hands On schedule: 10 minutes
Cook Time: 10 minutes
Serves: 2
- 3 cups new broccoli florets
- 1 tablespoon coconut oil
- ¼ teaspoon salt
- ½ cup destroyed sharp cheddar
- ¼ cup sharp cream
- 4 cuts cooked without sugar bacon, disintegrated
- 1 medium scallion, managed and cut on the predisposition

1. Spot broccoli into ungreased air fryer bushel, shower with coconut oil, and sprinkle with salt. Change the temperature to 350°F and set the clock for 8 minutes. Shake crate multiple times during cooking to stay away from consumed spots.
2. At the point when clock signals, sprinkle broccoli with Cheddar and set the clock for 2 extra minutes. When done, cheddar will be liquefied and broccoli will be delicate.
3. Serve warm in an enormous serving dish, finished off with harsh cream, disintegrated bacon, and scallion cuts.

Per serving Calories: 381 protein: 19g
Fiber: 4g net starches: 7g fat: 27g sodium: 917mg
starches: 11g sugar: 3g

RICH MUSHROOMS

This basic side packs as much flavor as it does medical advantages, including Nutrient D. These delicate, rich mushrooms make the ideal side dish to any of your most loved keto entrées.

Pantry Staples: Salt, ground dark pepper
Hands On schedule: 10 minutes
Cook Time: 10 minutes
Serves: 4
- 8 ounces cremini mushrooms, split
- 2 tablespoons salted spread, liquefied
- ¼ teaspoon salt
- ¼ teaspoon ground dark pepper

1. In a medium bowl, throw mushrooms with spread, at that point sprinkle with salt and pepper. Spot into ungreased air fryer bin.
2. Change the temperature to 400°F and set the clock for 10 minutes, shaking the bin part of the way through cooking. Mushrooms will be delicate when done. Serve warm.

Per serving Calories: 63
Protein: 1g fiber: 0g net starches: 3g
Fat: 5g sodium: 194mg starches: 3g
Sugar: 1g

"FALSE TATO" HASH

Crude radishes are regularly utilized in **Servings** of mixed greens for a light crunch, yet when cooked they take on a totally different flavor that is marginally peppery. This formula is the ideal expansion to any feast one may regularly combine with potatoes. You can likewise add your most loved go-to vegetable flavoring mix for considerably more flavor.

Pantry Staples: ground dark pepper, garlic powder
Hands On schedule: 10 minutes
Cook Time: 12 minutes
Serves: 4
- 1 pound radishes, closes eliminated, quartered
- ¼ medium yellow onion, stripped and diced
- ½ medium green chime pepper, cultivated and cleaved
- 2 tablespoons salted spread, liquefied
- ½ teaspoon garlic powder
- ¼ teaspoon ground dark pepper

1. In a huge bowl, join radishes, onion, and chime pepper. Throw with margarine.

2. Sprinkle garlic powder and dark pepper over blend in bowl, at that point spoon into ungreased air fryer bin.
3. Change the temperature to 320°F and set the clock for 12 minutes. Shake bin partially through cooking. Radishes will be delicate when done. Serve warm.

Per serving Calories: 69 protein: 1g
fiber: 2g net carbs: 2g fat: 5g
sodium: 73mg carbs: 4g sugar: 2g

MEDITERRANEAN ZUCCHINI BOATS

This dish exploits the flexible kind of zucchini, giving it a Greek-propelled wind. Take a stab at adding 2 tablespoons hacked kalamata olives to your filling for a wonderful explosion of tart flavor.

Pantry Staples: Salt
Hands On schedule: 5 minutes
Cook Time: 10 minutes
Serves: 4
- 1 enormous zucchini, closes eliminated, divided the long way
- 6 grape tomatoes, quartered
- ¼ teaspoon salt
- ¼ cup feta cheddar
- 1 tablespoon balsamic vinegar
- 1 tablespoon olive oil

1. Utilize a spoon to scoop out 2 tablespoons from focus of every zucchini half, making barely adequate room to load up with tomatoes and feta.
2. Spot tomatoes equitably in focuses of zucchini parts and sprinkle with salt. Spot into ungreased air fryer container. Change the temperature to 350°F and set the clock for 10 minutes. When done, zucchini will be delicate.
3. Move boats to a serving plate and sprinkle with feta, at that point shower with vinegar and olive oil. Serve warm.

Per serving Calories: 74
Protein: 2g fiber: 1g net carbs: 3g fat: 5g
Sodium: 238mg carbs: 4g sugar: 3g

BROILED BROCCOLI SALAD

This formula stops any discernments that broccoli is exhausting! Overflowing with exquisite flavors, a tad of tang, and the perfect measure of crunch, this serving of mixed greens is the ideal supplement to any supper.

Pantry Staples: Salt, ground dark pepper
Hands On schedule: 5 minutes
Cook Time: 7 minutes
Serves: 4

- 2 cups new broccoli florets, hacked
- 1 tablespoon olive oil
- ¼ teaspoon salt
- ⅛ teaspoon ground dark pepper
- ¼ cup lemon juice, partitioned
- ¼ cup destroyed Parmesan cheddar
- ¼ cup cut cooked almonds

1. In an enormous bowl, throw broccoli and olive oil together. Sprinkle with salt and pepper, at that point shower with 2 tablespoons lemon juice.
2. Spot broccoli into ungreased air fryer crate. Change the temperature to 350°F and set the clock for 7 minutes, shaking the container partially through cooking. Broccoli will be brilliant on the edges when done.
3. Spot broccoli into an enormous serving bowl and shower with outstanding lemon juice. Sprinkle with Parmesan and almonds. Serve warm.

Per serving Calories: 102 protein: 4g
Fiber: 2g net sugars: 4g Fat: 7g sodium: 245mg
sugars: 6g sugar: 1g

BACON-JALAPEÑO MESSY "BREADSTICKS"

The astounding taste of this formula could trick any carb darling! It's just about as simple as it appears, and surprisingly more flavorful. To make this an entrée, essentially add your number one pizza

Fixings , like cooked disintegrated sausage.
Pantry Staples: None
Hands On schedule: 10 minutes
Cook Time: 15 minutes
Yields 8 sticks

- 2 cups destroyed mozzarella cheddar
- ¼ cup ground Parmesan cheddar
- ¼ cup cleaved salted jalapeños
- 2 huge eggs, whisked
- 4 cuts cooked without sugar bacon, cleaved

1. Combine all Fixings as one in a huge bowl. Cut a piece of material paper to fit inside air fryer bin.
2. Hose your hands with a touch of water and press out blend into a circle to fit on ungreased material. You may have to isolate into two more modest circles, contingent upon the size of air fryer.
3. Spot material with cheddar blend into air fryer bin. Change the temperature to 320°F and set the clock for 15 minutes. Cautiously flip when 5 minutes stay on clock. The top will be brilliant earthy colored when done. Cut into eight sticks. Serve warm.

Per serving (2 sticks) calories: 275
Protein: 22g fiber: 0g net starches: 5g Fat: 16g
sodium: 783mg starches: 5g Sugar: 1g

SUPPER ROLLS

If you're an aficionado of multigrain moves, this formula is for you. The ground flax helps add a wheat-like flavor to the moves, making them the ideal keto bread substitution. They can likewise be delighted in as slider buns, or utilized with your #1 sandwich garnishes.

Pantry Staples: Preparing powder
Hands On schedule: 10 minutes
Cook Time: 12 minutes
Serves: 6

- 1 cup destroyed mozzarella cheddar
- 1 ounce cream cheddar, broken into little pieces
- 1 cup whitened finely ground almond flour
- ¼ cup ground flaxseed
- ½ teaspoon heating powder
- 1 enormous egg, whisked

1. Spot mozzarella, cream cheddar, and flour in an enormous microwave-safe bowl. Microwave on high 1 moment. Blend until smooth.
2. Add flaxseed, heating powder, and egg to combination until completely consolidated and smooth. Microwave an extra 15 seconds if mixture turns out to be excessively firm.
3. Separate batter into six equivalent pieces and fold each into a ball. Spot folds into ungreased air fryer container. Change the temperature to 320°F and set the clock for 12 minutes, turning rolls partially through cooking. Permit moves to cool totally prior to serving, around 5 minutes.

Per serving **Calories**: 235 protein: 11g
Fiber: 4g net starches: 3g fat: 18g
Sodium: 199mg starches: 7g sugar: 1g

PARMESAN SPICE RADISHES

While most root vegetables have an excessive number of carbs to handily find a way into a ketogenic diet, radishes have just around 2 grams of net carbs per cup. When cooked, radishes take on a slight peppery flavor and have a delicate chomp that fills in as a pleasant surface option in contrast to potatoes.

Pantry Staples: ground dark pepper, garlic powder
Hands On schedule: 10 minutes
Cook Time: 10 minutes
Serves: 6

- 1 pound radishes, closes eliminated, quartered
- 2 tablespoons salted spread, dissolved
- ½ teaspoon garlic powder
- ½ teaspoon dried parsley
- ¼ teaspoon dried oregano
- ¼ teaspoon ground dark pepper
- ¼ cup ground Parmesan cheddar

1. Spot radishes into a medium bowl and shower with spread. Sprinkle with garlic powder, parsley, oregano, and pepper, at that point place into ungreased air fryer crate.
2. Change the temperature to 350°F and set the clock for 10 minutes, shaking the crate multiple times during cooking. Radishes will be done when delicate and brilliant.
3. Spot radishes into a huge serving dish and sprinkle with Parmesan. Serve warm.

Per serving Calories: 59 protein: 2g
Fiber: 1g net starches: 2g fat: 5g
Sodium: 124mg starches: 3g sugar: 1g

FIRM GREEN BEANS

The air fryer permits green beans to hold more nutrients and flavor, rather than bubbling, which eliminates a ton of the supplements and can make the green beans taste watery. This dish tastes extraordinary with an additional shower of margarine, or joined by Caesar salad dressing for plunging.

Pantry Staples: Salt, ground dark pepper
Hands On schedule: 5 minutes

Cook Time: 8 minutes
Serves: 4

- 2 teaspoons olive oil
- ½ pound new green beans, closes managed
- ¼ teaspoon salt
- ¼ teaspoon ground dark pepper

1. In an enormous bowl, shower olive oil over green beans and sprinkle with salt and pepper.
2. Spot green beans into ungreased air fryer crate. Change the temperature to 350°F and set the clock for 8 minutes, shaking the crate multiple times during cooking. Green beans will be dull brilliant and firm at the edges when done. Serve warm.

Per serving Calories: 37 protein: 1g Fiber: 2g net carbs: 2g fat: 2g Sodium: 148mg carbs: 4g sugar: 2g

FLATBREAD SCOOPS

If you're getting a charge out of a rich soup or plunge, the ideal side dish is a crunchy scoop to help you relish each and every nibble. These Flatbread Scoops are like a slim level bread and have a gentle flavor that will not overwhelm your entrée. Also, with only three Fixings , you can get them ready in under 15 minutes!

Pantry Staples: None
Hands On schedule: 5 minutes
Cook Time: 8 minutes
Yields 12 triangles

- 1 cup destroyed mozzarella cheddar
- 1 ounce cream cheddar, broken into little pieces
- ½ cup whitened finely ground almond flour

1. Spot mozzarella into an enormous microwave-safe bowl. Add cream cheddar pieces. Microwave on high 60 seconds, at that point mix to consolidate. Add flour and mix until a delicate bundle of mixture structures.
2. Cut batter ball into two equivalent pieces. Slice a piece of material to find a way into air fryer container. Press every batter piece into a 5" round on ungreased material.
3. Spot material with mixture into air fryer bin. Change the temperature to 350°F and set the clock for 8 minutes. Cautiously flip the flatbread over partially through cooking. Flatbread will be brilliant earthy colored when done.
4. Allow flatbread to cool 5 minutes, at that point cut each round into six triangles. Serve warm.

Per serving (3 triangles)

Calories: 194 protein: 10g fiber: 2g
Net starches: 2g fat: 15g sodium: 218mg
Starches: 4g sugar: 1g

LITTLE SPINACH AND SWEET PEPPER POPPERS

These are a superb option to jalapeño poppers, particularly if zesty isn't your thing. They're slightly sweet yet pack a major crunch that sets consummately with the velvety garlic filling. The spinach is a simple method to get in your salad greens, however go ahead and preclude if you like.

Pantry Staples: Garlic powder
Hands On schedule: 10 minutes
Cook Time: 8 minutes
Yields 16 poppers
- 4 ounces cream cheddar, mellowed
- 1 cup cleaved new spinach leaves
- ½ teaspoon garlic powder
- 8 smaller than expected sweet ringer peppers, tops eliminated, cultivated, and divided longwise

1. In a medium bowl, blend cream cheddar, spinach, and garlic powder. Spot 1 tablespoon combination into every sweet pepper half and press down to smooth.
2. Spot poppers into ungreased air fryer bushel. Change the temperature to 400°F and set the clock for 8 minutes. Poppers will be done when cheddar is carmelized on top and peppers are delicate fresh. Serve warm.

Per serving (4 poppers)
Calories: 116 Protein: 3g fiber: 1g net carbs: 4g Fat: 8g sodium: 109mg carbs: 5g Sugar: 3g

COOKED BRUSSELS FLEDGLINGS

At the point when you broil vegetables, it draws out their characteristic pleasantness—and that is the same for Brussels sprouts. This simple dish meets up in only a couple minutes, and the caramelized, fresh edges of the leaves and delicate internal parts will make this a staple side to any protein.

Pantry Staples: Salt, ground dark pepper, garlic powder, coconut oil
Hands On schedule: 5 minutes
Cook Time: 10 minutes
Serves: 6
- 1 pound new Brussels grows, managed and divided
- 2 tablespoons coconut oil
- ½ teaspoon salt
- ¼ teaspoon ground dark pepper
- ½ teaspoon garlic powder
- 1 tablespoon salted margarine, liquefied

1. Spot Brussels sprouts into an enormous bowl. Shower with coconut oil and sprinkle with salt, pepper, and garlic powder.
2. Spot Brussels sprouts into ungreased air fryer bushel. Change the temperature to 350°F and set the clock for 10 minutes, shaking the crate multiple times during cooking. Brussels fledglings will be dull brilliant and delicate when done.
3. Spot cooked fledglings in a huge serving dish and sprinkle with margarine. Serve warm.

Per serving
Calories: 89 protein: 3g fiber: 3g Net carbs: 4g fat: 6g sodium: 227mg Carbs: 7g sugar: 2g

BROILED SALSA

Air fryers are an incredible method to prepare a supper without warming up your living region (like a traditional broiler frequently does). During the hotter months, when tomatoes are in season, this salsa makes a particularly tasty fixing to chicken thighs, taco bowls, or eggs.

Pantry Staples: Salt, coconut oil
Hands On schedule: 5 minutes
Cook Time: 30 minutes
Yields 2 cups
- 2 huge San Marzano tomatoes, cored and cut into enormous lumps
- ½ medium white onion, stripped and huge diced
- ½ medium jalapeño, cultivated and huge diced
- 2 cloves garlic, stripped and diced
- ½ teaspoon salt
- 1 tablespoon coconut oil
- ¼ cup new lime juice

1. Spot tomatoes, onion, and jalapeño into an ungreased 6" round nonstick preparing dish. Add garlic, at that point sprinkle with salt and shower with coconut oil.
2. Spot dish into air fryer crate. Change the temperature to 300°F and set the clock for 30

minutes. Vegetables will be dim earthy colored around the edges and delicate when done.

3. Empty combination into a food processor or blender. Add lime juice. Interaction on low speed 30 seconds until a couple of lumps remain.

4. Move salsa to a sealable compartment and refrigerate in any event 60 minutes. Serve chilled.

Per serving (¼ cup)
Calories: 28 protein: 1g
Fiber: 1g net carbs: 2g fat: 2g
Sodium: 148mg carbs: 3g sugar: 2g

Chicken is probably already one of the most commonly eaten meats in your household. It's hard to compete with its affordability and convenience, plus chicken is an excellent source of protein, and it can be a great source of fat too! The problem? Chicken can get a little boring. Luckily, this chapter is full of healthy and exciting ideas that will bring a whole new light to dinnertime. From Crispy Buffalo Chicken Tenders to Chicken Pizza Crust, you'll have no shortage of amazing meals to add to your weekly rotation!

CRISPY BUFFALO CHICKEN TENDERS

Your days of delicious crispy chicken aren't over just because you don't eat traditional breading! This recipe replaces the carb- filled, heavy wheat flour or bread crumbs you might be used to with an amazing zero-carb substitute: pork rinds! Serve these with ranch dressing or your favorite dipping sauce.

HandsOn Time: 15 minutes
Cook Time: 20 minutes
Serves 4

- 1 pound boneless, skinless chicken tenders
- 1/4 cup hot sauce 1
- 1/2 ounces pork rinds, finely ground
- 1 teaspoon chili powder
- 1 teaspoon garlic powder

Directions

- ✓ Place chicken tenders in large bowl and pour hot sauce over them. Toss tenders in hot sauce, evenly coating.
- ✓ In a separate large bowl, mix ground pork rinds with chili powder and garlic powder.
- ✓ Place each tender in the ground pork rinds, covering completely. Wet your hands with water and press down the pork rinds into the chicken.
- ✓ Place the tenders in a single layer into the air fryer basket.
- ✓ Adjust the temperature to 375°F and set the timer for 20 minutes.
- ✓ Serve warm.

Per serving
Calories: 160
Protein: 27.3 g fiber: 0.4 g
Net carbohydrates: 0.6 g fat: 4.4 g
Sodium: 387 mg carbohydrates: 1.0 g sugar: 0.1 g

TERIYAKI WINGS

These marinated wings are dripping with finger-licking flavor and are supereasy to prepare! The garlic and ginger give this recipe a bit of a kick while the teriyaki sauce adds some salt to bring out the wings' natural flavors. Before air frying, you toss the wings in baking powder for extra crispy skin rivaling traditional breaded wings!

HandsOn Time: 1 hour
Cook Time: 25 minutes
Serves 4

- 2 pounds chicken wings
- 1/2 cup sugar-free teriyaki sauce
- 2 teaspoons minced garlic
- 1/4 teaspoon ground ginger
- 2 teaspoons baking powder

Directions

- ✓ Place all ingredients except baking powder into a large bowl or bag and let marinade for 1 hour in the refrigerator.
- ✓ Place wings into the air fryer basket and sprinkle with baking powder. Gently rub into wings.
- ✓ Adjust the temperature to 400°F and set the timer for 25 minutes.
- ✓ Toss the basket two or three times during cooking.
- ✓ Wings should be crispy and cooked to at least 165°F internally when done. Serve immediately.

Per serving
Calories: 446 protein: 41.8 g fiber: 0.1 g
Net carbohydrates: 3.1 g fat: 29.8 g
Sodium: 1,034 mg carbohydrates: 3.2 g sugar: 0.0 g

LEMON THYME ROASTED CHICKEN

Who knew you could perfectly roast an entire chicken in your air fryer? In less time, and with more even convection cooking than a standard oven, it'll be tough to go back to your old way!

HandsOn Time: 10 minutes
Cook Time: 60 minutes
Serves 6

- 1 (4-pound) chicken
- 2 teaspoons dried thyme
- 1 teaspoon garlic powder
- 1/2 teaspoon onion powder

- 2 teaspoons dried parsley
- 1 teaspoon baking powder
- 1 medium lemon
- 2 tablespoons salted butter, melted

Directions

- ✓ Rub chicken with thyme, garlic powder, onion powder, parsley, and baking powder.
- ✓ Slice lemon and place four slices on top of chicken, breast side up, and secure with toothpicks. Place remaining slices inside of the chicken.
- ✓ Place entire chicken into the air fryer basket, breast side down.
- ✓ Adjust the temperature to 350°F and set the timer for 60 minutes.
- ✓ After 30 minutes, flip chicken so breast side is up.
- ✓ When done, internal temperature should be 165°F and the skin golden and crispy. To serve, pour melted butter over entire chicken.

Per serving

Calories: 504 protein: 32.0 g fiber: 0.3 g
Net carbohydrates: 1.1 g fat: 36.8 g sodium: 240 mg
Carbohydrates: 1.4 g sugar: 0.2 g

CILANTRO LIME CHICKEN THIGHS

Chicken thighs are a more affordable and fattier cut of chicken compared to chicken breasts—perfect for anyone following the keto diet! Along with the fat comes succulent flavor bursting through the skin. Paired with cilantro lime seasoning, this recipe is perfection.

HandsOn Time: 15 minutes
Cook Time: 22 minutes
Serves: 4

4 bone-in, skin-on chicken thighs
- 1 teaspoon baking powder
- 1/2 teaspoon garlic powder
- 2 teaspoons chili powder
- 1 teaspoon cumin
- 2 medium limes
- 1/4 cup chopped fresh cilantro

Directions

- ✓ Pat chicken thighs dry and sprinkle with baking powder.
- ✓ In a small bowl, mix garlic powder, chili powder, and cumin and sprinkle evenly over thighs, gently rubbing on and under chicken skin.
- ✓ Cut one lime in half and squeeze juice over thighs. Place chicken into the air fryer basket.

- ✓ Adjust the temperature to 380°F and set the timer for 22 minutes.
- ✓ Cut other lime into four wedges for serving and garnish cooked chicken with wedges and cilantro.

Per serving

Calories: 435 protein: 32.3 g fiber: 0.6 g
Net carbohydrates: 2.0 g fat: 29.1 g sodium: 317 mg
Carbohydrates: 2.6 g sugar: 0.3 g

LEMON PEPPER DRUMSTICKS

Lemon pepper is a popular coating for keto-friendly chicken because it's a simple, savory, dry-rub seasoning with no reason to add unnecessary carbs. When you crisp these drumsticks in your air fryer, that seasoning soaks into the chicken skin, giving each bite a zesty flair!

HandsOn Time: 5 minutes
Cook Time: 25 minutes
Yields 8 drumsticks (2 per serving)
- 2 teaspoons baking powder
- 2 teaspoon garlic powder
- 8 chicken drumsticks
- 4 tablespoons salted butter, melted
- 1 tablespoon lemon pepper seasoning

Directions

- ✓ Sprinkle baking powder and garlic powder over drumsticks and rub into chicken skin. Place drumsticks into the air fryer basket.
- ✓ Adjust the temperature to 375°F and set the timer for 25 minutes.
- ✓ Use tongs to turn drumsticks halfway through the cooking time.
- ✓ When skin is golden and internal temperature is at least 165°F, remove from fryer.
- ✓ In a large bowl, mix butter and lemon pepper seasoning. Add drumsticks to the bowl and toss until coated. Serve warm.

Per serving

Calories: 532 protein: 48.3 g fiber: 0.0 g
Net carbohydrates: 1.2 g fat: 32.3 g sodium: 706 mg
Carbohydrates: 1.2 g sugar: 0.0 g

FAJITA-STUFFED CHICKEN BREAST

This dish is so good you won't even miss the tortilla! The smoky spices create a flavorful crust on the chicken while the veggies brighten up your meal. For a cheesy twist, sprinkle a half cup of shredded Monterey jack cheese on top of the chicken rolls before baking.

HandsOn Time: 15 minutes
Cook Time: 25 minutes
Serves 4

- 2 (6-ounce) boneless, skinless chicken breasts
- 1/4 medium white onion, peeled and sliced
- 1 medium green bell pepper, seeded and sliced
- 1 tablespoon coconut oil
- 2 teaspoons chili powder
- 1 teaspoon ground cumin
- 1/2 teaspoon garlic powder

Directions

- ✓ Slice each chicken breast completely in half lengthwise into two even pieces. Using a meat tenderizer, pound out the chicken until it's about V4" thickness.
- ✓ Lay each slice of chicken out and place three slices of onion and four slices of green pepper on the end closest to you. Begin rolling the peppers and onions tightly into the chicken. Secure the roll with either toothpicks or a couple pieces of butcher's twine.
- ✓ Drizzle coconut oil over chicken. Sprinkle each side with chili powder, cumin, and garlic powder. Place each roll into the air fryer basket.
- ✓ Adjust the temperature to 350°F and set the timer for 25 minutes.
- ✓ Serve warm.

Per serving
Calories: 146
Protein: 19.8 g fiber: 1.2 g
Net carbohydrates: 2.0 g fat: 4.9 g Sodium: 78 mg
Carbohydrates: 3.2 g sugar: 1.1 g

<u>CHICKEN PARMESAN</u>

Chicken Parmesan is a popular Italian dish that is usually made with breaded chicken covered in tomato sauce and cheese, served over spaghetti. This recipe cuts not only the carbs from the breading but also the unnecessary sugar that is used in most tomato sauces.
HandsOn Time: 10 minutes
Cook Time: 25 minutes
Serves 4

- 2 (6-ounce) boneless, skinless chicken breasts
- 1/2 teaspoon garlic powder
- 1/4 teaspoon dried oregano
- 1/2 teaspoon dried parsley
- 4 tablespoons full-fat mayonnaise, divided
- 1 cup shredded mozzarella cheese, divided
- 1 ounce pork rinds, crushed
- 1/2 cup grated Parmesan cheese, divided
- 1 cup low-carb, no-sugar- added pasta sauce

Directions

- ✓ Slice each chicken breast in half lengthwise and pound out to 3/4" thickness. Sprinkle with garlic powder, oregano, and parsley.
- ✓ Spread 1 tablespoon mayonnaise on top of each piece of chicken, then sprinkle V4 cup mozzarella on each piece.
- ✓ In a small bowl, mix the crushed pork rinds and Parmesan. Sprinkle the mixture on top of mozzarella.
- ✓ Pour sauce into 6" round baking pan and place chicken on top. Place pan into the air fryer basket.
- ✓ Adjust the temperature to 320°F and set the timer for 25 minutes.
- ✓ Cheese will be browned and internal temperature of the chicken will be at least 165°F when fully cooked. Serve warm.

Per serving
Calories: 393 protein: 34.2 g fiber: 2.1 g
Net carbohydrates: 4.7 g fat: 22.8 g sodium: 983 mg
carbohydrates: 6.8 g sugar: 2.4 g

<u>CHICKEN CORDON BLEU CASSEROLE</u>

This ultra creamy casserole gives you all the flavors of traditional cordon bleu without the carbs! Crushed pork rinds give this dish a crunchy topping. Don't worry if you aren't a fan of pork rinds; you can use crushed pure cheese crisps! Just be sure there's no added flours in the crisps.
HandsOn Time: 15 minutes
Cook Time: 15 minutes
Serves 4

- 2 cups cubed cooked chicken thigh meat
- 1/2 cup cubed cooked ham
- 2 ounces Swiss cheese, cubed
- 4 ounces full-fat cream cheese, softened
- 1 tablespoon heavy cream
- 2 tablespoons unsalted butter, melted
- 2 teaspoons Dijon mustard
- 1 ounce pork rinds, crushed

Directions

- ✓ Place chicken and ham into a 6" round baking pan and toss so meat is evenly mixed. Sprinkle cheese cubes on top of meat.
- ✓ In a large bowl, mix cream cheese, heavy cream, butter, and mustard and then pour the mixture over the meat and cheese. Top with pork rinds. Place pan into the air fryer basket.

✓ Adjust the temperature to 350°F and set the timer for 15 minutes.
✓ The casserole will be browned and bubbling when done. Serve warm.

Per serving
Calories: 403 protein: 30.7 g fiber: 0.0 g
Net carbohydrates: 2.3 g fat: 28.2 g sodium: 660 mg
Carbohydrates: 2.3 g sugar: 1.2 g

JALAPENO POPPER HASSELBACK CHICKEN

This easy entree has plenty of jalapeno spice, but it's complemented by the cream cheese that also keeps the chicken moist and juicy. If you like jalapeno poppers, you'll love this upgraded version!
HandsOn Time: 20 minutes
Cook Time: 20 minutes
Serves 2

- 4 slices sugar-free bacon, cooked and crumbled
- 2 ounces full-fat cream cheese, softened
- 2 cup shredded sharp Cheddar cheese, divided
- 4 cup sliced pickled jalapenos
- 2 (6-ounce) boneless, skinless chicken breasts

Directions
✓ In a medium bowl, place cooked bacon, then fold in cream cheese, half of the Cheddar, and the jalapeno slices.
✓ Use a sharp knife to make slits in each of the chicken breasts about 3/4 of the way across the chicken, being careful not to cut all the way through. Depending on the size of the chicken breast, you'll likely have 6-8 slits per breast.
✓ Spoon the cream cheese mixture into the slits of the chicken. Sprinkle remaining shredded cheese over chicken breasts and place into the air fryer basket.
✓ Adjust the temperature to 350°F and set the timer for 20 minutes.
✓ Serve warm.

Per serving
Calories: 501 protein: 53.8 g fiber: 0.2 g
Net carbohydrates: 1.4 g fat: 25.3 g sodium: 860 mg
Carbohydrates: 1.6 g sugar: 1.0 g

CHICKEN ENCHILADAS

One great way to make smart swaps in keto recipes is to completely replace an optional high-carb ingredient with a low- carb ingredient that is a major part of the recipe. In this case we're swapping out tortillas for deli chicken so we can still get the full effect without any of the added carbs!
HandsOn Time: 20 minutes
Cook Time: 10 minutes
Serves 4

- 11/2 cups shredded cooked chicken
- 1/3 cup low-carb enchilada sauce, divided
- 1/2 pound medium-sliced deli chicken
- 1 cup shredded medium Cheddar cheese
- 1/2 cup shredded Monterey jack cheese
- 1/2 cup full-fat sour cream 1 medium avocado, peeled, pitted, and sliced

Directions
✓ In a large bowl, mix shredded chicken and half of the enchilada sauce. Lay slices of deli chicken on a work surface and spoon 2 tablespoons shredded chicken mixture onto each slice.
✓ Sprinkle 2 tablespoons of Cheddar onto each roll. Gently roll closed.
✓ In a 4-cup round baking dish, place each roll, seam side down. Pour remaining sauce over rolls and top with Monterey jack. Place dish into the air fryer basket.
✓ Adjust the temperature to 370°F and set the timer for 10 minutes.
✓ Enchiladas will be golden on top and bubbling when cooked. Serve warm with sour cream and sliced avocado.

Per serving
Calories: 416 protein: 34.2 g fiber: 2.3 g
Net carbohydrates: 4.2 g fat: 25.2 g sodium: 1,081 mg carbohydrates: 6.5 g sugar: 1.1 g

CHICKEN PIZZA CRUST

Using chicken as a pizza crust is a great way to replace carbs with protein! This highly customizable recipe can satisfy your pizza cravings while helping to keep your muscles strong. Even better, it crisps up so well in your air fryer that you can even pick it up just like a traditional slice!
HandsOn Time: 10 minutes
Cook Time: 25 minutes
Serves: 4

- 1 pound ground chicken thigh meat
- 1/4 cup grated Parmesan cheese
- 1/2 cup shredded mozzarella

Directions

- ✓ In a large bowl, mix all ingredients. Separate into four even parts.
- ✓ Cut out four (6") circles of parchment and press each portion of the chicken mixture out onto one of the circles. Place into the air fryer basket, working in batches as needed.
- ✓ Adjust the temperature to 375°F and set the timer for 25 minutes.
- ✓ Flip the crust halfway through the cooking time.
- ✓ Once fully cooked, you may top it with cheese and your favorite toppings and cook 5 additional minutes. Or, you may place crust into refrigerator or freezer and top when ready to eat.

Per serving

Calories: 230 Protein: 24.7 g fiber: 0.0 g
Net carbohydrates: 1.2 g fat: 12.8 g Sodium: 268 mg
carbohydrates: 1.2 g sugar: 0.2 g

BLACKENED CAJUN CHICKEN TENDERS

Blackening meat is a technique used to maximize flavor without needing to add any breading. The secret to this chicken is all of the delicious spices that will have you salivating while it cooks!

HandsOn Time: 10 minutes
Cook Time: 17 minutes
Serves 4

- 2 teaspoons paprika
- 1 teaspoon chili powder
- 1/2 teaspoon garlic powder
- 1/2 teaspoon dried thyme
- 1/4 teaspoon onion powder
- 1/8 teaspoon ground cayenne pepper
- 2 tablespoons coconut oil
- 1 pound boneless, skinless chicken tenders
- 1/4 cup full-fat ranch dressing

Directions

- ✓ In a small bowl, combine all seasonings.
- ✓ Drizzle oil over chicken tenders and then generously coat each tender in the spice mixture. Place tenders into the air fryer basket.
- ✓ Adjust the temperature to 375°F and set the timer for 17 minutes.
- ✓ Tenders will be 165°F internally when fully cooked. Serve with ranch dressing for dipping.

Per serving

Calories: 163 protein: 21.2 g fiber: 0.8 g
Net carbohydrates: 0.7 g fat: 7.5 g sodium: 132 mg
Carbohydrates: 1.5 g sugar: 0.2 g

SPINACH AND FETA STUFFED CHICKEN BREAST

Stuffing chicken is one of the easiest ways to elevate it. If you need to take your protein to the next level, this recipe is a great creamy and nutritious way to do just that! It comes out deliciously golden brown with hot, gooey, bubbly cheese.

HandsOn Time: 15 minutes
Cook Time: 25 minutes
Serves 2

- 1 tablespoon unsalted butter
- 5 ounces frozen spinach, thawed and drained
- 1/2 teaspoon garlic powder, divided
- 1/2 teaspoon salt, divided
- 1/4 cup chopped yellow onion
- 1/4 cup crumbled feta 2 (6-ounce) boneless, skinless chicken breasts
- 1 tablespoon coconut oil

Directions

- ✓ In a medium skillet over medium heat, add butter to the pan and saute spinach 3 minutes. Sprinkle V4 teaspoon garlic powder and V4 teaspoon salt onto spinach and add onion to the pan.
- ✓ Continue sauteing 3 more minutes, then remove from heat and place in medium bowl. Fold feta into spinach mixture.
- ✓ Slice a roughly 4" slit into the side of each chicken breast, lengthwise. Spoon half of the mixture into each piece and secure closed with a couple toothpicks. Sprinkle outside of chicken with remaining garlic powder and salt. Drizzle with coconut oil. Place chicken breasts into the air fryer basket.
- ✓ Adjust the temperature to 350°F and set the timer for 25 minutes.
- ✓ When completely cooked chicken should be golden brown and have an internal temperature of at least 165°F. Slice and serve warm.

Per serving

Calories: 393 Protein: 43.9 G
Fiber: 2.5 G Net Carbohydrates: 3.7 G Fat: 18.5 G
Sodium: 882 Mg Carbohydrates: 6.2 G Sugar: 2.1 G

SOUTHERN "FRIED" CHICKEN

An audible crunch, a juicy middle, and an overflow of flavor are all characteristics of the perfect bite of fried chicken. You'll get all the classic feel you're used to in this favorite without the carbs or the frying oil.
HandsOn Time: 15 minutes
Cook Time: 25 minutes
Serves 4

- 2 (6-ounce) boneless, skinless chicken breasts
- 2 tablespoons hot sauce
- 1 tablespoon chili powder
- 1/2 teaspoon cumin
- 1/4 teaspoon onion powder
- 1/4 teaspoon ground black pepper
- 2 ounces pork rinds, finely ground

Directions

- ✓ Slice each chicken breast in half lengthwise. Place the chicken into a large bowl and coat with hot sauce.
- ✓ In a small bowl, mix chili powder, cumin, onion powder, and pepper. Sprinkle over chicken.
- ✓ Place the ground pork rinds into a large bowl and dip each piece of chicken into the bowl, coating as much as possible. Place chicken into the air fryer basket.
- ✓ Adjust the temperature to 350°F and set the timer for 25 minutes.
- ✓ Halfway through the cooking time, carefully flip the chicken.
- ✓ When done, internal temperature will be at least 165°F and pork rind coating will be dark golden brown. Serve warm.

Per serving
Calories: 192 Protein: 27.8 G Fiber: 0.9 G
Net Carbohydrates: 0.7 G Fat: 6.9 G Sodium: 374 Mg
Carbohydrates: 1.6 G Sugar: 0.2 G

ALMOND-CRUSTED CHICKEN

This chicken comes with a nutty crunch because it's "breaded" with almonds. Not only are almonds a low-carb nut, they are also a fatty, filling food that helps support healthy brain function.
HandsOn Time: 15 minutes
Cook Time: 25 minutes
Serves 4

- 1/4 cup slivered almonds
- 2 (6-ounce) boneless, skinless chicken breasts
- 2 tablespoons full-fat mayonnaise
- 1 tablespoon Dijon mustard

Directions

- ✓ Pulse the almonds in a food processor or chop until finely chopped. Place almonds evenly on a plate and set aside.
- ✓ Completely slice each chicken breast in half lengthwise.
- ✓ Mix the mayonnaise and mustard in a small bowl and then coat chicken with the mixture.
- ✓ Lay each piece of chicken in the chopped almonds to fully coat. Carefully move the pieces into the air fryer basket.
- ✓ Adjust the temperature to 350°F and set the timer for 25 minutes.
- ✓ Chicken will be done when it has reached an internal temperature of 165°F or more. Serve warm.

Per serving
Calories: 195 protein: 20.9 g fiber: 0.8 g
Net carbohydrates: 1.0 g fat: 10.1 g sodium: 175 mg
Carbohydrates: 1.8 g sugar: 0.3 g

PEPPERONI AND CHICKEN PIZZA BAKE

This is a great way to have "pizza" for dinner while piling on the protein! Who could argue with a meal so tasty? This dish will definitely satisfy the whole family while helping to keep everyone's muscles strong!
HandsOn Time: 10 minutes
Cook Time: 15 minutes
Serves 4

- 2 cups cubed cooked chicken
- 20 slices pepperoni
- 1 cup low-carb, sugar-free pizza sauce
- 1 cup shredded mozzarella cheese
- 1/4 cup grated Parmesan cheese

Directions

- ✓ In a 4-cup round baking dish add chicken, pepperoni, and pizza sauce. Stir so meat is completely covered with sauce.
- ✓ Top with mozzarella and grated Parmesan. Place dish into the air fryer basket.
- ✓ Adjust the temperature to 375°F and set the timer for 15 minutes.
- ✓ Dish will be brown and bubbling when cooked. Serve immediately.

Per serving
Calories: 353 Protein: 34.4 G Fiber: 1.0 G
Net Carbohydrates: 6.5 G Fat: 17.4 G
Sodium: 754 Mg Carbohydrates: 7.5 G Sugar: 2.3 G

QUICK CHICKEN FAJITAS

Make all the yummy elements of chicken fajitas at the same time with this air fryer spin on a classic sheet pan meal. Serve these with your favorite toppings such as avocado and sour cream. Be sure to pair them with the Pork Rind Tortillas (Chapter 3) for the full effect!

HandsOn Time: 10 minutes
Cook Time: 15 minutes
Serves 2

- 10 ounces boneless, skinless chicken breast, sliced into 1/4" strips 2 tablespoons coconut oil, melted 1 tablespoon chili powder 1/2 teaspoon cumin 1/2 teaspoon paprika 1/2 teaspoon garlic powder 1/4 medium onion, peeled and sliced 1/2 medium green bell pepper, seeded and sliced 1/2 medium red bell pepper, seeded and sliced

Directions

- ✓ Place chicken and coconut oil into a large bowl and sprinkle with chili powder, cumin, paprika, and garlic powder. Toss chicken until well coated with seasoning. Place chicken into the air fryer basket.
- ✓ Adjust the temperature to 350°F and set the timer for 15 minutes.
- ✓ Add onion and peppers into the fryer basket when the timer has 7 minutes remaining.
- ✓ Toss the chicken two or three times during cooking. Vegetables should be tender and chicken fully cooked to at least 165°F internal temperature when finished. Serve warm.

Per serving
Calories: 326 protein: 33.5 g fiber: 3.2 g
Net carbohydrates: 5.2 g fat: 15.9 g sodium: 180 mg
carbohydrates: 8.4 g sugar: 3.2 g

CHICKEN PATTIES

What could be better on a warm summer evening than a juicy burger made from chicken and dredged in crushed pork rinds? This low-carb twist on a classic recipe will leave your whole family satisfied. It's also the perfect meal to prepare ahead of time and freeze for later!

HandsOn Time: 15 minutes
Cook Time: 12 minutes
Serves 4

- 1 pound ground chicken thigh meat
- 1/2 cup shredded mozzarella cheese
- 1 teaspoon dried parsley
- 1/2 teaspoon garlic powder
- 1/4 teaspoon onion powder
- 1 large egg
- 2 ounces pork rinds, finely ground

Directions

- ✓ In a large bowl, mix ground chicken, mozzarella, parsley, garlic powder, and onion powder. Form into four patties.
- ✓ Place patties in the freezer for 15-20 minutes until they begin to firm up.
- ✓ Whisk egg in a medium bowl. Place the ground pork rinds into a large bowl.
- ✓ Dip each chicken patty into the egg and then press into pork rinds to fully coat. Place patties into the air fryer basket.
- ✓ Adjust the temperature to 360°F and set the timer for 12 minutes.
- ✓ Patties will be firm and cooked to an internal temperature of 165°F when done. Serve immediately.

Per serving
Calories: 304 protein: 32.7 g fiber: 0.1 g
Net carbohydrates: 0.8 g fat: 17.4 g sodium: 406 mg
Carbohydrates: 0.9 g sugar: 0.2 g

GREEK CHICKEN STIR-FRY

This speedy stir-fry is perfect for a light lunch. For an even more filling meal, try the stir-fry over a bowl of steamed cauliflower!

HandsOn Time: 15 minutes
Cook Time: 15 minutes
Serves 2

- 1 (6-ounce) chicken breast, cut into 1" cubes
- 1/2 medium zucchini, chopped
- 1/2 medium red bell pepper, seeded and chopped
- 1/4 medium red onion, peeled and sliced
- 1 tablespoon coconut oil
- 1 teaspoon dried oregano
- 1/2 teaspoon garlic powder
- 1/4 teaspoon dried thyme

Directions

- ✓ Place all ingredients into a large mixing bowl and toss until the coconut oil coats the meat and vegetables. Pour the contents of the bowl into the air fryer basket.
- ✓ Adjust the temperature to 375°F and set the timer for 15 minutes.
- ✓ Shake the fryer basket halfway through the cooking time to redistribute the food. Serve immediately.

Per serving
Calories: 186 Protein: 20.4 g Fiber: 1.7 g
Net carbohydrates: 3.9 g fat: 8.0 g Sodium: 43 mg
Carbohydrates: 5.6 g sugar: 3.1 g

CHICKEN, SPINACH, AND FETA BITES

Combining protein-rich chicken with fiber-filled spinach and calcium-fortified feta cheese makes for a very well-rounded low- carb masterpiece!

HandsOn Time: 10 minutes
Cook Time: 12 minutes
Serves 4

- 1 pound ground chicken thigh meat
- 1/3 cup frozen spinach, thawed and drained
- 1/3 cup crumbled feta
- 1/4 teaspoon onion powder
- 1/2 teaspoon garlic powder
- 1/2 ounce pork rinds, finely ground

Directions

- ✓ Mix all ingredients in a large bowl. Roll into 2" balls and place into the air fryer basket, working in batches if needed.
- ✓ Adjust the temperature to 350°F and set the timer for 12 minutes.
- ✓ When done, internal temperature will be 165°F.
- ✓ Serve immediately.

Per serving
Calories: 220 Protein: 24.1 g Fiber: 0.4 g
Net carbohydrates: 1.1 g fat: 12.2 g
Sodium: 250 mg Carbohydrates: 1.5 g sugar: 0.6 g

BUFFALO CHICKEN CHEESE STICKS

Not only are these cheese sticks ridiculously simple, but they're also very filling. You can thank the added protein from the chicken for turning what is traditionally an appetizer into a satisfying meal.

HandsOn Time: 5 minutes
Cook Time: 8 minutes
Serves 2

- 1 cup shredded cooked chicken
- 4 cup buffalo sauce
- 1 cup shredded mozzarella cheese
- 1 large egg
- 4 cup crumbled feta

Directions

- ✓ In a large bowl, mix all ingredients except the feta. Cut a piece of parchment to fit your air fryer basket and press the mixture into a 1/2"-thick circle.
- ✓ Sprinkle the mixture with feta and place into the air fryer basket.
- ✓ Adjust the temperature to 400°F and set the timer for 8 minutes.
- ✓ After 5 minutes, flip over the cheese mixture.

- ✓ Allow to cool 5 minutes before cutting into sticks. Serve warm.

Per serving
Calories: 369 Protein: 35.7 g fiber: 0.0 g
Net carbohydrates: 2.2 g fat: 21.5 g
Sodium: 1,530 mg carbohydrates: 2.2 g sugar: 1.4 g

ITALIAN CHICKEN THIGHS

Chicken thighs are ideal for keto cooking. They're generally the most inexpensive part of the chicken and are full of the fat that gives loads of juicy flavor while helping to keep you full. Show off your air fryer's abilities with crispy thighs coated in Italian seasoning!

HandsOn Time: 5 minutes
Cook Time: 20 minutes
Serves 2

- 4 bone-in, skin-on chicken thighs
- 2 tablespoons unsalted butter, melted
- 1 teaspoon dried parsley
- 1 teaspoon dried basil
- 2 teaspoon garlic powder
- 4 teaspoon onion powder
- 4 teaspoon dried oregano

Directions

- ✓ Brush chicken thighs with butter and sprinkle remaining ingredients over thighs. Place thighs into the air fryer basket.
- ✓ Adjust the temperature to 380°F and set the timer for 20 minutes.
- ✓ Halfway through the cooking time, flip the thighs.
- ✓ When fully cooked, internal temperature will be at least 165°F and skin will be crispy. Serve warm.

Per serving
Calories: 596 protein: 68.3 g Fiber: 0.4 g
Net carbohydrates: 0.8 g fat: 30.9 g sodium: 292 mg
Carbohydrates: 1.2 g sugar: 0.1 g

AIR SINGED CHICKEN AND WAFFLES

Planning Time: 15 minutes
Cook Time: 30 minutes
Servings: 10
Fixings

- for the waffles
- 1/2 teaspoon salt
- 1 teaspoon preparing powder
- 1 cup hefty whipping cream
- 1 cup vanilla almond milk (unsweetened) with additional 1/4 teaspoon of vanilla
- 2 cups almond flour
- 4 tablespoons liquefied margarine

- 6 major eggs
- 15 drops fluid stevia, if wanted

for the chicken
- 1/4 teaspoon pepper
- 3/4 cup almond flour
- 1 tablespoon paprika
- 1 tablespoon coconut oil
- 1 teaspoon powdered garlic
- 1/2 teaspoon salt
- 2 1/2 pound skinless and boneless chicken thighs
- cayenne pepper, as wanted

Directions for the waffles
1. Warmth the waffle creator up to a high warmth then, at that point consolidate the salt, preparing powder and almond flour together in an enormous blending bowl until fused.
2. Utilizing another blending bowl, include the cream, eggs, spread and almond oil then, at that point whisk together until appropriately blended.
3. Delicately rush in the dry Fixings into the wet Fixings combination until very much blended.
4. Utilize a non stick shower to splash the waffle producer in include 1/2 cup of the hitter in, close and cook until the steam radiating from the waffle make decreases.
5. Cautiously open the waffle make then, at that point eliminate the pre-arranged waffles and rehash a similar interaction with the excess player.

For the chicken
1. Preheat the broiler to 375°F meanwhile consolidate the flavors along with the almond flour.
2. Coat every one of the chicken pieces with the almond blend then, at that point move into the air fryer crate and spritz with oil.
3. Cook the chicken thighs until done enemy 10-12 minutes each layer in turn.
4. Serve the waffles and top with the chicken and some other Fixings .

Nourishment Data
Calories: 448 | Complete Fat: 32.8g | Absolute Sugar: 8.2g | Protein: 33.2g

AIR SEARED CHICKEN PARMESAN

Planning Time: 10 minutes
Cook Time: 18 minutes
Servings: 4
Fixings
- 1/2 cup marinara
- 1 tablespoon dissolved spread
- 2 (8 oz. each) cut chicken bosom
- 2 tablespoons parmesan cheddar, ground
- 6 tablespoons breadcrumbs, prepared
- 6 tablespoons low fat mozzarella cheddar
- cooking splash

Directions
1. Set the air fryer to 360°F and warm awake for 9 minutes.
2. Gently splash the air fryer crate with the cooking shower.
3. Utilizing a blending bowl, add the parmesan cheddar, breadcrumbs and join together.
4. Utilize the softened spread to painstakingly rub the cut chicken bosom then, at that point dunk into the breadcrumb blend.
5. Spot the covered chicken into the air fryer crate then, at that point splash with the cooking shower.
6. Spot the crate into the air fryer and cook for 6 minutes then, at that point flip it and top with 1/2 tablespoon of mozzarella cheddar and 1 tablespoon sauce.
7. Keep on cooking until the cheddar is softened for 3 additional minutes.
8. Put the cooked chicken away while you rehash similar cycle with the leftover chicken pieces.

Sustenance Data
Calories: 251 | All out Fat: 9.5g | All out Sugars: 14g | Protein: 31.5g

SINGED BACON WRAPPED CHICKEN

Planning Time: 10 minutes
Cook Time: 8 minutes
Servings: 10
Fixings
- 3 (1.25 pounds) skinless and boneless chicken bosom, cleaved into 1" lumps
- 10 focus cut bacon cuts, cleaved into thirds
- Thai sweet stew sauce, if wanted

Guidance
1. Warmth the air fryer up to 400°F then, at that point wrap every chicken piece with a piece of bacon.

2. Hold the pieces along with a toothpick then, at that point place them in an even layer and cook in clusters for 8 minutes until seared.
3. Flip the pieces midway.
4. Utilize a paper towel to smear then, at that point serve and appreciate.

Sustenance Data
Calories: 98 | All out Fat: 3.5g | Absolute Sugars: 0g | Protein: 16g

AIR FRYER SWEET AND FIERY BACON WRAPPED CHICKEN

Planning Time: 10 minutes
Cook Time: 13 minutes
Servings: 4
Fixings
- 1/8 teaspoon cayenne pepper
- 1/2 tablespoon bean stew powder
- 1/3 cup earthy colored sugar
- 1 pound chicken bosom, slashed into 1" pieces
- 6 bacon cuts, cut into thirds

Guidelines
1. Warmth the air fryer up to 390°F.
2. Put a piece of chicken toward one side of every bacon piece then, at that point move it up and utilize a toothpick to hold it together.
3. Add the bean stew powder, earthy colored sugar and cayenne pepper into a blending bowl then, at that point mix to consolidate.
4. Utilize this combination to cover each piece of the bacon wrapped chicken then, at that point put them away.
5. Move the bacon wrapped pieces into the crate then the air fryer and cook for 13-15 minutes.

Nourishment Data
Calories: 781 | Complete Fat: 17g | Absolute Sugars: 15g | Protein: 132g

KETO AIR FRYER CHICKEN WINGS

Planning Time: 5 minutes
Cook Time: 25 minutes
Servings: 4
Fixings
- 1 tablespoon pepper
- 1 tablespoon garlic powder
- 3 tablespoons preparing salt
- 16 entire chicken wings

Guidelines
1. Preheat the air fryer for around 5 minutes to 370°F. Add every one of the flavors into a combining bowl and join everything as one.
2. Wash the chicken wings and wipe off then throw into the flavors blend to cover.
3. Move the covered chicken wings into the air fryer crate and fry until firm for 25 minutes.
4. Continually flip the chicken to keep it from staying.
5. Serve and appreciate

Sustenance Data
Calories 438 | All out Fat 30g | All out Sugars 2g | Protein 35g

AIR SINGED CHICKEN WITH COCONUT RICE

Planning Time: 5 minutes
Cook Time: 40 minutes
Servings: 6
Fixings
- for the marinade
- 1/4 teaspoon dried cilantro
- 1/4 teaspoon chile glue, if wanted
- 1/2 cup coconut cream
- 1 teaspoon cumin
- 1 lemon zing and juice
- 1 minced garlic clove
- 1/2 teaspoon coriander, ground
- 2 tablespoon soy sauce
- 2 teaspoon curry powder
- 2 tablespoon unadulterated maple syrup
- 3 tablespoons avocado oil
- 4 chicken bosoms
- a scramble cayenne
- lemon wedges, for serving

for the coconut rice
- 1 teaspoon salt
- 1 would coconut be able to cream
- 2 cups jasmine rice
- 2 1/4 cups water

Directions
Utilizing a major zip lock sack, include all the marinade Fixings then, at that point put away to marinate for 2 hours.
Preheat the air fryer to 370°F.
Add all the rice Fixings into a huge stock pot then, at that point heat to the point of boiling.
Cover the stock pot and stew for 15 minutes.
Spill the marinade out of the pack into a pan then, at

that point move the chicken bosom into the air fryer bushel and cook for 10-15 minutes.

Meanwhile, heat up the marinade over medium warmth for 10 minutes, sometimes blending.

Fill in as wanted and appreciate.

Nourishment Data

Calories: 839 | Absolute Fat: 14g | All out Sugars: 21g | Protein: 72g

AIR FRYER PARMESAN CHEDDAR CHICKEN

Planning Time: 5 minutes
Cook Time: 14 minutes
Servings: 2
Fixings

- 1/2 cup breadcrumbs
- 1/2 cup parmesan cheddar, ground
- 1 pound skinless and boneless chicken bosom tenderloins
- 2 beaten eggs

Guidelines

1. Preheat the air fryer to 360°F.
2. Utilizing a shallow heating dish, consolidate the breadcrumbs and parmesan cheddar together.
3. Plunge chicken bosom tenderloins in the beaten eggs then into the cheddar and breadcrumbs.
4. Utilizing a cooking splash, oil the fryer bushel then, at that point organize in the covered chicken bosom.
5. Fry the chicken for 12-14 minutes then, at that point serve and appreciate.

Nourishment Data

Calories: 437 | Absolute Fat: 13g | Complete Sugars: 11g | Protein: 59g

AIR FRYER CHICKEN BOSOM

Planning Time: 1 moment
Cook Time: 12 minutes
Servings: 2
Fixings

- 2 teaspoon olive oil
- 2 huge chicken bosom
- salt and pepper, to taste

Guidelines

1. Supplant the air fryer container with a barbecue dish then, at that point preheat to 350°F.
2. Orchestrate the chicken bosoms on the barbecue container then, at that point sprinkle with salt, pepper and a teaspoon of oil.
3. Cook the chicken for 12 minutes.
4. Once cooked, serve and appreciate.

Sustenance Data

Calories: 601 | All out Fat: 18.8g | Absolute Sugars: 1.5g | Protein: 100.3g

AIR TERMINATED FROZEN CHICKEN

Planning Time: 1 moment
Cook Time: 12 minutes
Servings: 4
Fixings

- a chicken wing pack

Guidelines

1. Warmth the air fryer up to 360°F.
2. Move the frozen chicken wings into the fryer bushel.
3. Cook the chicken for 12 minutes.
4. Once done, serve hot with any sauce of your decision.

Sustenance Data

Calories: 63 | All out Fat: 5g | Complete Sugars: 0g | Protein: 5g

MARINATED CHICKEN TIKKA

Planning Time: 3 minutes
Cook Time: 10 minutes
Servings: 4
Fixings

- 2 major chicken bosoms
- for the marinade
- 1/2 little onion, diced
- 1 lime skin and squeeze
- 1 teaspoon ginger, ground
- 2 teaspoons cumin
- 2 teaspoons paprika
- 2 teaspoons turmeric
- 2 teaspoons garlic puree
- 2 teaspoons garam masala
- 300 ml Greek yogurt
- a touch of bean stew

Directions

1. Utilize a medium estimated blending bowl to join all the marinade Fixings together.
2. Add the chicken bosoms into the marinade and permit to sit for the time being.
3. Warmth the air fryer up to 360°F.

4. Remove the chicken from the marinade and onto a level workstation.
5. Slash the marinated chicken into nibble shapes then, at that point organize on a barbecue skillet and spot inside the air fryer.
6. Cook for 10 minutes then, at that point serve hot and appreciate.

Nourishment Data
Calories: 210 | All out Fat: 5g | All out Starches: 7g | Protein: 32g

AIR SINGED SPATCHCOCK CHICKEN

Planning Time: 1 moment
Cook Time: 50 minutes
Servings: 4
Fixings
- 1 teaspoon blended spices
- 1 tablespoon garlic puree
- 2 teaspoons olive oil
- 2 pounds spatchcock chicken
- salt and pepper

Guidelines
1. Warmth the air fryer up to 360°F.
2. Add the blended spices, salt, pepper, garlic puree and olive oil together.
3. Altogether combine every one of the **Fixings** as one until a thick glue shaped.
4. Liberally cover the chicken with the thick glue.
5. Utilizing a barbecue container, place the covered chicken noticeable all around fryer and cook for 25 minutes for every side.
6. Serve close by some other dish of your decision and appreciate.

Nourishment Data
Calories: 400 | Absolute Fat: 28g | Complete Sugars: 1g | Protein: 32g

AIR SEARED CHEESED CHICKEN

Planning Time: 5 minutes
Cook Time: 20 minutes
Servings: 2
Fixings
- 1 little egg
- 3 major chicken bosom
- 10g pack trembles crisps

Directions
1. Warmth the air fryer up to 180°c.
2. Cut the chicken into strips then, at that point break the egg into a little blending bowl and beat.
3. Add the shakes crisps into another bowl then, at that point go through your hands to break them.
4. Plunge the chicken strips into the beaten eggs then into the wrecked trembles.
5. Move the covered chicken strips into the air fryer container and spot inside the air fryer.
6. Cook for 15 minutes then, at that point flip and cook for an additional 5 minutes.
7. Serve and appreciate.

Sustenance Data
Calories: 774 | All out Fat: 10g | Complete Starches: 3g | Protein: 159g

GREEK AIR SINGED CHICKEN SOUVLAKI

Planning Time: 5 minutes
Cook Time: 9 minutes
Servings: 2
Fixings
- 1 tablespoon oregano
- 1 enormous chicken bosom
- 1 teaspoon coconut oil
- 1 teaspoon Greek yogurt
- 1 little lime skin and squeeze
- 3 garlic cloves
- a squeeze thyme
- Greek sticks
- salt and pepper, to taste

Guidelines
1. Cut the chicken bosom into medium measured lumps.
2. Meagerly mince the garlic cloves then, at that point consolidate with the lime and preparing in a medium measured bowl.
3. Add the diced chicken into the blending bowl then, at that point utilize your hands to join everything together.
4. Move the blend into a bowl, cover then, at that point place inside the ice chest over the course of the evening.
5. Utilize the coconut oil to throw the chicken then the Greek yogurt.
6. Sew the covered chicken on the sticks then, at that point place into the 350°F preheated air fryer and cook for 9 minutes.
7. Flip the sticks part of the way through and cook until firm all finished.
8. Serve and appreciate with new oregano.

GARLIC LEMON PEPPER AIR FRYER CHICKEN WINGS

Planning Time: 7 minutes
Cook Time: 25 minutes
Servings: 4
Fixings

- 1 cup squeezed lime
- 1 tablespoon powdered garlic
- 2 tablespoons salt
- 2 pounds chicken bosom
- 2 tablespoons lime pepper

Directions

1. Utilize a medium estimated blending bowl to join the flavoring and squeezed lime together.
2. Move the blend into a cooler pack then, at that point include the chicken bosom and freeze to marinate.
3. Warmth the air fryer up to 370°F.
4. Spot the marinated chicken bosoms into the air fryer and cook until firm for 20-25 minutes.
5. Flip the chicken bosom part of the way through cooking to get every one of the sides fresh.
6. Serve and appreciate.

AIR SEARED WILD OX CHICKEN WINGS

Planning Time. 5 minutes
Cook Time: 35 minutes
Servings: 4
Fixings

- 1/4 cup spread
- 1/2 cup bison sauce
- 1/2 cup self-rising flour
- 1 teaspoon salt
- 2 pounds chicken wings
- celery, for serving
- blue cheddar dressing, for serving

Directions

1. Warmth the air fryer up to 360°F.
2. Add the salt and flour into a combining bowl then, at that point consolidate as one.

3. Throw the chicken wings in the flour combination until all around covered then shake off each abundance.
4. Move the covered chicken into the fryer bin and into the air fryer.
5. Cook the chicken until fresh and brilliant earthy colored for 30-35 minutes, mixing after like clockwork.
6. Move the cooked chicken into a serving place meanwhile; soften the spread in a little pot over medium warmth.
7. Whisk the bison sauce into the softened spread, then, at that point pour the blend over the chicken wings until covered.
8. Serve close by the celery and blue cheddar dressing.

BASIC WILD OX CHICKEN BOSOM

Planning Time: 5 minutes
Cook Time: 25 minutes
Servings: 5

Fixings

- 1/4 teaspoon stew powder
- 1/2 teaspoon paprika
- 1/2 teaspoon cayenne pepper
- 1 teaspoon nectar
- 1 pack chicken bosom
- 1 teaspoon garlic puree
- 1 tablespoon Worcester sauce
- 2 tablespoons white wine vinegar
- 4 tablespoons coconut oil
- 150ml hand crafted pureed tomatoes
- salt and pepper, to taste

Directions

1. Put the chicken bosom in a huge blending bowl then, at that point mope in 2 tbsps coconut oil, salt and pepper then, at that point blend well until the chicken is very much covered.
2. Warmth the air fryer up to 180°C then, at that point cook the chicken for 15 minutes.
3. Utilizing a different blending bowl, include the leftover **Fixings** then, at that point consolidate until all around joined.
4. When the chicken is done, plunge it into the **Fixings** combination and coat appropriately.
5. Envelop the covered chicken by silver foil then, at that point return it into the air fryer and cook at 160°C for 10 minutes.

6. Once done, serve and appreciate.

Nourishment Data
Calories: 126 | Complete Fat: 11g | Absolute Carbs:
5g | Protein: 0g

AIR SEARED CHICKEN BOSOM AND EGGS

Planning Time: 15 minutes
Cook Time: 14 minutes
Servings: 4
Fixings

- 1/2 teaspoon pepper
- 1/2 teaspoon ocean salt
- 3/4 cup almond flour
- 3/4 cup parmesan cheddar
- 3/4 cups pickle juice (aged), if wanted
- 2 beaten eggs
- 16 ounces chicken bosom
- avocado oil splash

Guidelines
1. Wash the chicken and spot in a zip lock pack.
2. Utilizing a moving pin, smash the chicken bosom into a uniform 1/2" thickness.
3. Move the squashed chicken into a blending bowl then, at that point pour the pickle juice over it.
4. Spot the covered chicken bosom in the fridge for 2 hours to salt water.
5. Warmth the air fryer up to 390°F.
6. Add the parmesan cheddar, almond flour, salt and pepper into a combining bowl then, at that point consolidate as one.
7. Add the eggs into a different bowl and beat together.
8. Channel the chicken of the pickle squeeze then, at that point use paper towels to wipe it off.
9. Residue the chicken bosom in the beaten egg then through the almond flour combination.
10. Saturate your hands then, at that point massage the flour and egg into the chicken bosom and splash with the oil.
11. Move the chicken bosom into the bushel then, at that point cook for 6-7 minutes.
12. Flip the chicken bosom over then shower again and cook until firm and brilliant for 6-7 minutes.
13. Serve and appreciate.

Nourishment Data
Calories: 351 | Absolute Fat: 20g | All out Starches:
5g | Protein: 36g

MUSHROOM CHICKEN PATTIES

Planning Time: 10 minutes
Cook Time: 10 minutes
Serves:: 5 **Servings**
Fixings

- 1 tbsp preparing sauce
- 6 medium (wash and shake abundance fluid off) new mushrooms (30g ea)
- 1 tsp onion powder
- 1 tsp garlic powder
- 1/2 tsp dark pepper, ground
- 1/2 tsp salt
- 500g chicken, ground additional lean.

Strategy
1. Add the washed mushrooms into a food processor and puree until a fine consistency is reached. Include the flavoring sauce, onion powder, garlic powder, ground dark pepper and salt into the food processor and cycle briefly.
2. Empty the food processor blend into a major bowl, and include the ground chicken. Utilize clean hands to blend until very much joined. Split combination into 5 parts and shape into 5 even patties. Make a space in every patty.
3. Coat avocado oil on each side of every patty. Move patties into the wire bushel of an air fryer in one layer. Cook until an interior temperature of 165°F is reached, for 10 minutes at 360°F.
4. Serve without a moment's delay and dive in.

Healthful Data/Serving
Calories 130 kcal, Protein 19.2g, Absolute Carbs
0.7g, Fat 9g

AIR FRYER CHICKEN STRIPS

Planning Time: 10 minutes
Cook Time: 15 minutes
Serves:: 6 **Servings**
Fixings

- 4 tablespoons avocado oil
- 1 (whisked) egg
- 100g almond flour
- 850g (cut into strips) chicken bosom
- 1/2 teaspoon garlic powder
- 1/2 teaspoon salt
- 1 teaspoon onion pieces

Strategy
Add avocado oil and egg into a bowl and speed until consolidated. Add onion, garlic, salt and almond

flour into a bowl and blend until consolidated. Inundate chicken strips into the avocado oil blend until completely covered.

Coat the wire crate of an air fryer with avocado oil. Include the chicken strips and cook for 10 minutes at 350ºF. Fill in as wanted.

Dietary Data/Serving

Calories 445 kcal, Protein 48.8g, Carbs 4.5g, Fat 25.5g

YUMMY CHICKEN DISH

Planning Time: 10 minutes
Cook Time: 50 minutes
Serves:: 6 **Servings**
Fixings
- 1 squeeze garlic salt
- Ground dark pepper
- 2 tbsps spread
- 1/3 cup salt
- 1/3 cup stevia powder
- 1 (3 lbs.) chicken bosom, defrosted
- 2 cups water

Strategy
1. Add 2 cups water into a pot over prescription warmth and bring to bubbling. Include pepper, Stevie powder and 1/3 cup salt and mix until joined. Take container off warmth and let sit for 30 minutes until entirely cool.
2. Add chicken into the skillet with brackish water until entirely covered, place top over bowl and refrigerate for 8 hours. Warmth up air fryer to 390ºF. Remove chicken from the brackish water and dispose of saline solution. Wipe off the chicken and smear with margarine.
3. Sprinkle pepper and garlic salt over covered chicken. Spot prepared chicken in the wire container of the preheated air fryer and cook for 15 minutes. Flip and sprinkle with garlic salt and pepper. Change air fryer temp to 360ºF.
4. Cook chicken for 15 additional minutes, flip and cook for 5 additional minutes. Change air fryer temperature to 390ºF, flip chicken again and cook for 15 additional minutes, until no pink remaining parts in the center. Allow chicken to sit for 5 minutes. Cut chicken and fill in as wanted.

Dietary Data/Serving

Calories 314 kcal, Protein 48g, Carbs 4g, Fat 9.8g

CHICKEN DRUMSTICKS

Planning Time: 5 minutes
Cook Time: 25 minutes
Serves:: 2 **Servings**
Fixings
- 2 tbsps (softened) ghee
- 2 pounds (eliminate skin) chicken drumsticks
- 1/4 cup hot sauce

Technique
1. Spread avocado oil into the container of an air fryer. For 2-3 minutes, heat up air fryer to 400ºF. Add drumsticks into the preheated air fryer and cook for 15 minutes. Turn chicken drumsticks and cook for 5 additional minutes.
2. Add hot sauce and softened ghee into a major bowl and blend until joined. Add chicken drumsticks into the large bowl of sauce and throw until completely covered. Move the covered chicken drumsticks into the air fryer container and top with the excess sauce.
3. Cook until an inside temperature of 165ºF is reached, for 5 additional minutes. Fill in as wanted.

Nourishing Data/Serving

Calories 983 kcal, Protein 110g, Carbs 5g, Fat 55g

MESSY TURKEY WING

Planning Time: 10 minutes
Cook Time: 15 minutes
Serves:: 4 **Servings**
Fixings
1. ½ cup parmesan cheddar, ground
2. 2 pounds (cut into drumettes and pads, and wipe off) turkey wings
3. 1 teaspoon Herbes de Provence
4. 1 teaspoon paprika
5. Avocado oil
6. Salt

Technique
1. Add turkey wings into a bowl and let sit. Add salt, herbes de Provence, paprika, and parmesan into a little bowl and blend until joined.
2. Add turkey wings into the cheddar blend until completely covered. Warmth up air fryer to 350ºF.
3. Coat the wire bin of an air fryer with avocado oil. Work in clusters, add turkey wings into the preheated air fryer, and cook for 15 minutes. Flip turkey wings halfway while cooking. Serve embellished as wanted with parmesan cheddar.

Nourishing Data/Serving
Calories 633 kcal, Fat 38.4g, Protein 65.6g, Carb 2g

TASTY TURKEY DRUMSTICKS

Planning Time: 10 minutes
Cook Time: 20 minutes
Serves:: 6 **Servings**
Fixings
- 1/4 cup coconut flour
- 2 1/2 pounds turkey drumsticks
- 1/4 tsp dark pepper
- 1/2 tsp ocean salt
- 1 cup pork skins morsels
- 2 eggs, enormous
- 1/2 teaspoon garlic powder
- 1 teaspoon paprika, smoked
- 1/4 teaspoon sage, dried

Technique
1. Add dark pepper, salt and coconut flour into a normal level lined bowl, mix to join and let sit. Break the eggs into another bowl, race to consolidate and let sit. Add dried sage, garlic powder, smoked paprika and pork skin morsels into another bowl and mix until joined.
2. Dunk turkey drumsticks into the flour combination until completely covered. Drench in the bowl with egg wash and shake to eliminate any overabundance. Press covered turkey pieces into the scrap combination until consolidated.
3. For 5 minutes, heat up air fryer to 400ºF. Coat the wired crate of the preheated air fryer softly. Add breaded turkey onto the pre-arranged air fryer container in one layer, leaving adequate space between each piece. Seal air fryer and cook until an inner temperature of 165ºF is reached, for 20 minutes.

Nourishing Data/Serving
Calories 273 kcal, Net Carbs 2g, Protein 28g, Fat 15g

PREP-DAY CHICKEN THIGHS

Chicken thighs are kind with the wallet, but at the same time are succulent and tasty. Make these and add them to Servings of mixed greens or soups during the week, or simply heat them up and eat them with no guarantees!
Involved Time: 5 minutes
CookTime: 35 minutes
Fixings | **Serves:**4
- 2 teaspoons olive oil
- 1¼ pounds boneless, skinless chicken thighs (around 6)
- ½ teaspoon salt
- ¼ teaspoon newly ground dark pepper

Technique
1. Brush oil softly over chicken. Season with salt and pepper.
2. Preheat air fryer at 350°F for 3 minutes.
3. Add chicken to fryer container and cook 35 minutes.
4. Utilizing a meat thermometer, guarantee that the chicken is at any rate 165°F. Move to a serving plate and let rest 5 minutes.
5. Slash and store canvassed in the fridge for a portion of your week's plans.

Per serving Calories: 207 | Fat: 9.9 g | Protein: 26.0 g | Sodium: 401 mg | Fiber: 0.0 g | Starches: 0.1 g | Sugar: 0.0 g

SALSA CHICKEN

This is totally the least demanding, most delicious, and most minimal calorie supper you can plan in minutes at the top of the hour. Trust your own warmth o-meter while picking your salsa, or make some natural product salsas all things considered.

Involved Time: 5 minutes
CookTime: 30 minutes
Fixings | **Serves:**2
- 1 pound boneless, skinless chicken thighs (around 4)
- 1 cup salsa of your decision

1. Preheat air fryer at 350°F for 3 minutes.
2. Spot chicken thighs in square cake barrel (frill). Cover with salsa.
3. Cook 30 minutes. Utilizing a meat thermometer, guarantee that the chicken is at any rate 165°F. Add one more moment to the cooking time if important.
4. Move to a serving plate and let rest 5 minutes. Serve warm.

Per serving Calories: 341 | Fat: 12.5 g | Protein: 43.3 g | Sodium: 671 mg | Fiber: 1.6 g | Starches: 8.1 g | Sugar: 0.0 g

133

These seared chicken legs are fresh outwardly and succulent within. The buttermilk loans a citrus quality, adding flavor just as the capacity to soften the meat and make a crispier skin.

Involved Time: 10 minutes
CookTime: a day and a half
Fixings | **Serves:**3
- 1¹/2 pounds boneless, skinless chicken legs (around 5–6)
- 1 cup buttermilk
- 1 cup plain bread morsels
- 1 teaspoon smoked paprika
- 1 teaspoon garlic powder
- Squeeze ground nutmeg
- 1 teaspoon salt
- 1 teaspoon newly ground dark pepper
- 3 tablespoons margarine, liquefied

Technique

1. In a medium bowl, place chicken legs and buttermilk and marinate in the fridge concealed 30 minutes to expedite.
2. Preheat air fryer at 350°F for 3 minutes.
3. Consolidate bread morsels, paprika, garlic powder, nutmeg, salt, and pepper in a shallow dish. Shake abundance buttermilk off chicken legs and dig in bread morsel combination. Put away.
4. Add half of chicken to delicately lubed fryer bushel and cook 10 minutes.
5. Brush delicately with liquefied spread. Flip chicken. Brush opposite side softly with margarine. Increment temperature to 400°F. Cook an extra 8 minutes. Utilizing a meat thermometer, guarantee that the chicken is in any event 165°F.
6. Move to a serving plate. Rehash cooking measure with staying chicken and serve warm.

Per serving Calories: 661 | Fat: 28.3 g | Protein: 71.2 g | Sodium: 904 mg | Fiber: 1.2 g | Starches: 18.0 g | Sugar: 3.8 g

By utilizing grill sauce rather than egg wash to clutch the bread morsel covering, you let these chicken legs hold the entirety of the flavor yet get a "seared" outside covering. Remember to serve some additional sauce as an afterthought for plunging!

Involved Time: 10 minutes
CookTime: a day and a half
Fixings | **Serves:**3
- 1¹/2 pounds chicken legs (roughly 5–6)
- 1 cup grill sauce of your decision
- 1 cup plain bread morsels
- 1 teaspoon salt
- 3 tablespoons margarine, liquefied

1. In a medium bowl, throw chicken legs with grill sauce. Refrigerate concealed 30 minutes or to expedite.
2. Preheat air fryer at 350°F for 3 minutes.
3. Consolidate bread pieces and salt in a shallow dish. Shake abundance sauce off of chicken legs and dig in bread morsel combination. Put away.
4. Delicately splash or brush fryer bushel with oil. Add half of chicken to fryer bushel and cook 10 minutes.
5. Brush chicken delicately with dissolved spread. Flip chicken. Brush opposite side daintily with spread. Increment temperature to 400°F. Cook an extra 8 minutes. Utilizing a meat thermometer, guarantee that the chicken is at any rate 165°F.
6. Move chicken to a serving plate. Rehash cooking measure with staying chicken and serve warm.

Per serving Calories: 965 | Fat: 36.7 g | Protein: 92.7 g | Sodium: 1,875 mg | Fiber: 1.9 g | Starches: 48.6 g | Sugar: 25.5 g

SESAME CHICKEN LEGS

The mix of soy sauce, nectar, sriracha, and lime meet up to loan a beautiful equilibrium of Asian flavors. The toasted sesame seed embellish has a little nuttiness and gives another layer of smash to these fresh chicken legs.

Involved Time: 5 minutes
CookTime: a day and a half
Fixings | **Serves:**3

- ¼ cup soy sauce
- ¼ cup nectar
- 1 tablespoon sriracha
- Juice of 1 little lime
- 1¹/2 pounds chicken legs (roughly 5–6)
- 1 cup plain bread pieces
- 1 teaspoon salt
- 3 tablespoons spread, softened
- 2 tablespoons toasted sesame seeds

1. In a medium bowl, consolidate soy sauce, nectar, sriracha, and lime juice. Throw chicken legs in sauce. Refrigerate concealed 30 minutes to expedite.
2. Preheat air fryer at 350°F for 3 minutes.
3. Consolidate bread pieces and salt in a shallow dish. Shake overabundance sauce off chicken legs and dig in bread morsel blend. Put away.
4. Delicately splash or brush fryer bushel with oil. Add half of chicken to fryer container and cook 10 minutes.
5. Brush delicately with dissolved spread. Flip chicken. Brush opposite side daintily with spread. Increment temperature to 400°F. Cook an extra 8 minutes. Utilizing a meat thermometer, guarantee that the chicken is at any rate 165°F.
6. Move to a serving plate. Rehash cooking measure with staying chicken.
7. Topping with toasted sesame seeds and serve warm.

Per serving Calories: 862 | Fat: 36.6 g | Protein: 92.7 g | Sodium: 1,270 mg | Fiber: 1.2 g | Carbs: 23.9 g | Sugar: 4.1 g

ELEGANT CHICKEN MEATBALLS

Ground chicken can will in general be somewhat dry, yet with the onions and the rich idea of the Ritz saltines, these meatballs are succulent and delightful.

Per serving Calories: 452 | Fat: 22.4 g | Protein: 37.4 g | Sodium: 1,572 mg | Fiber: 1.4 g | Starches: 21.8 g | Sugar: 3.4 g

Involved Time: 10 minutes
CookTime: 16 minutes
Fixings | **Serves:**2

- 1 pound ground chicken
- 1 enormous egg
- ³/4 cup squashed Ritz saltines
- ¼ cup finely diced yellow onion
- 1 teaspoon Italian flavoring
- 1 teaspoon salt
- ¹/2 teaspoon newly ground dark pepper
- ¼ cup cleaved new parsley

1. Preheat air fryer at 350°F for 3 minutes.
2. In a medium bowl, join chicken, egg, saltines, onion, Italian flavoring, salt, and pepper. Structure into eighteen meatballs, around 2 tablespoons each.
3. Add half of meatballs to fryer bin and cook 6 minutes. Flip meatballs. Cook an extra 2 minutes. Move to serving dish.
4. Rehash with residual meatballs and topping with cleaved parsley.

MEXICAN CHICKEN BURGERS

Enhanced with cumin and stew powder, these burgers get their dampness from the red onion and diced green chilies. They're extraordinary served alone, or you can soften queso fresco on the patties, add a cut of tomato and some Sriracha Mayonnaise, and eat on a bun.

Active Time: 10 minutes
CookTime: 26 minutes
Fixings | **Serves:**4

- 1 pound ground chicken
- 2 tablespoons minced red onion
- 1 huge egg white
- ¼ cup panko bread scraps
- 2 tablespoons canned diced green chilies
- 1 tablespoon stew powder
- ¹/2 teaspoon ground cumin
- Squeeze salt

1. Preheat air fryer at 350°F for 3 minutes.
2. In a medium bowl, consolidate every one of the Fixings and structure into four patties, making a slight space in every burger.
3. Add two patties to delicately lubed fryer crate and cook 6 minutes. Flip burgers and cook an extra 7 minutes or until wanted doneness. Rehash with residual burgers.
4. Move to a serving plate and serve warm.

ITALIAN STUFFED CHICKEN BOSOMS

The air fryer and breading give this chicken a beautiful covering and guarantee that the chicken remaining parts delicate.

Involved Time: 10 minutes
CookTime: 18 minutes
Fixings | Serves:4

- 1 huge egg
- 1¹/2 cups entire milk
- 1 cup plain bread pieces
- 1 tablespoon Italian flavoring
- 2 boneless, skinless chicken bosoms (roughly 1 pound)
- ¹/4 teaspoon salt
- ¹/4 teaspoon newly ground dark pepper
- 2 tablespoons cream cheddar
- 2 teaspoons Dijon mustard
- 4 cuts jostled simmered red peppers
- 4 (1-ounce) cuts shop ham
- 2 tablespoons spread, softened

1. In a medium bowl, whisk together egg and milk.
2. In a shallow dish, consolidate bread morsels and Italian flavoring.
3. Between two bits of material paper, pound chicken bosoms to ¹/4" thickness. Season with salt and pepper.
4. Spread a layer of a large portion of the cream cheddar and afterward a large portion of the mustard on every chicken bosom. Add 2 pepper cuts and 2 ham cuts on each. Roll firmly from short finish to short end.
5. Preheat air fryer at 375°F for 3 minutes.
6. Cautiously dunk chicken moves in egg combination. Dig in bread morsels. Shake off any overabundance.
7. Add moved chicken to air fryer crate. Cook 10 minutes. Brush tops with softened spread. Cook an extra 8 minutes.
8. Move to a cutting board. Let rest 5 minutes. Cut each bosom into four adjusts and serve warm.

Per serving Calories: 362 | Fat: 15.4 g | Protein: 34.5 g | Sodium: 1,147 mg | Fiber: 1.5 g | Carbs: 18.5 g | Sugar: 3.1 g

WILD RICE AND PESTO-STUFFED CHICKEN BOSOMS

You can pay jostled pesto off the racks of most supermarkets. This formula is magnificent presented with a side serving of mixed greens and a fresh, chilled glass of Pinot Grigio.

Active Time: 10 minutes
CookTime: 18 minutes
Fixings | Serves:2

- 1 huge egg
- 1¹/2 cups entire milk
- 1 cup plain bread pieces
- 1 tablespoon dried basil
- 2 boneless, skinless chicken bosoms (roughly 1 pound)
- ¹/4 teaspoon salt
- ¹/4 teaspoon newly ground dark pepper
- ¹/4 cup Conventional Pesto
- ¹/4 cup cooked wild rice
- 2 tablespoons spread, softened

1. In a medium bowl, whisk together egg and milk.
2. In a shallow dish, consolidate bread morsels and dried basil.
3. Between two bits of material paper, pound chicken bosoms to ¹/4" thickness. Season with salt and pepper.
4. Spread a layer of a large portion of the Conventional Pesto on every chicken bosom. Add a large portion of the rice to each. Roll firmly from short finish to short end.
5. Preheat air fryer at 375°F for 3 minutes.
6. Cautiously dunk chicken moves in egg combination. Dig in bread morsels. Shake off any abundance.
7. Add moved chicken to air fryer bushel. Cook 10 minutes. Brush tops with liquefied spread. Cook an extra 8 minutes.
8. Move to a cutting board. Let rest 5 minutes. Cut each bosom into four adjusts and serve warm.

Per serving Calories: 362 | Fat: 29.3 g | Protein: 21.5 g | Sodium: 747 mg | Fiber: 3.5 g | Carbs: 42.8 g | Sugar: 6.3 g

Marinating these chicken chomps in the nectar mustard and afterward utilizing a portion of the unused sauce for plunging gets serious about the sweet and appetizing flavor blend.

Active Time: 10 minutes
CookTime: 18 minutes
Fixings | **Serves:**2
- 1 enormous egg
- 2 tablespoons nectar
- 2 tablespoons Dijon mustard
- 1 teaspoon apple juice vinegar
- 2 boneless, skinless chicken bosoms (roughly 1 pound), cut into 1" blocks
- 1 cup plain bread pieces
- 1 teaspoon salt
- 1 teaspoon newly ground dark pepper

1. In a medium bowl, whisk together egg, nectar, mustard, and vinegar. Throw in chicken 3D shapes. Refrigerate concealed 30 minutes or to expedite.
2. Preheat air fryer at 350°F for 3 minutes.
3. In a shallow dish, consolidate bread morsels, salt, and pepper. Shake overabundance marinade off each piece of chicken and afterward dig in bread scrap combination.
4. Add chicken 3D shapes in two bunches to air fryer bushel. Cook 4 minutes. Shake delicately. Cook an extra 5 minutes. Check the chicken utilizing a meat thermometer to guarantee the inner temperature is in any event 165°F.
5. Move chicken to a serving plate and serve warm.

Per serving Calories: 413 | Fat: 8.6 g | Protein: 54.0 g | Sodium: 1,334 mg | Fiber: 1.4 g | Carbs: 29.2 g | Sugar: 10.4 g

S E S A M E - O R A N G E C H I C K E N

This Sesame-Orange Chicken is sound, efficient, and moderate. To reduce down on expense considerably more, you can utilize chicken thighs. They are similarly as brilliant.

Active Time: 10 minutes
CookTime: 18 minutes
Fixings | **Serves:**4
- $^1/_3$ cup newly crushed squeezed orange
- 2 tablespoons sesame oil
- $^1/_4$ cup nectar

137

- 2 tablespoons soy sauce
- 1 teaspoon stripped and minced new ginger
- 1 teaspoon sriracha
- 2 boneless, skinless chicken bosoms (around 1 pound), cut into 1" 3D shapes
- $1^1/_2$ cups plain bread pieces
- 1 teaspoon salt
- 4 cups cooked rice
- $^1/_4$ cup slashed new cilantro

1. In a medium bowl, whisk together squeezed orange, oil, nectar, soy sauce, ginger, and sriracha. Empty portion of blend into a little bowl and put away.
2. Throw chicken blocks in the medium bowl with sauce blend and refrigerate covered 30 minutes.
3. In a shallow dish, consolidate bread morsels and salt. Shake overabundance marinade off each piece of chicken and afterward dig in bread scrap blend.
4. Preheat air fryer at 350°F for 3 minutes.
5. Add chicken chomps in two groups to air fryer bin. Cook 4 minutes. Shake tenderly and flip chicken. Cook an extra 5 minutes. Check the chicken utilizing a meat thermometer to guarantee the inner temperature is at any rate 165°F.
6. Move to a serving plate and shower with outstanding marinade.
7. Serve chicken warm over rice and embellishment with cilantro.

Per serving Calories: 465 | Fat: 7.3 g | Protein: 30.7 g | Sodium: 821 mg | Fiber: 1.4 g | Carbs: 68.4 g | Sugar: 14.5 g

C H I C K E N P L A T E O F M I X E D G R E E N S W I T H S T R A W B E R R I E S A N D W A L N U T S

Regardless of whether you serve this on bread, in lettuce wraps, or straight off the spoon, the strawberries add a new contort on this exemplary plate of mixed greens. The mash from the walnuts gives a textural component that adds another unforeseen pleasure!

Active Time: 10 minutes
CookTime: 18 minutes
Fixings | **Serves:**4
- 2 boneless, skinless chicken bosoms (roughly 1 pound), cut into 1" 3D squares
- 1 teaspoon salt
- $^1/_4$ teaspoon newly ground dark pepper
- $^3/_4$ cup mayonnaise

- 1 tablespoon new lime juice
- ¹/2 cup hacked walnuts
- ¹/2 cup finely hacked celery
- ¹/2 cup diced strawberries

1. Preheat air fryer at 350°F for 3 minutes.
2. Season chicken with salt and pepper.
3. Add chicken solid shapes in two bunches to air fryer container. Cook 4 minutes. Shake delicately and flip chicken. Cook an extra 5 minutes. Check the chicken utilizing a meat thermometer to guarantee the inward temperature is at any rate 165°F.
4. Move to a plate and cool.
5. Cleave chicken and add to a medium bowl. Add remaining Fixings and join well. Refrigerate covered until prepared to eat.

Per serving Calories: 504 | Fat: 42.4 g | Protein: 26.0 g | Sodium: 1,028 mg | Fiber: 1.9 g | Carbs: 4.4 g | Sugar: 1.9 g

CHICKEN TACO BOWL

Taco Tuesday just tracked down another formula. Despite the fact that there are leafy greens at the lower part of this stacked bowl, it is unquestionably a stage up from a drained supper salad. A shower of natively constructed Cilantro-Jalapeño Farm Plunge arranges everything!

Active Time: 15 minutes
CookTime: 15 minutes
Fixings | Serves:4
- 1 tablespoon avocado oil
- 1 teaspoon stew powder
- ¹/2 teaspoon ground cumin
- ¹/8 teaspoon garlic powder
- ¹/8 teaspoon smoked paprika
- ¹/8 teaspoon salt
- Squeeze cayenne pepper
- 1 pound boneless, skinless chicken thighs, daintily cut into 1" strips
- 4 cups blended greens
- 1 cup yellow corn portions
- 1 cup dark beans, washed and depleted
- 1 huge avocado, stripped, pitted, and diced
- 2 medium Roma tomatoes, cultivated and diced
- 16 tortilla chips
- ¹/2 cup Cilantro-Jalapeño Farm Plunge (see Section 15)

1. In a medium bowl, whisk together avocado oil, stew powder, cumin, garlic powder, paprika, salt, and cayenne pepper. Add chicken and throw. Refrigerate covered 30 minutes.
2. Preheat air fryer at 350°F for 3 minutes.
3. Add chicken to air fryer crate. Cook 6 minutes. Throw. Cook an additional 6 minutes. Throw. Cook 3 minutes more.
4. To gather bowls, circulate blended greens among four dishes. Top with chicken, corn, dark beans, avocado, and tomatoes. Squash 4 chips over each bowl. Sprinkle with Cilantro-Jalapeño Farm Plunge.

Per serving Calories: 858 | Fat: 60.5 g | Protein: 32.9 g | Sodium: 1,325 mg | Fiber: 9.8 g | Carbs: 41.9 g | Sugar: 6.5 g

CHICKEN-PIMIENTO PUFFS

These eminent pockets are dissolve in-your-mouth heavenly. Serve either for supper, as a tidbit, or as a starter for visitors.

Active Time: 15 minutes
CookTime: 20 minutes
Fixings | Serves:4
- 2 tablespoons universally handy flour, isolated
- 1 cup slashed cooked chicken
- 4 ounces mascarpone cheddar
- 1 (2-ounce) container pimientos, depleted
- 1 teaspoon herbes de Provence
- ¹/4 cup diced sweet onion
- ¹/2 teaspoon salt
- ¹/4 teaspoon newly ground dark pepper
- 2 sheets puff baked good, defrosted to room temperature
- 1 cnormous egg, whisked

1. Utilize 1 tablespoon flour to sprinkle on a level, clean surface. Put away the other tablespoon for your hands when you begin working with the batter, just as for the surface if required.
2. Preheat air fryer at 375°F for 3 minutes.
3. In a medium bowl, join chicken, cheddar, pimientos, herbes de Provence, onion, salt, and pepper.
4. Spot a sheet of puff baked good on floured surface. Cut the sheet into six equivalent square shapes. Spot 1 tablespoon of chicken blend in every square shape. Overlay over short side to short side and delicately squeeze the crease edges, utilizing the prongs of a fork

to get the seal. Rehash to make twelve puff pockets. Brush the highest points of each with whisked egg.

5. Add three chicken puffs to softly lubed air fryer bin. Cook 5 minutes. Move to a plate. Rehash until all are cooked and serve warm.

Per serving Calories: 350 | Fat: 21.2 g | Protein: 19.0 g | Sodium: 630 mg | Fiber: 0.9 g | Carbs: 18.3 g | Sugar: 2.0 g

CHICKEN QUESADILLAS

Because of its capacity to equitably cook tortillas, the air fryer is the ideal apparatus for quesadillas. These Chicken Quesadillas are delectable all alone however balance a supper when presented with harsh cream, guacamole, destroyed lettuce, and a side of rice and dark beans.

Active Time: 10 minutes
CookTime: 12 minutes
Fixings | **Serves:**4

- 2 medium Roma tomatoes, cultivated and diced
- 1 teaspoon stew powder
- $^{1}/2$ teaspoon salt
- 3 tablespoons spread, dissolved
- 8 (6") flour tortillas
- 2 cups destroyed cooked chicken
- 2 cups ground Mexican cheddar mix

1. In a little bowl, throw diced tomatoes with bean stew powder and salt. Put away.
2. Preheat air fryer at 350°F for 3 minutes.
3. Gently brush liquefied spread on one side of a tortilla. Spot tortilla margarine side down in air fryer bushel. Layer $^{1}/4$ of the destroyed chicken on tortilla, trailed by $^{1}/4$ of the tomatoes and $^{1}/4$ of the cheddar. Top with second tortilla. Delicately spread top of tortilla.
4. Cook 3 minutes. Put away and keep on making three additional quesadillas.
5. Cut every quesadilla like a pie into six segments. Serve warm.

Per serving Calories: 608 | Fat: 30.5 g | Protein: 41.5 g | Sodium: 967 mg | Fiber: 2.1 g | Carbs: 33.4 g | Sugar: 3.6 g

CHICKEN AND GREEN OLIVE PIZZADILLAS

Pizza + quesadilla = pizzadilla! The intriguing blend of Fixings combined with the crisp astounding taste will make you return for additional!

Active Time: 10 minutes
CookTime: 12 minutes
Fixings | **Serves:**4

- 2 cups destroyed cooked chicken
- 1 teaspoon garlic powder
- 3 tablespoons spread, softened
- 8 (6") flour tortillas
- 1 cup Very Simple Romesco Sauce
- 2 cups ground mozzarella cheddar
- 1 cup cut pitted green olives
- 2 teaspoons new thyme leaves

In a little bowl, throw chicken with garlic powder. Preheat air fryer at 350°F for 3 minutes.
Delicately brush dissolved margarine on one side of a tortilla. Spot tortilla margarine side down in air fryer crate. Spread $^{1}/4$ of Very Simple Romesco Sauce on tortilla in container. Layer $^{1}/4$ of the chicken, $^{1}/4$ of the cheddar, $^{1}/4$ of the olives, and $^{1}/4$ of the thyme leaves. Top with second tortilla. Gently margarine top of tortilla. Cook 3 minutes. Put away and keep on making the other three pizzadillas.
Cut each pizzadilla into six segments. Serve warm.

Per serving Calories: 724 | Fat: 40.5 g | Protein: 43.0 g | Sodium: 1,844 mg | Fiber: 4.3 g | Carbs: 40.5 g | Sugar: 3.4 g

FIERY PRETZEL CHICKEN PIECES

There's no compelling reason to add salt to this treat; the squashed pretzels loan a pungency and an unmistakable flavor separate from plain bread pieces. If you don't need the warmth, avoid the sriracha.

Active Time: 10 minutes
CookTime: 18 minutes
Fixings | **Serves:**4

- 1 enormous egg
- 1 tablespoon sriracha
- 1 tablespoon yellow mustard
- 1 tablespoon mayonnaise
- 2 boneless, skinless chicken bosoms (around 1 pound), cut into 1" blocks
- 1 cup panko bread morsels
- 1 cup squashed pretzels

1. In a medium bowl, whisk together egg, sriracha, yellow mustard, and mayonnaise. Throw in chicken blocks. Refrigerate concealed 30 minutes or to expedite.
2. Preheat air fryer at 350°F for 3 minutes.
3. In a shallow dish, join bread pieces and squashed pretzels. Shake abundance marinade off each piece of chicken and afterward dig in bread scrap blend.
4. Add half of chicken chomps to air fryer container. Cook 4 minutes. Shake tenderly. Cook an extra 5 minutes. Check the chicken utilizing a meat thermometer to guarantee the interior temperature is in any event 165°F. Rehash with staying chicken.
5. Move to a plate and serve warm.

Per serving Calories: 243 | Fat: 6.4 g | Protein: 27.8 g | Sodium: 490 mg | Fiber: 0.4 g | Carbs: 18.9 g | Sugar: 1.1 g

BROILED CORNISH HEN

An entire chicken is a regular standard decision, however when it is scaled down into a Cornish hen it turns into a provocative supper for two or an extravagant dish for visitors. You'll cherish this basic and flavorful dish.

Active Time: 10 minutes
CookTime: 28 minutes
Fixings | **Serves:**2
- 1 teaspoon salt
- ¹/2 teaspoon newly ground dark pepper
- ¹/2 teaspoon smoked paprika
- ¹/2 teaspoon ground fennel powder
- 2 teaspoons olive oil
- 1 (roughly 2-pound) Cornish hen
- ¹/2 medium lime, split
- 2 cloves garlic, split

1. In a little bowl, join salt, pepper, paprika, and fennel powder.
2. Preheat air fryer at 350°F for 3 minutes.
3. Rub oil over and inside Cornish hen. Sprinkle hen with preparing blend. Stuff lime and garlic into the hen's pit.
4. Spot hen on air fryer bushel. Cook 10 minutes. Flip hen. Cook 10 additional minutes. Flip hen and cook an extra 8 minutes. Utilizing a meat thermometer, check to guarantee inner temperature is in any event 165°F. If half-cooked, cook an extra 2 minutes and check again until temperature is reached.
5. Move hen to a cutting board and let rest 5 minutes. Dispose of lime and garlic cloves.

Chop down the spine of the hen to split and serve warm.

Per serving Calories: 376 | Fat: 25.9 g | Protein: 28.8 g | Sodium: 1,244 mg | Fiber: 0.6 g | Starches: 0.9 g | Sugar: 0.1 g

LEMON ROSEMARY CHICKEN

Fixings
- 1 pound chicken (350 g)

For the Marinate:
- 1 tablespoon soy sauce
- ½ tablespoon olive oil
- 1 teaspoon minced ginger

For the Sauce:
- 3 tablespoons earthy colored sugar
- 1 tablespoon clam sauce
- ½ wedge-cut lemon in skins
- Discretionary: 15 g (0.5 ounces) new rosemary

Guidelines
1. Leave the skin on the rosemary and cleave.
2. Mix the entirety of the marinade segments. Pour over the chicken. Allow them to chill in the cooler for around thirty minutes.
3. Spot the marinade and chicken in a heating dish, and prepare for six minutes in the AF at 392°F.
4. Mix the entirety of the sauce **Fixings** (short the lemon).
5. Pour the combination over the chicken when it is about crazy.
6. Spot the lemon wedges in the skillet uniformly and crush so the zing will elevate the kind of the chicken. Keep heating for an extra 13 minutes going to guarantee the entirety of the pieces are cooked equitably.
7. Note: You can overlook the rosemary.

JAMAICAN CHICKEN MEATBALLS

Fixings
- 1 huge stripped and diced onion
- 2 huge chicken bosoms
- 1 teaspoon stew powder
- 2 tablespoons nectar
- Pepper and salt to taste
- 3 tablespoons soy sauce

1 tablespoon each:
- Dry mustard

- Cumin
- Thyme
- Basil
- Discretionary: 2 teaspoons Jerk Glue

Directions
1. Utilizing a blender—mince the chicken; add the onion and mince; blend well. Throw in the Jamaican flavors and mix once more. Make ten medium balls.
2. Spot on the preparing mat in the AF and cook at 356ºF or 180ºC.
3. Put them on a stick when done cooking and some utilization of the additional sauce over the meatballs.
4. Add a few spices on the top, serve, and appreciate.

Yields: Ten Servings
Note: in the event that you don't know; jerk glue is a mix of earthy colored flavors, ginger, peppers, and thyme.

PREP-DAY CHICKEN THIGHS

Chicken thighs are kind with the wallet, but on the other hand are succulent and heavenly. Make these and add them to plates of mixed greens or soups during the week, or simply heat them up and eat them with no guarantees!

Involved Time: 5 minutes
CookTime: 35 minutes
Fixings | **Serves:**4
- 2 teaspoons olive oil
- $1^1/4$ pounds boneless, skinless chicken thighs (around 6)
- $^1/2$ teaspoon salt
- $^1/4$ teaspoon newly ground dark pepper

Directions
1. Brush oil gently over chicken. Season with salt and pepper.
2. Preheat air fryer at 350°F for 3 minutes.
3. Add chicken to fryer bin and cook 35 minutes.
4. Utilizing a meat thermometer, guarantee that the chicken is at any rate 165°F. Move to a serving plate and let rest 5 minutes.
5. Slash and store shrouded in the fridge for a portion of your week's plans.

Per serving Calories: 207 | Fat: 9.9 g | Protein: 26.0 g | Sodium: 401 mg | Fiber: 0.0 g | Starches: 0.1 g | Sugar: 0.0 g

SALSA CHICKEN

This is totally the simplest, most delicious, and least calorie feast you can get ready in minutes at the top of the hour. Trust your own warmth o-meter while picking your salsa, or make some organic product salsas all things considered.

Active Time: 5 minutes
CookTime: 30 minutes
Fixings | **Serves:**2
- 1 pound boneless, skinless chicken thighs (roughly 4)
- 1 cup salsa of your decision

1. Preheat air fryer at 350°F for 3 minutes.
2. Spot chicken thighs in square cake barrel (extra). Cover with salsa.
3. Cook 30 minutes. Utilizing a meat thermometer, guarantee that the chicken is in any event 165°F. Add one more moment to the cooking time if essential.
4. Move to a serving plate and let rest 5 minutes. Serve warm.

Per serving Calories: 341 | Fat: 12.5 g | Protein: 43.3 g | Sodium: 671 mg | Fiber: 1.6 g | Carbs: 8.1 g | Sugar: 0.0 g

BUTTERMILK SOUTHERN-SEARED CHICKEN LEGS

These seared chicken legs are fresh outwardly and succulent within. The buttermilk loans a citrus quality, adding flavor just as the capacity to soften the meat and make a crispier skin.

Active Time: 10 minutes
CookTime: a day and a half
Fixings | **Serves:**3
- $1^1/2$ pounds boneless, skinless chicken legs (roughly 5–6)
- 1 cup buttermilk
- 1 cup plain bread pieces
- 1 teaspoon smoked paprika
- 1 teaspoon garlic powder
- Squeeze ground nutmeg
- 1 teaspoon salt
- 1 teaspoon newly ground dark pepper
- 3 tablespoons margarine, liquefied

1. In a medium bowl, place chicken legs and buttermilk and marinate in the fridge concealed 30 minutes to expedite.
2. Preheat air fryer at 350°F for 3 minutes.

3. Join bread morsels, paprika, garlic powder, nutmeg, salt, and pepper in a shallow dish. Shake abundance buttermilk off chicken legs and dig in bread morsel combination. Put away.
4. Add half of chicken to daintily lubed fryer bin and cook 10 minutes.
5. Brush daintily with dissolved spread. Flip chicken. Brush opposite side softly with margarine. Increment temperature to 400°F. Cook an extra 8 minutes. Utilizing a meat thermometer, guarantee that the chicken is in any event 165°F.
6. Move to a serving plate. Rehash cooking measure with staying chicken and serve warm.

Per serving Calories: 661 | Fat: 28.3 g | Protein: 71.2 g | Sodium: 904 mg | Fiber: 1.2 g | Carbs: 18.0 g | Sugar: 3.8 g

BAR-B-QUE BREADED CHICKEN LEGS

By utilizing grill sauce rather than egg wash to clutch the bread piece covering, you let these chicken legs hold the entirety of the flavor yet get a "seared" outside covering. Remember to serve some additional sauce as an afterthought for plunging!

Active Time: 10 minutes
CookTime: a day and a half
Fixings | **Serves:**3
- 1¹/2 pounds chicken legs (roughly 5–6)
- 1 cup grill sauce of your decision
- 1 cup plain bread pieces
- 1 teaspoon salt
- 3 tablespoons spread, softened

1. In a medium bowl, throw chicken legs with grill sauce. Refrigerate concealed 30 minutes or to expedite.
2. Preheat air fryer at 350°F for 3 minutes.
3. Consolidate bread morsels and salt in a shallow dish. Shake abundance sauce off of chicken legs and dig in bread piece blend. Put away.
4. Delicately shower or brush fryer bin with oil. Add half of chicken to fryer bushel and cook 10 minutes.
5. Brush chicken delicately with softened margarine. Flip chicken. Brush opposite side delicately with spread. Increment temperature to 400°F. Cook an extra 8 minutes. Utilizing a meat thermometer, guarantee that the chicken is at any rate 165°F.

6. Move chicken to a serving plate. Rehash cooking measure with staying chicken and serve warm.

Per serving Calories: 965 | Fat: 36.7 g | Protein: 92.7 g | Sodium: 1,875 mg | Fiber: 1.9 g | Carbs: 48.6 g | Sugar: 25.5 g

SESAME CHICKEN LEGS

The blend of soy sauce, nectar, sriracha, and lime meet up to loan a beautiful equilibrium of Asian flavors. The toasted sesame seed decorate has a little nuttiness and gives another layer of mash to these firm chicken legs.
Involved Time: 5 minutes
Fixings | **Serves:**3
- ¹/4 cup soy sauce
- ¹/4 cup nectar
- 1 tablespoon sriracha
- Juice of 1 little lime
- 1¹/2 pounds chicken legs (around 5–6)
- 1 cup plain bread scraps
- 1 teaspoon salt
- 3 tablespoons margarine, softened
- 2 tablespoons toasted sesame seeds

1. In a medium bowl, join soy sauce, nectar, sriracha, and lime juice. Throw chicken legs in sauce. Refrigerate concealed 30 minutes to expedite.
2. Preheat air fryer at 350°F for 3 minutes.
3. Join bread scraps and salt in a shallow dish. Shake abundance sauce off chicken legs and dig in bread morsel combination. Put away.
4. Softly shower or brush fryer bin with oil. Add half of chicken to fryer container and cook 10 minutes.
5. Brush softly with liquefied margarine. Flip chicken. Brush opposite side daintily with margarine. Increment temperature to 400°F. Cook an extra 8 minutes. Utilizing a meat thermometer, guarantee that the chicken is at any rate 165°F.
6. Move to a serving plate. Rehash cooking measure with staying chicken.
7. Embellishment with toasted sesame seeds and serve warm.

Per serving Calories: 862 | Fat: 36.6 g | Protein: 92.7 g | Sodium: 1,270 mg | Fiber: 1.2 g | Starches: 23.9 g | Sugar: 4.1 g

<u>**ELEGANT CHICKEN MEATBALLS**</u>

Ground chicken can will in general be somewhat dry, however with the onions and the rich idea of the Ritz wafers, these meatballs are succulent and flavorful.

Involved Time: 10 minutes
CookTime: 16 minutes
Fixings | **Serves:**2

- 1 pound ground chicken
- 1 enormous egg
- 3/4 cup squashed Ritz saltines
- 1/4 cup finely diced yellow onion
- 1 teaspoon Italian flavoring
- 1 teaspoon salt
- 1/2 teaspoon newly ground dark pepper
- 1/4 cup slashed new parsley

1. Preheat air fryer at 350°F for 3 minutes.
2. In a medium bowl, join chicken, egg, saltines, onion, Italian flavoring, salt, and pepper. Structure into eighteen meatballs, around 2 tablespoons each.
3. Add half of meatballs to fryer bin and cook 6 minutes. Flip meatballs. Cook an extra 2 minutes. Move to serving dish.
4. Rehash with outstanding meatballs and topping with cleaved parsley.
5.
   Per serving Calories: 452 | Fat: 22.4 g | Protein: 37.4 g | Sodium: 1,572 mg | Fiber: 1.4 g | Starches: 21.8 g | Sugar: 3.4 g

<u>**MEXICAN CHICKEN BURGERS**</u>

Seasoned with cumin and bean stew powder, these burgers get their dampness from the red onion and diced green chilies. They're extraordinary served alone, or you can liquefy queso fresco on the patties, add a cut of tomato and some Sriracha Mayonnaise, and eat on a bun.

Active Time: 10 minutes
CookTime: 26 minutes
Fixings | **Serves:**4

- 1 pound ground chicken
- 2 tablespoons minced red onion
- 1 huge egg white
- 1/4 cup panko bread pieces
- 2 tablespoons canned diced green chilies
- 1 tablespoon stew powder
- 1/2 teaspoon ground cumin
- Squeeze salt

1. Preheat air fryer at 350°F for 3 minutes.
2. In a medium bowl, consolidate every one of the Fixings and structure into four patties, making a slight space in every burger.
3. Add two patties to softly lubed fryer container and cook 6 minutes. Flip burgers and cook an extra 7 minutes or until wanted doneness. Rehash with residual burgers.
4. Move to a serving plate and serve warm.

   Per serving Calories: 207 | Fat: 9.3 g | Protein: 22.1 g | Sodium: 216 mg | Fiber: 1.2 g | Carbs: 7.9 g | Sugar: 1.0 g

<u>**ITALIAN STUFFED CHICKEN BOSOMS**</u>

The air fryer and breading give this chicken a beautiful covering and guarantee that the chicken remaining parts delicate.
Involved Time: 10 minutes
CookTime: 18 minutes
Fixings | **Serves:**4

- 1 enormous egg
- 1 1/2 cups entire milk
- 1 cup plain bread scraps
- 1 tablespoon Italian flavoring
- 2 boneless, skinless chicken bosoms (around 1 pound)
- 1/4 teaspoon salt
- 1/4 teaspoon newly ground dark pepper
- 2 tablespoons cream cheddar
- 2 teaspoons Dijon mustard
- 4 cuts jolted cooked red peppers
- 4 (1-ounce) cuts store ham

1. 2 tablespoons margarine, liquefied
2. In a medium bowl, whisk together egg and milk.
3. In a shallow dish, join bread pieces and Italian flavoring.
4. Between two bits of material paper, pound chicken bosoms to 1/4" thickness. Season with salt and pepper.
5. Spread a layer of a large portion of the cream cheddar and afterward a large portion of the mustard on every chicken bosom. Add 2 pepper cuts and 2 ham cuts on each. Roll firmly from short finish to short end.
6. Preheat air fryer at 375°F for 3 minutes.
7. Cautiously plunge chicken moves in egg combination. Dig in bread morsels. Shake off any overabundance.
8. Add moved chicken to air fryer crate. Cook 10 minutes. Brush tops with softened margarine. Cook an extra 8 minutes.

9. Move to a cutting board. Let rest 5 minutes. Cut each bosom into four adjusts and serve warm.

Per serving Calories: 362 | Fat: 15.4 g | Protein: 34.5 g | Sodium: 1,147 mg | Fiber: 1.5 g | Starches: 18.5 g | Sugar: 3.1 g

NECTAR MUSTARD CHICKEN NIBBLES

Marinating these chicken nibbles in the nectar mustard and afterward utilizing a portion of the unused sauce for plunging gets serious about the sweet and appetizing flavor blend.

Involved Time: 10 minutes
CookTime: 18 minutes
Fixings | **Serves:**2

- 1 enormous egg
- 2 tablespoons nectar
- 2 tablespoons Dijon mustard
- 1 teaspoon apple juice vinegar
- 2 boneless, skinless chicken bosoms (around 1 pound), cut into 1" solid shapes
- 1 cup plain bread scraps
- 1 teaspoon salt
- 1 teaspoon newly ground dark pepper

1. In a medium bowl, whisk together egg, nectar, mustard, and vinegar. Throw in chicken solid shapes. Refrigerate concealed 30 minutes or to expedite.
2. Preheat air fryer at 350°F for 3 minutes.
3. In a shallow dish, join bread scraps, salt, and pepper. Shake overabundance marinade off each piece of chicken and afterward dig in bread scrap blend.
4. Add chicken solid shapes in two groups to air fryer bushel. Cook 4 minutes. Shake tenderly. Cook an extra 5 minutes. Check the chicken utilizing a meat thermometer to guarantee the interior temperature is at any rate 165°F.
5. Move chicken to a serving plate and serve warm.

Per serving Calories: 413 | Fat: 8.6 g | Protein: 54.0 g | Sodium: 1,334 mg | Fiber: 1.4 g | Starches: 29.2 g | Sugar: 10.4 g

SESAME-ORANGE CHICKEN

This Sesame-Orange Chicken is solid, efficient, and reasonable. To reduce down on expense considerably more, you can utilize chicken thighs. They are similarly as great.

Involved Time: 10 minutes
CookTime: 18 minutes
Fixings | **Serves:**4

- ^{1}/3 cup newly crushed squeezed orange
- 2 tablespoons sesame oil
- ^{1}/4 cup nectar
- 2 tablespoons soy sauce
- 1 teaspoon stripped and minced new ginger
- 1 teaspoon sriracha
- 2 boneless, skinless chicken bosoms (around 1 pound), cut into 1" 3D squares
- 1^1/2 cups plain bread morsels
- 1 teaspoon salt
- 4 cups cooked rice
- ^{1}/4 cup slashed new cilantro

1. In a medium bowl, whisk together squeezed orange, oil, nectar, soy sauce, ginger, and sriracha. Empty portion of combination into a little bowl and put away.
2. Throw chicken shapes in the medium bowl with sauce combination and refrigerate covered 30 minutes.
3. In a shallow dish, join bread scraps and salt. Shake abundance marinade off each piece of chicken and afterward dig in bread scrap combination.
4. Preheat air fryer at 350°F for 3 minutes.
5. Add chicken nibbles in two clumps to air fryer container. Cook 4 minutes. Shake tenderly and flip chicken. Cook an extra 5 minutes. Check the chicken utilizing a meat thermometer to guarantee the inside temperature is in any event 165°F.
6. Move to a serving plate and sprinkle with residual marinade.
7. Serve chicken warm over rice and enhancement with cilantro.

Per serving Calories: 465 | Fat: 7.3 g | Protein: 30.7 g | Sodium: 821 mg | Fiber: 1.4 g | Starches: 68.4 g | Sugar: 14.5 g

Regardless of whether you serve this on bread, in lettuce wraps, or straight off the spoon, the strawberries add a new bend on this exemplary plate of mixed greens. The smash from the walnuts gives a textural component that adds another unforeseen pleasure!

Involved Time: 10 minutes
CookTime: 18 minutes
Fixings | Serves:4
- 2 boneless, skinless chicken bosoms (around 1 pound), cut into 1" shapes
- 1 teaspoon salt
- 1/4 teaspoon newly ground dark pepper
- 3/4 cup mayonnaise
- 1 tablespoon new lime juice
- 1/2 cup hacked walnuts
- 1/2 cup finely hacked celery
- 1/2 cup diced strawberries

1. Preheat air fryer at 350°F for 3 minutes.
2. Season chicken with salt and pepper.
3. Add chicken 3D squares in two groups to air fryer bin. Cook 4 minutes. Shake delicately and flip chicken. Cook an extra 5 minutes. Check the chicken utilizing a meat thermometer to guarantee the inner temperature is in any event 165°F.
4. Move to a plate and cool.
5. Hack chicken and add to a medium bowl. Add remaining Fixings and consolidate well. Refrigerate covered until prepared to eat.

Per serving Calories: 504 | Fat: 42.4 g | Protein: 26.0 g | Sodium: 1,028 mg | Fiber: 1.9 g | Starches: 4.4 g | Sugar: 1.9 g

CHICKEN TACO BOWL

Taco Tuesday just tracked down another formula. In spite of the fact that there are leafy greens at the lower part of this stacked bowl, it is unquestionably a stage up from a drained supper salad. A sprinkle of hand crafted Cilantro-Jalapeño Farm Plunge arranges everything!

Involved Time: 15 minutes
CookTime: 15 minutes
Fixings | Serves:4
- 1 tablespoon avocado oil
- 1 teaspoon bean stew powder
- 1/2 teaspoon ground cumin
- 1/8 teaspoon garlic powder
- 1/8 teaspoon smoked paprika
- 1/8 teaspoon salt
- Squeeze cayenne pepper
- 1 pound boneless, skinless chicken thighs, meagerly cut into 1" strips
- 4 cups blended greens
- 1 cup yellow corn pieces
- 1 cup dark beans, washed and depleted
- 1 huge avocado, stripped, pitted, and diced
- 2 medium Roma tomatoes, cultivated and diced
- 16 tortilla chips
- 1/2 cup Cilantro-Jalapeño Farm Plunge (see Section 15)

1. In a medium bowl, whisk together avocado oil, stew powder, cumin, garlic powder, paprika, salt, and cayenne pepper. Add chicken and throw. Refrigerate covered 30 minutes.
2. Preheat air fryer at 350°F for 3 minutes.
3. Add chicken to air fryer bushel. Cook 6 minutes. Throw. Cook an additional 6 minutes. Throw. Cook 3 minutes more.
4. To gather bowls, disperse blended greens among four dishes. Top with chicken, corn, dark beans, avocado, and tomatoes. Pulverize 4 chips over each bowl. Shower with Cilantro-Jalapeño Farm Plunge.

Per serving Calories: 858 | Fat: 60.5 g | Protein: 32.9 g | Sodium: 1,325 mg | Fiber: 9.8 g | Starches: 41.9 g | Sugar: 6.5 g

CHICKEN-PIMIENTO PUFFS

These wonderful pockets are dissolve in-your-mouth heavenly. Serve either for supper, as a bite, or as a hors d'oeuvre for visitors.

Active Time: 15 minutes
CookTime: 20 minutes
Fixings | Serves:4
- 2 tablespoons generally useful flour, separated
- 1 cup hacked cooked chicken
- 4 ounces mascarpone cheddar
- 1 (2-ounce) container pimientos, depleted
- 1 teaspoon herbes de Provence
- 1/4 cup diced sweet onion
- 1/2 teaspoon salt
- 1/4 teaspoon newly ground dark pepper
- 2 sheets puff cake, defrosted to room temperature

- 1 huge egg, whisked

1. Utilize 1 tablespoon flour to sprinkle on a level, clean surface. Put away the other tablespoon for your hands when you begin working with the batter, just as for the surface if required.
2. Preheat air fryer at 375°F for 3 minutes.
3. In a medium bowl, consolidate chicken, cheddar, pimientos, herbes de Provence, onion, salt, and pepper.
4. Spot a sheet of puff cake on floured surface. Cut the sheet into six equivalent square shapes. Spot 1 tablespoon of chicken blend in every square shape. Overlay over short side to short side and daintily squeeze the crease edges, utilizing the prongs of a fork to get the seal. Rehash to make twelve puff pockets. Brush the highest points of each with whisked egg.
5. Add three chicken puffs to delicately lubed air fryer bushel. Cook 5 minutes. Move to a plate. Rehash until all are cooked and serve warm.

Per serving Calories: 350 | Fat: 21.2 g | Protein: 19.0 g | Sodium: 630 mg | Fiber: 0.9 g | Carbs: 18.3 g | Sugar: 2.0 g

CHICKEN QUESADILLAS

Because of its capacity to uniformly cook tortillas, the air fryer is the ideal machine for quesadillas. These Chicken Quesadillas are scrumptious all alone however balance a feast when presented with harsh cream, guacamole, destroyed lettuce, and a side of rice and dark beans.

Involved Time: 10 minutes
CookTime: 12 minutes
Fixings | **Serves:**4
- 2 medium Roma tomatoes, cultivated and diced
- 1 teaspoon bean stew powder
- $1/2$ teaspoon salt
- 3 tablespoons margarine, dissolved
- 8 (6") flour tortillas
- 2 cups destroyed cooked chicken
- 2 cups ground Mexican cheddar mix

1. In a little bowl, throw diced tomatoes with bean stew powder and salt. Put away.
2. Preheat air fryer at 350°F for 3 minutes.
3. Daintily brush softened spread on one side of a tortilla. Spot tortilla spread side down in air fryer crate. Layer $1/4$ of the destroyed chicken on tortilla, trailed by $1/4$ of the tomatoes and $1/4$

of the cheddar. Top with second tortilla. Softly spread top of tortilla.
4. Cook 3 minutes. Put away and keep on making three additional quesadillas.
5. Cut every quesadilla like a pie into six areas. Serve warm.

Per serving Calories: 608 | Fat: 30.5 g | Protein: 41.5 g | Sodium: 967 mg | Fiber: 2.1 g | Starches: 33.4 g | Sugar: 3.6 g

ZESTY PRETZEL CHICKEN PIECES

There's no compelling reason to add salt to this treat; the squashed pretzels loan a pungency and a particular flavor separate from plain bread pieces. If you don't need the warmth, skirt the sriracha.

Active Time: 10 minutes
CookTime: 18 minutes
Fixings | **Serves:**4
- 1 huge egg
- 1 tablespoon sriracha
- 1 tablespoon yellow mustard
- 1 tablespoon mayonnaise
- 2 boneless, skinless chicken bosoms (roughly 1 pound), cut into 1" 3D shapes
- 1 cup panko bread pieces
- 1 cup squashed pretzels

1. In a medium bowl, whisk together egg, sriracha, yellow mustard, and mayonnaise. Throw in chicken 3D shapes. Refrigerate concealed 30 minutes or to expedite.
2. Preheat air fryer at 350°F for 3 minutes.
3. In a shallow dish, consolidate bread morsels and squashed pretzels. Shake abundance marinade off each piece of chicken and afterward dig in bread morsel blend.
4. Add half of chicken nibbles to air fryer crate. Cook 4 minutes. Shake delicately. Cook an extra 5 minutes. Check the chicken utilizing a meat thermometer to guarantee the interior temperature is at any rate 165°F. Rehash with staying chicken.
5. Move to a plate and serve warm.

Per serving Calories: 243 | Fat: 6.4 g | Protein: 27.8 g | Sodium: 490 mg | Fiber: 0.4 g | Starches: 18.9 g | Sugar: 1.1 g

SALT AND PEPPER WINGS

Sauces and rubs are delightful, yet don't disparage the force of straightforward flavors. These wings are extra crunchy and turn out extraordinary for dinner prep, since they stay firm when warmed. Go ahead and pair them with your #1 sauce, for example, low-carb grill or buttermilk farm.

Pantry Staples: Salt, ground dark pepper
Hands On schedule: 5 minutes
Cook Time: 25 minutes
Serves: 4

- 2 pounds bone-in chicken wings, isolated at joints
- 1 teaspoon salt
- ½ teaspoon ground dark pepper

1. Sprinkle wings with salt and pepper, then, at that point place into ungreased air fryer bin in a solitary layer, working in groups if required.
2. Change the temperature to 400°F and set the clock for 25 minutes, shaking the bin like clockwork during cooking. Wings ought to have an inner temperature of at any rate 165°F and be brilliant earthy colored when done.
3. Serve warm.

Per serving calories: 316 protein: 29g
Fiber: 0g net carbs: 0g fat: 22g sodium: 720mg carbs: 0g sugar: 0g

GARLIC DILL WINGS

Made for the most part with wash room staples, this formula is extraordinary when you need an extremely late dinner that will not be lacking in flavor. The dill lights up the wings to make a flavor that helps you to remember farm blend. These wings pair well with a tart Greek yogurt–based sauce, for example, tzatziki for plunging.

Pantry Staples: Salt, ground dark pepper, garlic powder
Hands On schedule: 5 minutes
Cook Time: 25 minutes
Serves: 4

- 2 pounds bone-in chicken wings, isolated at joints
- ½ teaspoon salt
- ½ teaspoon ground dark pepper
- ½ teaspoon onion powder
- ½ teaspoon garlic powder
- 1 teaspoon dried dill

1. In an enormous bowl, throw wings with salt, pepper, onion powder, garlic powder, and dill until equally covered. Spot wings into ungreased air fryer container in a solitary layer, working in bunches if required.
2. Change the temperature to 400°F and set the clock for 25 minutes, shaking the bin like clockwork during cooking. Wings ought to have an inward temperature of in any event 165°F and be brilliant earthy colored when done. Serve warm.

Per serving Calories: 319 protein: 29g
Fiber: 0g net starches: 1g fat: 22g
Sodium: 430mg starches: 1g sugar: 0g

CHICKEN FAJITA POPPERS

These poppers are scrumptious and simple to make, however they likewise warm effectively in the microwave in only 1 moment on high, making them ideal for feast prep. To add more fat and flavor to this dinner, essentially pair with your most loved plunging sauce like acrid cream or guacamole.

Hands On schedule: 10 minutes
Cook Time: 20 minutes
Yields 18 poppers

- 1 pound ground chicken thighs
- ½ medium green ringer pepper, cultivated and finely cleaved
- ¼ medium yellow onion, stripped and finely cleaved
- ½ cup destroyed pepper jack cheddar
- (1-ounce) parcel without gluten fajita preparing

1. In a huge bowl, join all Fixings . Structure blend into eighteen 2" balls and spot in a solitary layer into ungreased air fryer crate, working in clumps if required.
2. Change the temperature to 350°F and set the clock for 20 minutes. Cautiously use utensils to turn poppers partially through cooking. At the point when 5 minutes stay on clock, increment temperature to 400°F to give the poppers a dim brilliant earthy colored tone.
3. Shake air fryer crate again when 2 minutes stay on clock. Serve warm.

Per serving (3 poppers)
Calories: 164 protein: 16g Fiber: 0g net sugars: 5g fat: 8g sodium:397mg Sugars: 5g sugar: 0g

At the point when you consider ground meat, you may initially consider hamburger and turkey. In any case, remember about ground chicken! It is the ideal gentle material for an assortment of flavors. The matching of chicken and pesto in this formula is mouthwateringly heavenly and will not cause you to feel torpid.

Pantry Staples: Salt, ground dark pepper
Hands On schedule: 10 minutes
Cook Time: 12 minutes
Serves: 4

- 1 pound ground chicken thighs
- ¼ teaspoon salt
- ⅛ teaspoon ground dark pepper
- ¼ cup basil pesto
- 1 cup destroyed mozzarella cheddar
- 4 grape tomatoes, cut

1. Cut four squares of material paper to find a way into your air fryer crate.
2. Spot ground chicken in a huge bowl and blend in with salt and pepper. Gap blend into four equivalent areas.
3. Wet your hands with water to forestall staying, then, at that point press each segment into a 6" circle onto a piece of ungreased material. Spot every chicken outside layer into air fryer bushel, working in bunches if required.
4. Change the temperature to 350°F and set the clock for 10 minutes, turning hulls partially through cooking.
5. At the point when the clock signals, spread 1 tablespoon pesto across the highest point of each outside layer, then, at that point sprinkle with ¼ cup mozzarella and top with 1 cut tomato.
6. Keep cooking at 350°F for 2 minutes. Cheddar will be dissolved and earthy colored when done. Serve warm.

Per serving
Calories: 318 protein: 28g fiber: 0g
Net sugars: 4g fat: 19g sodium: 546mg Sugars: 4g

Chicken bosom meat is low in fat and as such can without much of a stretch get dried out, however the mayonnaise utilized in this dish seals in dampness. Twofold this dinner for extras and warm noticeable all around fryer at 370°F for 8 minutes.

Pantry Staples: Salt, ground dark pepper, garlic powder
Hands On schedule: 15 minutes
Cook Time: 20 minutes
Serves: 4

- 2 ounces cream cheddar, mollified
- 1 cup slashed new broccoli, steamed
- ½ cup destroyed sharp cheddar
- 4 (6-ounce) boneless, skinless chicken bosoms
- 2 tablespoons mayonnaise
- ¼ teaspoon salt
- ¼ teaspoon garlic powder
- ⅛ teaspoon ground dark pepper

1. In a medium bowl, consolidate cream cheddar, broccoli, and Cheddar. Cut a 4" pocket into every chicken bosom. Equitably split combination between chicken bosoms; stuff the pocket of every chicken bosom with the blend.
2. Spread ¼ tablespoon mayonnaise per side of every chicken bosom, then, at that point sprinkle the two sides of bosoms with salt, garlic powder, and pepper.
3. Spot stuffed chicken bosoms into ungreased air fryer bin with the goal that the open creases face up. Change the temperature to 350°F and set the clock for 20 minutes, turning chicken part of the way through cooking. At the point when done, chicken will be brilliant and have an inward temperature of at any rate 165°F. Serve warm.

Per serving
Calories: 364 protein: 43g fiber: 1g
Net carbs: 2g fat: 16g sodium: 415mg
Carbs: 3g sugar: 1g

PICKLE-TENDERIZED SEARED CHICKEN

The firm external covering in this dish is the ideal difference to the succulent internal parts, making it an extraordinary solace food supper for quickly. You can likewise cleave the chicken into 2" 3D squares prior to covering to make scaled down firm chunks—essentially diminish the Cook Time to 12 minutes.

Pantry Staples: Salt, ground dark pepper
Hands On schedule: 1 hour 15 minutes
Cook Time: 20 minutes
Serves: 4

- (4-ounce) boneless, skinless chicken thighs
- ⅓ cup dill pickle juice
- 1 enormous egg
- 2 ounces plain pork skins, squashed
- ½ teaspoon salt
- ¼ teaspoon ground dark pepper

1. Spot chicken thighs in an enormous sealable bowl or pack and pour pickle juice over them. Spot fixed bowl or sack into cooler and permit to marinate at any rate 1 hour up to expedite.
2. In a little bowl, whisk egg. Spot pork skins in a different medium bowl.
3. Eliminate chicken thighs from marinade. Shake off overabundance pickle squeeze and wipe thighs off with a paper towel. Sprinkle with salt and pepper.
4. Plunge every thigh into egg and tenderly shake off overabundance. Press into pork skins to cover each side. Spot thighs into ungreased air fryer bin. Change the temperature to 400°F and set the clock for 20 minutes. At the point when chicken thighs are done, they will be brilliant and firm outwardly with an inward temperature of at any rate 165°F. Serve warm.

Per serving
Calories: 344 protein: 44g Fiber: 0g net starches: 0g fat: 16g Sodium: 711mg starches: 0g sugar: 0g

FLAVOR SCOURED CHICKEN THIGHS

You don't require customary breading to get firm chicken—the skin alone can become ultracrispy noticeable all around fryer. The fat in the skin assists it with crisping up, while the remainder of the chicken stays delicious. The brilliance and stimulating flavor from the lime juice makes the whole dish.

Pantry Staples: Salt, paprika, garlic powder
Hands On schedule: 10 minutes
Cook Time: 25 minutes
Serves: 4

- (4-ounce) bone-in, skin-on chicken thighs
- ½ teaspoon salt
- ½ teaspoon garlic powder
- 2 teaspoons stew powder
- 1 teaspoon paprika
- 1 teaspoon ground cumin
- 1 little lime, split

Wipe chicken thighs off and sprinkle with salt, garlic powder, bean stew powder, paprika, and cumin. Press juice from ½ lime over thighs. Spot thighs into ungreased air fryer crate. Change the temperature to 380°F and set the clock for 25 minutes, turning thighs partially through cooking. Thighs will be fresh and carmelized with an inward temperature of in any event 165°F when done.
Move thighs to a huge serving plate and shower with residual lime juice. Serve warm.

Per serving
Calories: 255 Protein: 34g Fiber: 1g Net carbs: 1g Fat: 10g Sodium: 475mg Sugars: 2g

FIERY PORK SKIN SINGED CHICKEN

This dish is ideal for the individuals who love a touch of warmth. Feel free to prepare stage 1 AM before you head out for the day to save time. For extras, warm rapidly noticeable all around fryer at 400°F for 8 minutes to get back that firm outside layer.

Pantry Staples: Ground dark pepper, paprika, garlic powder
Hands On schedule: 40 minutes
Cook Time: 20 minutes
Serves: 4

- ¼ cup bison sauce
- (4-ounce) boneless, skinless chicken bosoms
- ½ teaspoon paprika
- ½ teaspoon garlic powder
- ¼ teaspoon ground dark pepper
- 2 ounces plain pork skins, finely squashed

1. Empty bison sauce into an enormous sealable bowl or pack. Add chicken and throw to cover. Spot fixed bowl or sack into cooler and let marinate in any event 30 minutes up to expedite.
2. Eliminate chicken from marinade yet don't shake overabundance sauce off chicken.

Sprinkle the two sides of thighs with paprika, garlic powder, and pepper.

3. Spot pork skins into a huge bowl and press every chicken bosom into pork skins to cover equally on the two sides.
4. Spot chicken into ungreased air fryer crate. Change the temperature to 400°F and set the clock for 20 minutes, turning chicken partially through cooking. Chicken will be brilliant and have an interior temperature of in any event 165°F when done. Serve warm.

Per serving Calories: 185
Protein: 27g fiber: 0g net starches: 1g Fat: 7g sodium: 731mg starches: 1g Sugar: 0g

CHIPOTLE DRUMSTICKS

These dark red drumsticks sneak up suddenly. They're smoky with a touch of tang, like a chipotle-enlivened grill sauce. They're additionally incredible for dinner prep and toward the end in the fridge for as long as 5 days.

Pantry Staples: Salt, ground dark pepper, garlic powder
Hands On schedule: 5 minutes
Cook Time: 25 minutes
Serves: 4

- 1 tablespoon tomato glue
- ½ teaspoon chipotle powder
- ¼ teaspoon apple juice vinegar
- ¼ teaspoon garlic powder
- 8 chicken drumsticks
- ½ teaspoon salt
- ⅛ teaspoon ground dark pepper

1. In a little bowl, consolidate tomato glue, chipotle powder, vinegar, and garlic powder.
2. Sprinkle drumsticks with salt and pepper, then, at that point place into a huge bowl and pour in tomato glue combination. Throw or mix to uniformly cover all drumsticks in blend.
3. Spot drumsticks into ungreased air fryer bin. Change the temperature to 400°F and set the clock for 25 minutes, turning drumsticks part of the way through cooking. Drumsticks will be dim red with an inward temperature of in any event 165°F when done. Serve warm.

Per serving
Calories: 432 protein: 48g fiber: 0g Net starches: 1g fat: 22g sodium: 623mg starches: 1g sugar: 0g

GARLIC PARMESAN DRUMSTICKS

Drumsticks are spending cordial and brimming with flavor. These dull brilliant Garlic Parmesan Drumsticks are covered in a light, rich sauce however never lose that delectable fresh skin. It's a supper the entire family will adore.

Pantry Staples: Salt, ground dark pepper, garlic powder
Hands On schedule: 5 minutes
Cook Time: 25 minutes
Serves: 4

- 8 (4-ounce) chicken drumsticks
- ½ teaspoon salt
- ⅛ teaspoon ground dark pepper
- ½ teaspoon garlic powder
- 2 tablespoons salted margarine, softened
- ½ cup ground Parmesan cheddar
- 1 tablespoon dried parsley

Sprinkle drumsticks with salt, pepper, and garlic powder. Spot drumsticks into ungreased air fryer bin. Change the temperature to 400°F and set the clock for 25 minutes, turning drumsticks part of the way through cooking. Drumsticks will be brilliant and have an inner temperature of in any event 165°F when done.
Move drumsticks to a huge serving dish. Pour spread over drumsticks, and sprinkle with Parmesan and parsley. Serve warm.

Per serving
Calories: 533 protein: 52g fiber: 0g
Net carbs: 3g fat: 30g sodium: 845mg
Carbs: 3g sugar: 0g

WALNUT CRUSTED CHICKEN TENDERS

Walnuts are an amazing wellspring of fat and extraordinary to appreciate with some restraint when on a keto diet. They can be sweet yet in addition pair well with more flavorful sauces like those made with Dijon mustard. Balance the supper with a fresh green serving of mixed greens.
Pantry Staples: Salt, ground dark pepper
Hands On schedule: 10 minutes
Cook Time: 12 minutes
Serves: 4

- 2 tablespoons mayonnaise
- 1 teaspoon Dijon mustard
- 1 pound boneless, skinless chicken tenders
- ½ teaspoon salt
- ¼ teaspoon ground dark pepper

- ½ cup cleaved simmered walnuts, finely ground

1. In a little bowl, whisk mayonnaise and mustard until joined. Brush blend onto chicken tenders on the two sides, then, at that point sprinkle tenders with salt and pepper.
2. Spot walnuts in a medium bowl and press each delicate into walnuts to cover each side.
3. Spot tenders into ungreased air fryer container in a solitary layer, working in bunches if required.
4. Change the temperature to 375°F and set the clock for 12 minutes, turning tenders part of the way through cooking. Tenders will be brilliant brown and have an interior temperature of at any rate 165°F when done. Serve warm.

Per serving calories: 237 protein: 22g fiber: 1g net starches: 1g fat: 15g sodium: 469mg starches: 2g sugar: 1g

DARKENED CHICKEN TENDERS

This profoundly prepared dinner is incredible if you love a touch of warmth. The formula is named after darkening flavoring, which is zesty and like Cajun flavors. For a darkened style plunging sauce, blend ¼ teaspoon Cajun preparing in ¼ cup farm dressing and serve as an afterthought.

Pantry Staples: Salt, ground dark pepper, paprika, garlic powder, coconut oil
Hands On schedule: 5 minutes
Cook Time: 12 minutes
Serves: 4
- 1 pound boneless, skinless chicken tenders
- 2 tablespoons coconut oil, softened
- 1 teaspoon paprika
- ½ teaspoon bean stew powder
- ½ teaspoon salt
- ¼ teaspoon ground dark pepper
- ¼ teaspoon garlic powder
- ¼ teaspoon cayenne pepper

1. In an enormous bowl, throw chicken tenders in coconut oil. Sprinkle each side of chicken tenders with paprika, stew powder, salt, dark pepper, garlic powder, and cayenne pepper.
2. Spot tenders into ungreased air fryer crate. Change the temperature to 375°F and set the clock for 12 minutes. Tenders will be dim brown and have an inner temperature of in any event 165°F when done. Serve warm.

Per serving Calories: 156
Protein: 21g fiber: 0g net carbs: 1g
Fat: 7g sodium: 404mg carbs: 1g
Sugar: 0g

MARGARINE AND BACON CHICKEN

This feast isn't just simple yet in addition brimming with flavor. The pungent bacon seasons the chicken, so you'll enjoy each chomp. Use extras in chicken plate of mixed greens or destroyed in taco bowls.

Pantry Staples: Salt, ground dark pepper, garlic powder
Hands On schedule: 10 minutes
Cook Time: 65 minutes
Serves: 6
- 1 (4-pound) entire chicken
- 2 tablespoons salted margarine, mellowed
- 1 teaspoon dried thyme
- ½ teaspoon garlic powder
- 1 teaspoon salt ½ teaspoon ground dark pepper
- 6 cuts sans sugar bacon

1. Wipe chicken off with a paper towel, then, at that point rub with margarine on all sides. Sprinkle thyme, garlic powder, salt, and pepper over chicken.
2. Spot chicken into ungreased air fryer container, bosom side up. Lay pieces of bacon over chicken and secure with toothpicks.
3. Change the temperature to 350°F and set the clock for 65 minutes. Partially through cooking, eliminate and put away bacon and flip chicken over. Chicken will be done when the skin is brilliant and firm and the inside temperature is at any rate 165°F. Serve warm with bacon.

Per serving
Calories: 416 protein: 36g fiber: 0g Net starches: 0g fat: 26g sodium: 666mg Starches: 0g sugar: 0g

CHICKEN CORDON BLEU

Customarily, this formula calls for breading, however with delightful **Fixings** like Dijon mustard and Swiss cheddar, you will not miss it. When purchasing ham, ensure you pick one that has a "no sugar added" mark. Present with a side of Simmered Broccoli Salad

Pantry Staples: Salt, ground dark pepper
Hands On schedule: 15 minutes
Cook Time: 25 minutes

Serves: 4

- 4 (6-ounce) boneless, skinless chicken bosoms
- 4 (1-ounce) cuts Swiss cheddar
- 4 (1-ounce) cuts no-sugar-added ham
- ¼ cup Dijon mustard
- ½ teaspoon salt
- ¼ teaspoon ground dark pepper

1. Cut a 5"- since a long time ago cut in the side of every chicken bosom. Spot a cut of Swiss and a cut of ham inside each cut.
2. Brush chicken with mustard, then, at that point sprinkle with salt and pepper on the two sides.
3. Spot chicken into ungreased air fryer crate. Change the temperature to 375°F and set the clock for 25 minutes, turning chicken partially through cooking. Chicken will be brilliant brown and have an interior temperature of in any event 165°F when done. Serve warm.

Per serving
Calories: 388 protein: 53g fiber: 0g Net starches: 3g fat: 14g sodium: 1,154mg Starches: 3g sugar: 0g

MESSY CHICKEN CHUNKS

Who can prevent the exemplary flavors from getting chicken chunks? They may bring back cherished recollections, or they may be your exacting child's #1 thing to eat at the present time.
In any case, this formula is a compelling low-carb wind on the conventional breaded pieces.

Pantry Staples: Salt, garlic powder
Hands On schedule: 10 minutes
Cook Time: 15 minutes
Serves: 4

- 1 pound ground chicken thighs
- ½ cup destroyed mozzarella cheddar
- 1 enormous egg, whisked
- ½ teaspoon salt
- ¼ teaspoon dried oregano
- ¼ teaspoon garlic powder

1. In an enormous bowl, join all Fixings . Structure combination into twenty piece shapes, around 2 tablespoons each.
2. Spot chunks into ungreased air fryer bin, working in clusters if required. Change the temperature to 375°F and set the clock for 15 minutes, turning chunks part of the way through cooking. Let cool 5 minutes prior to serving.

Per serving Calories: 222 protein: 25g
Fiber: 0g net starches: 1g fat: 12g Sodium: 472mg starches: 1g sugar: 0g

GARLIC GINGER CHICKEN

This formula is delightful alone, yet in addition makes an incredible base for a pan fried food. The ginger adds a warmth and flavor that go with an assortment of vegetables, from mushrooms to cauliflower rice. This formula utilizes soy sauce, yet go ahead and trade for fluid aminos if you like.

Pantry Staples: Salt
Hands On schedule: 30 minutes
Cook Time: 12 minutes
Serves: 4

- 1 pound boneless, skinless chicken thighs, cut into 1" pieces
- ¼ cup soy sauce
- 2 cloves garlic, stripped and finely minced
- 1 tablespoon minced ginger
- ¼ teaspoon salt

Spot all Fixings in an enormous sealable bowl or sack. Spot fixed bowl or pack into cooler and let marinate at any rate 30 minutes up to expedite. Eliminate chicken from marinade and spot into ungreased air fryer bin. Change the temperature to 375°F and set the clock for 12 minutes, shaking the bin twice during cooking. Chicken will be brilliant and have an inner temperature of at any rate 165°F when done. Serve warm.

Per serving Calories: 140
Protein: 20g fiber: 0g net carbs: 0g
Fat: 6g sodium: 184mg carbs: 0g sugar: 0g

CHIPOTLE AIOLI WINGS

A significant advantage of making wings at home is knowing precisely what's going into your bunch, so you can stay away from the carb-filled flavors and sauces frequently utilized in eatery alternatives. These wings absorb the kind of the sauce, and the air fryer concocts them rapidly, so there's no compelling reason to marinate to get the ideal nibble without fail.

Pantry Staples: Salt, ground dark pepper
Hands On schedule: 5 minutes
Cook Time: 25 minutes
Serves: 6

- 2 pounds bone-in chicken wings
- ½ teaspoon salt
- ¼ teaspoon ground dark pepper
- 2 tablespoons mayonnaise
- 2 teaspoons chipotle powder
- 2 tablespoons lemon juice

1. In an enormous bowl, throw wings in salt and pepper, then, at that point place into ungreased

air fryer bin. Change the temperature to 400°F and set the clock for 25 minutes, shaking the bin twice while cooking. Wings will be done when brilliant and have an inward temperature of at any rate 165°F.

2. In a little bowl, whisk together mayonnaise, chipotle powder, and lemon juice. Spot cooked wings into an enormous serving bowl and sprinkle with aioli. Throw to cover. Serve warm.

Per serving Calories: 243 protein: 19g Fiber: 0g net carbs: 0g fat: 18g Sodium: 368mg carbs: 0g sugar: 0g

CAJUN-BREADED CHICKEN CHOMPS

Pork skins make an incredible option to carb-filled panko bread pieces when you need breading however don't have any desire to undermine your keto diet. You can without much of a stretch equilibrium out your fat macros by adding a plunging sauce like farm or fiery mayonnaise.

Pantry Staples: Salt, ground dark pepper
Hands On schedule: 10 minutes
Cook Time: 12 minutes
Serves: 4
* 1 pound boneless, skinless chicken bosoms, cut into 1" solid shapes
* ½ cup hefty whipping cream
* ½ teaspoon salt
* ¼ teaspoon ground dark pepper
* 1 ounce plain pork skins, finely squashed
* ¼ cup unflavored whey protein powder
* ½ teaspoon Cajun preparing

1. Spot chicken in a medium bowl and pour in cream. Mix to cover. Sprinkle with salt and pepper.
2. In a different enormous bowl, join pork skins, protein powder, and Cajun preparing. Eliminate chicken from cream, shaking off any overabundance, and throw in dry blend until completely covered.
3. Spot chomps into ungreased air fryer bushel. Change the temperature to 400°F and set the clock for 12 minutes, shaking the bin twice during cooking. Nibbles will be done when brilliant brown and have an interior

temperature of in any event 165°F. Serve warm.

Per serving Calories: 285
Protein: 34g fiber: 0g Net starches: 1g fat: 16g Sodium: 497mg starches: 1g sugar: 1g

JERK CHICKEN KEBABS

Air fryer kebabs are delectable and loaded with flavor. The edges get dull earthy colored and caramelized, giving vegetables a better broiled taste. You can likewise do without the sticks and prepare the cooked **Fixings** into a plate of mixed greens or serve over cauliflower rice.

Pantry Staples: Salt, coconut oil
Hands On schedule: 10 minutes
Cook Time: 14 minutes
Serves: 4
* 8 ounces boneless, skinless chicken thighs, cut into 1" 3D shapes
* 2 tablespoons jerk preparing
* 2 tablespoons coconut oil
* ½ medium red ringer pepper, cultivated and cut into 1" pieces
* ¼ medium red onion, stripped and cut into 1" pieces
* ½ teaspoon salt

1. Spot chicken in a medium bowl and sprinkle with jerk preparing and coconut oil. Throw to cover on all sides.
2. Utilizing eight 6" sticks, fabricate sticks by rotating chicken, pepper, and onion pieces, around three redundancies for every stick.
3. Sprinkle salt over sticks and spot into ungreased air fryer crate. Change the temperature to 370°F and set the clock for 14 minutes, turning sticks part of the way through cooking.
4. Chicken will be brilliant and have an interior temperature of at any rate 165°F when done. Serve warm.

Per serving Calories: 138 Protein: 10g fiber: 0g net starches: 2g Fat: 7g sodium: 550mg starches: 2g sugar: 1g

Beef and pork are two meats, already bursting with flavor, that you can make even better with your air fryer. Who would've thought it would be possible to achieve juicy, tender pork chops in minutes? These versatile meats can be used to create classics in a flash, as well as new and exciting dishes full of healthy protein and fat. With recipes ranging from Bacon Cheeseburger Casserole to Easy Juicy Pork Chops, this chapter will help you beef up your culinary repertoire in no time!

CLASSIC MINI MEATLOAF

It seems like meatloaf has been served on dinner tables since the beginning of time. It's a classic dish that many of us remember from childhood. It's also a very easy meal that can be used to hide veggies (for the pickier eaters) without sacrificing a juicy and delicious bite every time.

HandsOn Time: 10 minutes
Cook Time: 25 minutes
Serves: 6
- 1 pound 80/20 ground beef
- 1/4 medium yellow onion, peeled and diced
- 1/2 medium green bell pepper, seeded and diced
- 1 large egg
- 3 tablespoons blanched finely ground almond flour
- 1 tablespoon Worcestershire sauce
- 1/2 teaspoon garlic powder
- 1 teaspoon dried parsley
- 2 tablespoons tomato paste
- 1/4 cup water
- 1 tablespoon powdered erythritol

Direections
- ✓ In a large bowl, combine ground beef, onion, pepper, egg, and almond flour. Pour in the Worcestershire sauce and add the garlic powder and parsley to the bowl. Mix until fully combined.
- ✓ Divide the mixture into two and place into two (4") loaf baking pans.
- ✓ In a small bowl, mix the tomato paste, water, and erythritol. Spoon half the mixture over each loaf.
- ✓ Working in batches if necessary, place loaf pans into the air fryer basket.

- ✓ Adjust the temperature to 350°F and set the timer for 25 minutes or until internal temperature is 180°F.
- ✓ Serve warm.

Per serving Calories: 170 protein: 14.9 g fiber: 0.9 g Net carbohydrates: 2.6 g sugar alcohol: 1.5 g fat: 9.4 g sodium: 85 mg Carbohydrates: 5.0 g sugar: 1.5 g

CHORIZO AND BEEF BURGER

Take burgers to the next level by adding chorizo to the mix! These juicy burgers will be ready to eat in just minutes. If you really miss having them with a bun, you can cut open Dinner Rolls (Chapter 4) and put the burgers inside! Serve these with your favorite burger toppings.

HandsOn Time: 10 minutes
Cook Time: 15 minutes
Serves 4
3/4 pound 80/20 ground beef
- 1/4 pound Mexican-style ground chorizo
- 1/4 cup chopped onion
- 5 slices pickled jalapenos, chopped
- 2 teaspoons chili powder
- 1 teaspoon minced garlic
- 1/4 teaspoon cumin

Direections
- ✓ In a large bowl, mix all ingredients. Divide the mixture into four sections and form them into burger patties.
- ✓ Place burger patties into the air fryer basket, working in batches if necessary.
- ✓ Adjust the temperature to 375°F and set the timer for 15 minutes.
- ✓ Flip the patties halfway through the cooking time. Serve warm.

Per serving
Calories: 291 protein: 21.6 g fiber: 0.9 g
Net carbohydrates: 3.8 g fat: 18.3 g sodium: 474 mg
Carbohydrates: 4.7 g sugar: 2.5 g

CRISPY BRATS

Bratwursts are such a classic summertime lunch, whether you're having a picnic in the backyard or watching a game at the ballpark. And with this recipe you won't even miss the bun! Getting the crunchy, juicy bite that they're known for is easier than ever with your air fryer!

HandsOn Time: 5 minutes
Cook Time: 15 minutes
Serves 4
* 4 (3-ounce) beef bratwursts

Direections
✓ Place brats into the air fryer basket.
✓ Adjust the temperature to 375°F and set the timer for 15 minutes.
✓ Serve warm.

Per serving
Calories: 286
Protein: 11.8 G Fiber: 0.0 G Net Carbohydrates: 0.0 G Fat: 24.8 G Sodium: 50 Mg Carbohydrates: 0.0 G

TACO-STUFFED PEPPERS

You don't have to say goodbye to Taco Tuesday just because you don't eat taco shells anymore. These zesty peppers pack all that classic taco flavor into a pepper instead!

HandsOn Time: 15 minutes
Cook Time: 15 minutes
Serves 4
* 1 pound 80/20 ground beef
* 1 tablespoon chili powder
* 2 teaspoons cumin
* 1 teaspoon garlic powder 1 teaspoon salt
* 1/4 teaspoon ground black pepper
* 1 (10-ounce) can diced tomatoes and green chiles, drained
* 4 medium green bell peppers
* 1 cup shredded Monterey jack cheese, divided

Direections
✓ In a medium skillet over medium heat, brown the ground beef about 7-10 minutes. When no pink remains, drain the fat from the skillet.
✓ Return the skillet to the stovetop and add chili powder, cumin, garlic powder, salt, and black pepper. Add drained can of diced tomatoes and chiles to the skillet. Continue cooking 3-5 minutes.
✓ While the mixture is cooking, cut each bell pepper in half. Remove the seeds and white membrane. Spoon the cooked mixture evenly into each bell pepper and top with a V4 cup cheese. Place stuffed peppers into the air fryer basket.
✓ Adjust the temperature to 350°F and set the timer for 15 minutes.
✓ When done, peppers will be fork tender and cheese will be browned and bubbling. Serve warm.

Per serving
Calories: 346 Protein: 27.8 g
Fiber: 3.5 g Net carbohydrates: 7.2 g fat: 19.1 g Sodium: 991 mg Carbohydrates: 10.7 g sugar: 4.9 g

ITALIAN STUFFED BELL PEPPERS

Italian seasonings can enhance any dish, and they do just that in these stuffed peppers! With the zesty sausage, the spicy cheese, and the perfect seasonings, this low-carb dish will have your palate pleased!

HandsOn Time: 15 minutes
Cook Time: 15 minutes
Serves 4
* 1 pound ground pork Italian sausage
* 1/2 teaspoon garlic powder
* 1/2 teaspoon dried parsley
* 1 medium Roma tomato, diced
* 1/4 cup chopped onion
* 4 medium green bell peppers
* 1 cup shredded mozzarella cheese, divided

Direections
✓ In a medium skillet over medium heat, brown the ground sausage about 7-10 minutes or until no pink remains. Drain the fat from the skillet.
✓ Return the skillet to the stovetop and add garlic powder, parsley, tomato, and onion. Continue cooking 3-5 minutes.
✓ Slice peppers in half and remove the seeds and white membrane.
✓ Remove the meat mixture from the stovetop and spoon evenly into pepper halves. Top with mozzarella. Place pepper halves into the air fryer basket.
✓ Adjust the temperature to 350°F and set the timer for 15 minutes.
✓ When done, peppers will be fork tender and cheese will be golden. Serve warm.

Per serving
Calories: 358 protein: 21.1 g fiber: 2.6 g
Net carbohydrates: 8.7 g fat: 24.1 g sodium: 1,029 mg Carbohydrates: 11.3 g sugar: 4.8 g

BACON CHEESEBURGER CASSEROLE

Casseroles are often a favorite for busy people who don't have a lot of time to think about dinner. That's because you can pretty much just put all of the ingredients in a dish and set it to bake. This burger casserole still packs all the flavor of the handheld version. Even better, your air fryer can get this done in a fraction of the time you're used to!

HandsOn Time: 15 minutes
Cook Time: 20 minutes
Serves 4

- 1 pound 80/20 ground beef
- 1/4 medium white onion, peeled and chopped
- 1 cup shredded Cheddar cheese, divided
- 1 large egg
- 4 slices sugar-free bacon, cooked and crumbled 2 pickle spears, chopped

Direections
- ✓ Brown the ground beef in a medium skillet over medium heat about 7-10 minutes. When no pink remains, drain the fat. Remove from heat and add ground beef to large mixing bowl.
- ✓ Add onion, V2 cup Cheddar, and egg to bowl. Mix ingredients well and add crumbled bacon.
- ✓ Pour the mixture into a 4-cup round baking dish and top with remaining Cheddar. Place into the air fryer basket.
- ✓ Adjust the temperature to 375°F and set the timer for 20 minutes.
- ✓ Casserole will be golden on top and firm in the middle when fully cooked. Serve immediately with chopped pickles on top.

Per serving
Calories: 369 Protein: 31.0 g fiber: 0.2 g Net carbohydrates: 1.0 g fat: 22.6 g Sodium: 454 mg carbohydrates: 1.2 g sugar: 0.5 g

PULLED PORK

Pulled pork is a barbecue classic. There's nothing better than tender shredded pork slathered in tangy barbecue sauce! Pulled pork is often a slow cooker recipe, with some methods taking more than 8 hours, but if you're short on time, cooking it in your air fryer is the perfect gateway to fast, succulent pork!

HandsOn Time: 10 minutes
Cook Time: 2V2 hours
Serves: 8

- 2 tablespoons chili powder
- 1 teaspoon garlic powder
- 1/2 teaspoon onion powder
- 1/2 teaspoon ground black pepper
- 1/2 teaspoon cumin 1 (4-pound) pork shoulder

Direections
- ✓ In a small bowl, mix chili powder, garlic powder, onion powder, pepper, and cumin. Rub the spice mixture over the pork shoulder, patting it into the skin. Place pork shoulder into the air fryer basket.
- ✓ Adjust the temperature to 350°F and set the timer for 150 minutes.
- ✓ Pork skin will be crispy and meat easily shredded with two forks when done. The internal temperature should be at least 145°F.

Per serving Calories: 537 Protein: 42.6 g fiber: 0.8 g Net carbohydrates: 0.7 g fat: 35.5 g Sodium: 180 mg carbohydrates: 1.5 g sugar: 0.2 g

BACON-WRAPPED HOT DOG

An easy favorite for the family! For a fun twist, try cutting a slit in the top of the hot dog and adding a little cheese before wrapping with the bacon!

HandsOn Time: 5 minutes
Cook Time: 10 minutes
Serves 4

- 4 beef hot dogs
- 4 slices sugar-free bacon

Direections
- ✓ Wrap each hot dog with slice of bacon and secure with toothpick. Place into the air fryer basket.
- ✓ Adjust the temperature to 370°F and set the timer for 10 minutes.
- ✓ Flip each hot dog halfway through the cooking time. When fully cooked, bacon will be crispy. Serve warm.

Per serving
Calories: 197 Protein: 9.2 g fiber: 0.0 g net carbohydrates: 1.3 g fat: 15.0 g sodium: 571 mg carbohydrates: 1.3 g sugar: 0.6 g

EASY JUICY PORK CHOPS

Pork chops are truly one of the easiest main dishes to cook in your air fryer. This cooking technique seals in all the flavorful juices while crisping up the outside for a succulent bite every time. You're just minutes away from pork chop perfection with this recipe!

HandsOn Time: 5 minutes
Cook Time: 15 minutes
Serves 2

- 1 teaspoon chili powder
- 1/2 teaspoon garlic powder
- 1/2 teaspoon cumin
- 1/4 teaspoon ground black pepper
- 1/4 teaspoon dried oregano 2 (4-ounce) boneless pork chops
- 2 tablespoons unsalted butter, divided

Direections

- ✓ In a small bowl, mix chili powder, garlic powder, cumin, pepper, and oregano. Rub dry rub onto pork chops. Place pork chops into the air fryer basket.
- ✓ Adjust the temperature to 400°F and set the timer for 15 minutes.
- ✓ The internal temperature should be at least 145°F when fully cooked. Serve warm, each topped with 1 tablespoon butter.

Per serving Calories: 313 Protein: 24.4 g Fiber: 0.7 g Net carbohydrates: 1.1 g fat: 22.6 g Sodium: 117 mg Carbohydrates: 1.8 g sugar: 0.1 g

SEASONING TIP!
If you're not sure how to season your meat, you can find lots of flavorful dry rubs in your grocery store. Just be sure to check the ingredients carefully as many of these seasonings are loaded with sugar!

REVERSE SEARED RIBEYE

The two main components of a tasty ribeye steak are the juicy inside and the dark sear on the outside. Who would've thought you'd be able to get both in no time with no maintenance at all? This recipe will get you the perfect medium steak, but be sure to adjust the cook time if you prefer yours more or less done!

HandsOn Time: 5 minutes
Cook Time: 45 minutes
Serves 2

- 1 (8-ounce) ribeye steak
- 2 teaspoon pink Himalayan salt
- 4 teaspoon ground peppercorn
- 1 tablespoon coconut oil
- 1 tablespoon salted butter, softened
- 4 teaspoon garlic powder
- 2 teaspoon dried parsley
- 4 teaspoon dried oregano

Direections

- ✓ Rub steak with salt and ground peppercorn. Place into the air fryer basket.
- ✓ Adjust the temperature to 250°F and set the timer for 45 minutes.

- ✓ After timer beeps, begin checking doneness and add a few minutes until internal temperature is your personal preference.
- ✓ In a medium skillet over medium heat, add coconut oil. When oil is hot, ☐uickly sear outside and sides of steak until crisp and browned. Remove from heat and allow steak to rest.
- ✓ In a small bowl, whip butter with garlic powder, parsley, and oregano.
- ✓ Slice steak and serve with herb butter on top.

Per serving Calories: 377 protein: 22.6 g fiber: 0.2 g Net carbohydrates: 0.4 g fat: 30.7 g sodium: 490 mg Carbohydrates: 0.6 g sugar: 0.0 g

PUB-STYLE BURGER

This burger is just bursting with flavor, and it will easily rival any restaurant favorite! After just one bite you'll be ready to kiss those long drive-through lanes goodbye because you'll be able to make your own delicious, much higher-☐uality burger at home in minutes, thanks to your air fryer!

HandsOn Time: 10 minutes
Cook Time: 10 minutes
Serves 4

- 1 pound ground sirloin
- 1/2 teaspoon salt
- 1/4 teaspoon ground black pepper
- 2 tablespoons salted butter, melted
- 1/2 cup full-fat mayonnaise
- 2 teaspoons sriracha
- 1/4 teaspoon garlic powder
- 8 large leaves butter lettuce
- 4 Bacon- Wrapped Onion Rings (Chapter 3)
- 8 slices pickle

Direections

- ✓ In a medium bowl, combine ground sirloin, salt, and pepper. Form four patties. Brush each with butter and then place into the air fryer basket.
- ✓ Adjust the temperature to 380°F and set the timer for 10 minutes.
- ✓ Flip the patties halfway through the cooking time for a medium burger. Add an additional 3-5 minutes for well-done.
- ✓ In a small bowl, mix mayonnaise, sriracha, and garlic powder. Set aside.
- ✓ Place each cooked burger on a lettuce leaf and top with onion ring, two pickles, and dollop of your prepared burger sauce. Wrap another lettuce leaf around tightly to hold. Serve warm.

PIGS IN A BLANKET

This take on a childhood favorite adds more substance to a plain old hot dog and is the perfect match for your air fryer. Instead of a regular hot dog, which often contains a mixture of poor-quality meats, this recipe uses 100 percent beef sausage, still very low in carbs but a whole lot better for your overall health!

HandsOn Time: 10 minutes
Cook Time: 7 minutes
Serves 2

- 1/2 cup shredded mozzarella cheese
- 2 tablespoons blanched finely ground almond flour
- 1 ounce full-fat cream cheese
- 2 (2-ounce) beef smoked sausages
- 1/2 teaspoon sesame seeds

Direections
- ✓ Place mozzarella, almond flour, and cream cheese in a large microwave-safe bowl. Microwave for 45 seconds and stir until smooth. Roll dough into a ball and cut in half.
- ✓ Press each half out into a 4" x 5" rectangle. Roll one sausage up in each dough half and press seams closed. Sprinkle the top with sesame seeds.
- ✓ Place each wrapped sausage into the air fryer basket.
- ✓ Adjust the temperature to 400°F and set the timer for 7 minutes.
- ✓ The outside will be golden when completely cooked. Scrve immediately.

CRISPY BEEF AND BROCCOLI STIR-FRY

You might be surprised to learn that your air fryer is perfect for cooking stir-fry! Temporarily removing your fryer basket and giving it a good shake is a great way to ensure even cooking, or "stir" your dish while it's still cooking.

HandsOn Time: 1 hour
Cook Time: 20 minutes
Serves 2

- 1/2 pound sirloin steak, thinly sliced
- 2 tablespoons soy sauce (or liquid aminos)
- 1/4 teaspoon grated ginger
- 1/4 teaspoon finely minced garlic
- 1 tablespoon coconut oil
- 2 cups broccoli florets
- 1/4 teaspoon crushed red pepper
- 1/8 teaspoon xanthan gum
- 1/2 teaspoon sesame seeds

Direections
- ✓ To marinate beef, place it into a large bowl or storage bag and add soy sauce, ginger, garlic, and coconut oil. Allow to marinate for 1 hour in refrigerator.
- ✓ Remove beef from marinade, reserving marinade, and place beef into the air fryer basket.
- ✓ Adjust the temperature to 320°F and set the timer for 20 minutes.
- ✓ After 10 minutes, add broccoli and sprinkle red pepper into the fryer basket and shake.
- ✓ Pour the marinade into a skillet over medium heat and bring to a boil, then reduce to simmer. Stir in xanthan gum and allow to thicken.
- ✓ When air fryer timer beeps, quickly empty fryer basket into skillet and toss. Sprinkle with sesame seeds. Serve immediately.

EMPANADAS

Empanadas are savory Latin American-style pastries usually filled with a Mexican seasoned meat. Serve these with your favorite dipping sauces.

HandsOn Time: 15 minutes
Cook Time: 10 minutes
Yields 4 empanadas (1 per serving)

- 1 pound 80/20 ground beef
- 1/4 cup water
- 1/4 cup diced onion
- 2 teaspoons chili powder
- 1/2 teaspoon garlic powder
- 1/4 teaspoon cumin
- 1/2 cups shredded mozzarella cheese
- 1/2 cup blanched finely ground almond flour
- 2 ounces full-fat cream cheese

- 1 large egg

Direections

- ✓ 1 In a medium skillet over medium heat, brown the ground beef about 7-10 minutes. Drain the fat. Return skillet to stove.
- ✓ 2 Add water and onion to the skillet. Stir and sprinkle with chili powder, garlic powder, and cumin. Reduce heat and simmer an additional 3-5 minutes. Remove from heat and set aside.
- ✓ 3 In a large microwave-safe bowl, add mozzarella, almond flour, and cream cheese. Microwave for 1 minute. Stir until smooth. Form the mixture into a ball.
- ✓ 4 Place dough between two sheets of parchment and roll out to V4" thickness. Cut the dough into four s□uares. Place V4 of ground beef onto the bottom half of each s□uare. Fold the dough over and roll the edges up or press with a wet fork to close.
- ✓ 5 Crack egg into small bowl and whisk. Brush egg over empanadas.
- ✓ 6 Cut a piece of parchment to fit your air fryer basket and place the empanadas on the parchment. Place into the air fryer basket.
- ✓ 7 Adjust the temperature to 400°F and set the timer for 10 minutes.
- ✓ 8 Flip the empanadas halfway through the cooking time. Serve warm.

Per serving Calories: 463 protein: 33.3 g fiber: 2.2 g Net carbohydrates: 4.3 g fat: 30.8 g sodium: 426 mg carbohydrates: 6.5 g sugar: 1.9 g

PEPPERCORN-CRUSTED BEEF TENDERLOIN

This buttery beef tenderloin is deliciously tender and perfectly seasoned with a blend of crushed peppercorns. It's the perfect elevated dish for a special occasion, even though it takes just minutes to prepare!

HandsOn Time: 10 minutes
Cook Time: 25 minutes
Serves 6

- 2 tablespoons salted butter, melted
- 2 teaspoons minced roasted garlic
- 3 tablespoons ground 4-peppercorn blend
- 1 (2-pound) beef tenderloin, trimmed of visible fat

Direections

- ✓ In a small bowl, mix the butter and roasted garlic. Brush it over the beef tenderloin.

- ✓ Place the ground peppercorns onto a plate and roll the tenderloin through them, creating a crust. Place tenderloin into the air fryer basket.
- ✓ Adjust the temperature to 400°F and set the timer for 25 minutes.
- ✓ Turn the tenderloin halfway through the cooking time.
- ✓ Allow meat to rest 10 minutes before slicing.

Per serving Calories: 289 protein: 34.7 g fiber: 0.9 g Net carbohydrates: 1.6 g fat: 13.8 g sodium: 96 mg Carbohydrates: 2.5 g sugar: 0.0 g

BREADED PORK CHOPS

Southern-style pork chops aren't complete without a crispy breading. While you wouldn't use flour and bread crumbs on a keto diet, you can definitely make a coating out of more pork . . . pork rinds! It tastes great and adds zero carbs to your delicious meal!

HandsOn Time: 10 minutes
Cook Time: 15 minutes
Serves 4

- 1/2 ounces pork rinds, finely ground
- 1 teaspoon chili powder
- 1/2 teaspoon garlic powder
- 1 tablespoon coconut oil, melted
- 4 (4-ounce) pork chops

Direections

- ✓ 1 In a large bowl, mix ground pork rinds, chili powder, and garlic powder.
- ✓ 2 Brush each pork chop with coconut oil and then press into the pork rind mixture, coating both sides. Place each coated pork chop into the air fryer basket.
- ✓ 3 Adjust the temperature to 400°F and set the timer for 15 minutes.
- ✓ 4 Flip each pork chop halfway through the cooking time.
- ✓ 5 When fully cooked the pork chops will be golden on the outside and have an internal temperature of at least 145°F.

Per serving Calories: 292 protein: 29.5 g fiber: 0.3 g Net carbohydrates: 0.3 g fat: 18.5 g sodium: 268 mg Carbohydrates: 0.6 g sugar: 0.1 g

EASY LASAGNA CASSEROLE

Forget the layers! This easy casserole is especially for the on- the-go chef who doesn't have time for anything too fancy. You don't miss out on a single lasagna flavor by baking all of the ingredients together, and nobody will know the difference!

HandsOn Time: 15 minutes
Cook Time: 15 minutes
Serves 4

- 3/4 cup low-carb no-sugar-added pasta sauce
- 1 pound 80/20 ground beef, cooked and drained
- 1/2 cup full-fat ricotta cheese
- 1/4 cup grated Parmesan cheese
- 1/2 teaspoon garlic powder
- 1 teaspoon dried parsley
- 1/2 teaspoon dried oregano
- 1 cup shredded mozzarella cheese

Direections

✓ In a 4-cup round baking dish, pour V4 cup pasta sauce on the bottom of the dish. Place V4 of the ground beef on top of the sauce.

✓ In a small bowl, mix ricotta, Parmesan, garlic powder, parsley, and oregano. Place dollops of half the mixture on top of the beef.

✓ Sprinkle with V3 of the mozzarella. Repeat layers until all beef, ricotta mixture, sauce, and mozzarella are used, ending with the mozzarella on top.

✓ Cover dish with foil and place into the air fryer basket.

✓ Adjust the temperature to 370°F and set the timer for 15 minutes.

✓ In the last 2 minutes of cooking, remove the foil to brown the cheese. Serve immediately.

Per serving
Calories: 371 protein: 31.4 g fiber: 1.6 g
Net carbohydrates: 4.2 g fat: 21.4 g sodium: 633 mg
Carbohydrates: 5.8 g sugar: 1.9 g

FAJITA FLANK STEAK ROLLS

Weekday dinner doesn't have to be boring! These steak rolls come together ☐uickly and can even be prepped the night before. Feel free to switch up the filling with your own favorites, such as spinach with provolone or even Parmesan and asparagus spears.

HandsOn Time: 20 minutes
Cook Time: 15 minutes
Serves 6

- 2 tablespoons unsalted butter
- 1/4 cup diced yellow onion
- 1 medium red bell pepper, seeded and sliced into strips
- 1 medium green bell pepper, seeded and sliced into strips
- 2 teaspoons chili powder 1 teaspoon cumin

- 1/2 teaspoon garlic powder
- 2 pounds flank steak
- 4 (1-ounce) slices pepper jack cheese

Direections

✓ In a medium skillet over medium heat, melt butter and begin sauteing onion, red bell pepper, and green bell pepper. Sprinkle with chili powder, cumin, and garlic powder. Saute until peppers are tender, about 5-7 minutes.

✓ Lay flank steak flat on a work surface. Spread onion and pepper mixture over entire steak rectangle. Lay slices of cheese on top of onions and peppers, barely overlapping.

✓ With the shortest end toward you, begin rolling the steak, tucking the cheese down into the roll as necessary. Secure the roll with twelve toothpicks, six on each side of the steak roll. Place steak roll into the air fryer basket.

✓ Adjust the temperature to 400°F and set the timer for 15 minutes.

✓ Rotate the roll halfway through the cooking time.

✓ Add an additional 1-4 minutes depending on your preferred internal temperature (135°F for medium).

✓ When timer beeps, allow roll to rest 15 minutes, then slice into six even pieces. Serve warm.

Per serving
Calories: 439 protein: 38.0 g fiber: 1.2 g
Net carbohydrates: 2.5 g fat: 26.6 g sodium: 226 mg
Carbohydrates: 3.7 g sugar: 1.8 g

GROUND BEEF TACO ROLLS

This fun and meaty dish is a Mexican-style spin on an egg roll! Dip these rolls in salsa, sour cream, and guacamole, all low-carb sauces that will enhance the flavor!

HandsOn Time: 20 minutes
Cook Time: 10 minutes
Serves 4

- 1/2 pound 80/20 ground beef
- 1/3 cup water
- 1 tablespoon chili powder
- 2 teaspoons cumin
- 1/2 teaspoon garlic powder
- 1/4 teaspoon dried oregano
- 1/4 cup canned diced tomatoes and chiles, drained
- 2 tablespoons chopped cilantro
- 1/2 cups shredded mozzarella cheese

- 1/2 cup blanched finely ground almond flour
- 2 ounces full-fat cream cheese
- 1 large egg

Direections

✓ In a medium skillet over medium heat, brown the ground beef about 7-10 minutes. When meat is fully cooked, drain.

✓ Add water to skillet and stir in chili powder, cumin, garlic powder, oregano, and tomatoes with chiles. Add cilantro. Bring to a boil, then reduce heat to simmer for 3 minutes.

✓ In a large microwave-safe bowl, place mozzarella, almond flour, cream cheese, and egg. Microwave for 1 minute. Stir the mixture □uickly until smooth ball of dough forms.

✓ Cut a piece of parchment for your work surface.

✓ Press the dough into a large rectangle on the parchment, wetting your hands to prevent the dough from sticking as necessary. Cut the dough into eight rectangles.

✓ On each rectangle place a few spoons of the meat mixture. Fold the short ends of each roll toward the center and roll the length as you would a burrito.

✓ Cut a piece of parchment to fit your air fryer basket. Place taco rolls onto the parchment and place into the air fryer basket.

✓ Adjust the temperature to 360°F and set the timer for 10 minutes.

✓ Flip halfway through the cooking time.

✓ Allow to cool 10 minutes before serving.

Per serving Calories: 380 Protein: 24.8 g
Fiber: 2.5 g Net carbohydrates: 4.5 g fat: 26.5 g
Sodium: 452 mg Carbohydrates: 7.0 g Sugar: 2.0 g

CRISPY PORK CHOP SALAD

It's nearly impossible to overstate the importance of vegetables on a keto diet. They contain key nutrients that help keep your body healthy and functioning properly. One of the best ways to make a salad filling is by adding mouthwatering protein to it. This crispy pork chop salad does just that, and it's something you're going to want to eat every day!

HandsOn Time: 15 minutes
Cook Time: 8 minutes
Serves 2

- 1 tablespoon coconut oil
- 2 (4-ounce) pork chops, chopped into 1" cubes
- 2 teaspoons chili powder
- 1 teaspoon paprika
- 1/2 teaspoon garlic powder
- 1/4 teaspoon onion powder
- 4 cups chopped romaine
- 1 medium Roma tomato, diced
- 1/2 cup shredded Monterey jack cheese
- 1 medium avocado, peeled, pitted, and diced
- 1/4 cup full-fat ranch dressing
- 1 tablespoon chopped cilantro

Direections

✓ In a large bowl, drizzle coconut oil over pork. Sprinkle with chili powder, paprika, garlic powder, and onion powder. Place pork into the air fryer basket.

✓ Adjust the temperature to 400°F and set the timer for 8 minutes.

✓ Pork will be golden and crispy when fully cooked.

✓ In a large bowl, place romaine, tomato, and crispy pork. Top with shredded cheese and avocado. Pour ranch dressing around bowl and toss the salad to evenly coat.

✓ Top with cilantro. Serve immediately.

Per serving Calories: 526 Protein: 34.4 g Fiber: 8.6 g
Net carbohydrates: 5.2 g fat: 37.0 g Sodium: 354 mg
Carbohydrates: 13.8 g sugar: 3.1 g

OVERSIZED BBQ MEATBALLS

These aren't your average meatballs! Supersized, savory, and stuffed with sizzling bacon, they make a filling dinner to satisfy any flavor-loving carnivore!

HandsOn Time: 10 minutes
Cook Time: 14 minutes
Serves 4

- 1 pound 80/20 ground beef
- 1/4 pound ground Italian sausage
- 1 large egg
- 1/4 teaspoon onion powder
- 1/2 teaspoon garlic powder
- 1 teaspoon dried parsley
- 4 slices sugar-free bacon, cooked and chopped
- 1/4 cup chopped white onion
- 1/4 cup chopped pickled jalapenos
- 1/2 cup low-carb, sugar-free barbecue sauce

Direections

✓ In a large bowl, mix ground beef, sausage, and egg until fully combined. Mix in all remaining ingredients except barbecue sauce. Form into eight meatballs. Place meatballs into the air fryer basket.

- ✓ Adjust the temperature to 400°F and set the timer for 14 minutes.
- ✓ Turn the meatballs halfway through the cooking time.
- ✓ When done, meatballs should be browned on the outside and have an internal temperature of at least 180°F.
- ✓ Remove meatballs from fryer and toss in barbecue sauce. Serve warm.

Per serving

Calories: 336 protein: 28.1 g fiber: 0.4 g
Net carbohydrates: 4.0 g fat: 19.5 g sodium: 761 mg
Carbohydrates: 4.4 g sugar: 0.7 g

FILET MIGNON STEAK STICKS

Planning Time: 10 minutes
Cook Time: 12 minutes
Serves:: 4 **Servings**
Fixings

- ¼ cup avocado oil
- 1 pound (cut into 1" lumps) filet mignon steak
- 1 tablespoon minced garlic
- ¼ cup soy sauce
- ½ teaspoon cumin, ground
- 1 teaspoon stevia
- 8 ounces (eliminate stems) child bella mushrooms
- ¼ teaspoon dark pepper
- 1 (slash into 1" pieces) green ringer pepper
- 1 (cleave into 1" pieces) red onion
- Salt and pepper, as important

Technique

1. Add dark pepper, salt, cumin, garlic, stevia, soy sauce, avocado oil and steak into a major bowl, blend until very much joined, and let sit for 30 minutes until marinated.
2. Alternatingly string red onion, green pepper, mushrooms and the meat onto pre-drenched bamboo sticks. Warmth up air fryer to 390ºF. Include the steak sticks to the bin of the preheated air fryer and cook for 5-6 minutes.
3. Flip sticks and cook for 5-6 additional minutes.

Dietary Data/Serving

Calories 320 kcal, Fat 18g, Protein 28g, Carbs 9g

MUSHROOM STEAK PIECES

Planning Time: 10 minutes
Cook Time: 20 minutes
Serves:: 4 **Servings**
Fixings

- 8 ounces (clean, wash and cut into equal parts) mushrooms
- 1 pound (cut into 1" 3D squares and wipe off) steaks
- 1 tsp Worcestershire sauce
- 2 tbsp dissolved margarine
- Salt and dark pepper, as fundamental
- 1/2 tsp garlic powder

Trimming with
New minced cilantro

Strategy

1. Add mushrooms and cubed meats into a bowl and blend until consolidated. Add liquefied margarine into the meat blend until throw until covered. Sprinkle pepper, salt, garlic powder and Worcestershire sauce over blend over combination. For 4 minutes, heat up air fryer to 400ºF.
2. Add the mushroom-meat blend into the crate of the preheated air fryer in one layer. Cook for 10-18 minutes at 400ºF. Flip and shake air fryer bushel threefold while cooking. Check for doneness and cook for 2-5 additional minutes, if essential.
3. Serve warm, embellished with new minced cilantro.

Healthful Data/Serving
Calories 198 kcal, Protein 23.9g, Carbs 3.5g, Fat 9.8g

YUMMY MEAT SATAY WITH COOKED PISTACHIOS

Planning Time: 5 minutes
Cook Time: 8 minutes
Serves:: 2 **Servings**
Fixings

- 2 tbsps avocado oil
- 1 lb. (cut into slender long strips) meat flank steak
- 1 tbsp soy sauce
- 1 tbsp fish sauce
- 1 tbsp garlic, minced
- 1 tbsp ginger, minced
- 1 tsp sriracha sauce
- 1 tbsp fluid stevia
- 1/2 cup (partitioned) parsley, slashed

- 1 tsp coriander, ground
- 1/4 cup (cooked) pistachios, cleaved

Technique

Add hamburger into a major bowl. Add 1/4 cup parsley, coriander, sriracha, stevia, garlic, ginger, soy sauce, fish sauce and avocado oil into the enormous bowl and blend until joined.

Refrigerate hamburger combination for 30 minutes until marinated. Move hamburger into the wire bin of an air fryer in one single layer. Dispose of abundance marinade. Cook hamburger for 8 minutes at 360ºF. Turn hamburger halfway while cooking. Move into a platter and top with simmered pistachios and 1/4 cup cleaved parsley.

Serve and delve in.

Nourishing Data/Serving

Calories 582 kcal, Fat 34g, Protein 56g, Carbs 12g

CARNE ASADA WITH GRAPEFRUIT

Planning Time: 10 minutes
Cook Time: 8 minutes
Serves:: 4 Servings
Fixings

- 1 medium (stripped and cultivated) grapefruit
- 2 medium (squeezed) limes
- 1 (diced) jalapeño pepper
- 1 cup parsley
- 2 tbsps white vinegar
- 2 tbsps avocado oil
- 1 tsps stevia
- 2 tsps ancho chile powder
- 1 tsp cumin seeds
- 1 tsp salt
- 1/2 lbs. skirt steak
- 1 tsp coriander seeds

Technique

1. Add each fixing into a high velocity electric blender, barring the skirt steak. Mix blend until a smooth consistency is reached. Cut steak into 4 segments and move into a Ziploc sack.
2. Add the mixed marinade into the Ziploc pack, shake and refrigerate for 1-8 hours until marinated. Warmth up air fryer to 400ºF. Work in clusters, move the marinated steaks into the wire bushel of an air fryer in a solitary layer.
3. Cook until steak arrives at an inward temperature of 145ºF, for 8 minutes. Let sit to cool prior to serving.

Dietary Data/Serving Calories 330 kcal, Fat 19g, Protein 37g, Carbs 1g

DELICIOUS HAMBURGER PORTION SLIDERS

Planning Time: 10 minutes
Cook Time: 10 minutes
Serves:: 8 Servings
Fixings

- 2 (beaten) eggs
- 1 pound ground meat
- 1 minced garlic clove
- ¼ cup (cleaved finely) onion
- ¼ cup coconut flour
- ½ cup (extra-fine) almond flour, whitened
- ½ teaspoon ocean salt
- ¼ cup ketchup
- 1 tablespoon Worcestershire Sauce
- ½ teaspoon dark pepper
- ½ teaspoon dried dill
- 1 teaspoon Italian flavoring

Strategy

1. Add each fixing into a major bowl and blend until all around joined. Structure 1" thick and 2" wide patties from the blend. Move patties into a cooler for 10 minutes to solidify. Warmth up air fryer to 360ºF. Work in bunches, include patties into the air fryer container.
2. Seal the cover and air fry for 10 minutes. Halfway during cooking, check the patties. Rehash measure with the leftover patties. Present with broiled vegetables or keto salad.

Dietary Data/Serving

Calories 228 kcal, Protein 13g, Carbs 4g, Fat 5g

HAMBURGER STEAK NIBBLES

Planning Time: 15 minutes
Cook Time: 20 minutes
Serves:: 4 **Servings**
Fixings

- 1 egg, enormous
- 1 lb. (cut into lumps) hamburger steak
- Avocado oil

Farm Plunge

- 1/4 cup harsh cream
- 1/4 cup mayo
- 1/2 tsp farm dressing
- 1 tsp chipotle glue

- 1/4 (squeezed) lemon, medium

Breading
- 1/2 cup pork skin
- 1/2 cup parmesan cheddar, ground
- 1/2 tsp prepared salt

Technique
1. Add each farm plunge fixing into a bowl and blend until very much joined. Spot blend into a fridge for 30 minutes-7 days. Add prepared salt, parmesan cheddar and pork skin into a bowl, join and let sit.
2. Warmth up air fryer to 400ºF. Add 1 egg into a bowl and beat well. Submerge steak pieces into the egg wash and plunge into the pork skin bowl until completely covered. Move breaded steak lumps onto a heating skillet fixed with material paper.
3. Move skillet with steak into a cooler for 30 minutes. Coat the wired bin of an air fryer with avocado oil and add the chilled lumps of steaks in a solitary layer. Seal air fryer lead and cook for 5 minutes. Flip takes and cook for 2-3 additional minutes.
4. Season with additional salt, let sit to cool and present with farm plunge.

Nourishing Data/Serving
Calories 350 kcal, Fat 20g, Protein 40g, Carbs 1g

HAMBURGER BULGOGI WITH SCALLION-MAYO SAUCE

Planning Time: 15 minutes
Cook Time: 10 minutes
Serves:: 4 **Servings**
Fixings (hamburger)
- 2 tbsp gochujang
- 1 lb. ground hamburger, lean
- 2 tsp garlic, minced
- 1 tbsp dim soy sauce
- 2 tsp stevia
- 2 tsp ginger, minced
- 1/4 cup green onions
- 1 tbsp sesame Oil
- 1/2 teaspoon salt

Scallion-Mayo Sauce
- 1 tbsp gochujang
- 1/4 cup mayonnaise
- 2 tsp sesame seeds
- 1 tbsp sesame oil
- 1/4 cup (slashed) scallions

Technique
1. Add salt, slashed onions, sesame oil, stevia, ginger, garlic, soy sauce, gochujang and ground meat into a major bowl, blend until consolidated and refrigerate for 1-8 hours.
2. Structure blend into 4 round patties and make a space in the focal point of every patty. Move patties into the wire crate of an air fryer in one layer, and cook for 10 minutes at 360ºF.
3. Meanwhile, add each mayo sauce fixing into a bowl and blend until all around consolidated. Serve hamburger bulgogi with scallion-mayo sauce over keto burgers or with no guarantees.

Healthful Data/Serving
Calories 392 kcal, Fat 29g, Protein 24g, Cards 7g

RIBEYE STEAK WITH SPICE SPREAD

Planning Time: 20 minutes
Cook Time: 15 minutes
Serves:: 2 **Servings**
Fixings
- Salt and newly broke dark pepper
- 2 (8 ounces) Ribeye steak, at room temperature
- Avocado oil

Herbed Margarine
- 2 tablespoons new slashed cilantro
- 1 stick (relaxed) margarine, unsalted
- 1 teaspoon Worcestershire Sauce
- 2 teaspoons minced garlic
- 1/2 teaspoon salt

Technique
1. Add each element for the spice spread into a bowl and blend until very much joined. Add into a material sheet and move until a log is framed. Spot in a fridge to chill prior to serving.
2. Coat steak with avocado oil until uniformly covered on the two sides and sprinkle with newly broke dark pepper and salt. Coat the wired container of an air fryer and warmth up to 400ºF. Add steak into the preheated air fryer bin.
3. Seal the top and cook for 6 minutes, flip and cook for 6 additional minutes, for medium cooked steak.

Nourishing Data/Serving
Calories 579 kcal, Protein 29.5g, All out Carbs 2.5g, Fat 49.5g

FIERY THROW STEAK WITH COCOA

Planning Time: 20 minutes
Cook Time: 10 minutes
Serves:: 2 **Servings**
Fixings

- 1/2 teaspoons ocean salt, coarse
- 1 pound toss steak
- 1/2 teaspoon espresso, ground
- 1 teaspoon earthy colored sugar
- 1/4 teaspoon bean stew powder
- 1/2 teaspoon dark pepper
- 1/4 teaspoon onion powder
- 1/4 teaspoon garlic powder
- 1/4 teaspoon chipotle powder
- 1/4 teaspoon paprika
- 1/8 teaspoon cocoa powder
- 1/8 teaspoon coriander

Technique

Add each zest into a little bowl, including cocoa and espresso and speed until separated and consolidated. Pour a liberal measure of the zest blend onto a platter. Coat and rub steak into the zest combination until uniformly covered.

Turn steak over and coat well on the opposite side. Coat the wired container of an air fryer with avocado oil. For 3 minutes, heat up air fryer to 390ºF. Spot steak in the pre-arranged air fryer bushel, seal and cook for 9 minutes. Note: don't open container or flip all through the cooking.

Eliminate the cooked steak, let sit for 5 minutes, cut and serve.

Dietary Data/Serving

Calories 495 kcal, Fay 32g, Protein 46g, Carbs 5g

BABY BACK RIBS

Planning Time: 15 minutes
Cook Time: 35 minutes
Serves:: 4 **Servings**
Fixings

- 1 tbsp avocado oil
- 1 rack (dispose of film from the back; wipe off and cut into 4 lumps) baby back ribs
- 1 tbsp stevia powder
- 1 tbsp fluid smoke
- 1/2 tsp dark pepper, ground
- 1/2 tsp salt
- 1/2 tsp onion powder
- 1/2 tsp garlic powder
- 1 cup bar-b-que sauce
- 1/2 tsp bean stew powder

Technique

1. Add fluid smoke and avocado oil into a little bowl and consolidate. Coat ribs uniformly with the fluid smoke blend. Add stew powder, onion powder, garlic pow-der, pepper, salt and stevia powder into a bowl and consolidate.
2. Sprinkle preparing blend over ribs until entirely covered on each side. Allow ribs to sit until flavors are implanted, for 30 minutes. Warmth up air fryer to 375ºF. Spot the prepared ribs in a single layer on the wire container of the air fryer.
3. Cook ribs for 15 minutes. Turn ribs and cook for 10 additional minutes. Take out ribs from the air fryer and coat bone-side of baby back ribs with 1/2 cup bar-b-que sauce. Return ribs into the air fryer bushel, cook for 5 minutes prior to flipping.
4. Coat the turned rib side (meat side) with the held 1/2 cup bar-b-que sauce and cook until singed as wanted, for 5 additional minutes.

Wholesome Data/Serving

Calories 445 kcal, Protein 18.2g, Carbs 26.8g, Fat 29g

GARLIC PORK SLASHES WITH CHEDDAR

Planning Time: 10 minutes
Cook Time: 15 minutes
Serves:: 6 **Servings**
Fixings

- 1/2 teaspoons garlic powder
- 1/2 cup parmesan cheddar, ground
- 1 teaspoon sage, dried
- 1 tablespoon cilantro, dried
- 3/4 teaspoon salt
- 1 teaspoon paprika
- 1/2 teaspoon onion powder
- 1/2 teaspoon pepper
- 1/8 teaspoon basil
- 1/4 teaspoon stew powder
- 4 pork hacks
- 1 tablespoon avocado oil

Strategy

1. Warmth up air fryer to 380ºF. Coat the bushel of the air fryer with avocado oil. Add flavors and parmesan cheddar into a level lined bowl and race until all around joined.
2. Add avocado oil into a major skillet over medications heat. Sprinkle flavor combination over pork until entirely covered. Cook until pork is singed on the two sides. Move the burned pork into the preheated air fryer and cook until all around cooked, for around 10-14 minutes at 380ºF. Flip once during cooking.

Healthful Data/Serving
Calories 423 kcal, Protein 59.8g, Carbs 4g, Fat 17.2g

SOGGY PORK HACKS

Planning Time: 2 minutes
Cook Time: 15 minutes
Serves:: 4 **Servings**
Fixings
- Salt and pepper, as essential
- 4 (boneless; thick) pork cleaves

Strategy
1. Sprinkle pepper and salt over pork cleaves until generously prepared. Move pork cleaves into the wire bin of an air fryer in one layer. Cook for until pork cleaves are very much cooked, for 10-15 minutes. Turn pork cleaves halfway during cooking.

Nourishing Data/Serving
Calories 328 kcal, Protein 40g, Carbs 0g, Fat 17g

PORK THIT NUONG

Planning Time: 20 minutes
Cook Time: 10 minutes
Serves:: 4 **Servings**
Fixings (marinade)
- 2 tbsps avocado oil
- 1/4 cup onions, minced
- 2 tsps dim soy sauce
- 1 tbsp splenda
- 1 tbsp fish sauce
- 1 tbsp garlic, minced
- 1/2 tsp pepper
- 1 tbsp (locally acquired) minced lemongrass glue
- 1 lb. (cut slight into little scaled down pieces) pork shoulder

Embellishment with
- 2 tbsps new hacked parsley
- 1/4 cup cooked peanuts, disintegrated

Strategy
2. Add pepper, lemongrass glue, fish sauce, garlic, avocado oil, soy sauce, splenda and onions into a bowl and speed to join. Add pork pieces into the marinade, throw until covered and let sit for 30 minutes or more until marinated.
3. Spot marinated pork into the fryer container in one layer. Cook pork for 5 minutes at 400°. Flip pork and cook for 5 minutes until wanted doneness is reached.

4. Serve pork, embellished with new cleaved parsley and disintegrated peanuts.

Wholesome Data/Serving
Calories 231 kcal, Protein 16g, Dietary Fiber 1g, Carbs 4g, Fat 16g

THICK-CUT BACON WITH CABBAGE

Planning Time: 10 minutes
Cook Time: 25 minutes
Serves:: 6 **Servings**
Fixings
- 6 thick-cut bacon strips
- 1 (dispose of the external layer prior to cutting cabbage into wedges) green cabbage head, little
- 1 teaspoon garlic powder
- 1 teaspoon onion powder
- 1/4 teaspoon stew chips
- 1/2 teaspoon fennel seeds
- Salt and pepper, as essential
- 3 tablespoons avocado oil

Strategy
1. Generously cover the wire crate of an air fryer with avocado oil. Add cuts of bacon into the air fryer bushel and cook for 10 minutes at 360°F. Cut cooked bacon cuts into little pieces and let sit.
2. Add pepper, salt, bean stew pieces, fennel seeds, onion powder and garlic powder into a little bowl and blend until consolidated. Spill avocado oil over cabbage and season with the garlic powder blend until uniformly covered.
3. Generously oil the wire crate of an air fryer bushel with avocado oil. Add in the prepared cabbage wedges into the pre-arranged air fryer crate and cook for 8 minutes at 400°F. Flip cabbage wedges, cover with additional avocado oil and cook for 6 additional minutes.
4. Eliminate and let sit to cool. Serve, finished off with hacked bacon.

Nourishing Data/Serving
Calories 123 kcal, Protein 4g, Carbs 2g, Fat 11g

DELICIOUS PORK HACKS

Planning Time: 5 minutes
Cook Time: 15 minutes
Serves:: 3 Servings
Fixings
- 2 tsps avocado oil
- 3 (6 oz.) {rinse and pat dry} pork cleaves
- Dark pepper, as essential
- Salt, as essential
- 1 tsp smoked paprika, or to taste
- 1 tsp garlic powder, or to taste

Technique
1. Coat the pork cleaves gently with avocado oil. Sprinkle smoked paprika, garlic powder, pepper and salt over pork cleaves to prepare. Move pork slashes into the wire bin of an air fryer, and cook for 5-7 minutes at 380ºF.
2. Turn the pork cleave and cook until very much cooked, for 5-7 additional minutes. Let sit to cool marginally prior to serving.

Dietary Data/Serving
Calories 227 kcal, Protein 34.8g, Complete Carbs 2.7g, Fat 9.8g

AIR FRYER PORK STOMACH

Planning Time: 10 minutes
Cook Time: 30 minutes
Serves:: 4 Servings
Fixings
- 3 cups water
- 1 lb. (cut into 3 pieces) pork stomach
- 1 tsp dark pepper, ground
- 1 tsp salt
- 2 cove leaves
- 2 tbsps soy sauce
- 6 garlic cloves

Technique
1. Add each fixing into a pan, place cover over dish and cook until a knife penetrates the skin-side effectively, for 60 minutes. Take out meat, let sit for 10 minutes to dry and deplete.
2. Cut each piece of pork gut into 2 long cuts. Move pork cuts into the wire container of an air fryer. Cook until pork gut fat is firm, for 15 minutes at 400ºF.
Serve and appreciate.

Dietary Data/Serving
Calories 594 kcal, Fat 21g, Fat 60g, Protein 11g

RIB STEAK

Fixings
- 1 Tablespoon of steak rub
- 2 pounds rib steaks
- 1 Tablespoon of olive oil

Directions
1. Before the time has come to cook; preheat the Air Fryer to 400ºF.
2. Flavor the meat on all spaces with the oil and rub.
3. Put it in the bushel for 14 minutes, flipping following seven minutes.
4. Allow it to rest for in any event ten minutes before you cut and serve.

Yields: Two Servings

STROMBOLI

Fixings
- 1 (12-ounce) refrigerated pizza covering
- ¾ cup Mozzarella destroyed cheddar
- 3 cups destroyed cheddar
- 1 tablespoon milk
- 1 egg yolk
- 1/3 pound cut cooked ham
- 3 ounces cooked red chime peppers

Guidelines
Preheat the Air Fryer at 360ºF.
Roll the batter until it is around ¼-inch thick.
Layer in the peppers, ham, and cheddar on one side of the batter and crease to seal.
Consolidate the milk and eggs to brush the mixture.
Put the Stromboli in the crate and set the clock for 15 minutes. Check it at regular intervals or somewhere in the vicinity—flip the Stromboli to the opposite side for careful cooking.

Yields: Four Servings

HAMBURGER RIB STEAK

Fixings
- 1 Tablespoon of steak rub
- 2 pounds rib steaks
- 1 Tablespoon of olive oil

Directions
1. Before the time has come to cook; preheat the Air Fryer to 400ºF.
2. Flavor the meat on all spaces with the oil and rub.
3. Put it in the crate for 14 minutes, flipping following seven minutes.
4. Allow it to rest for in any event ten minutes before you cut and serve.

Yields: Two Servings

Fixings
- 1 clove of garlic
- 1 Tbsp. olive oil
- Pepper and salt
- 1 ¾ pounds - rack of sheep
- Elements for the Outside
- 3 ounces Macadamia nuts (unsalted)
- 1 tablespoon each
- Fresh rosemary
- Breadcrumbs
- 1 egg

Directions
1. Preheat the Air Fryer to 220ºF.
2. Cleave the garlic clove into smidgens. Make the garlic oil by consolidating the garlic and oil. Brush the sheep and flavor with salt and pepper.
3. Cleave the nuts to a fine consistency in a bowl and mix in the rosemary and breadcrumbs. Beat/whip the egg in another dish.
4. Dig the meat through the egg blend and coat with the macadamia outside fixing.
5. Spot the rack of sheep Noticeable all around Fryer bin—setting the clock for 30 minutes.
6. After the time is slipped by; raise the warmth to 390ºF—setting the ideal opportunity for an extra five minutes.
7. Take the meat from the fryer and let it rest for around ten minutes covered with some aluminum foil.

FRESH TOFU

Fixings
- 2 tsp. toasted sesame oil

Simmered Rack of Sheep with a Macadamia Outside
- 1 clove of garlic
- 1 Tbsp. olive oil
- Pepper and salt
- 1 ¾ pounds - rack of sheep

Elements for the Covering
- 3 ounces Macadamia nuts (unsalted)
- 1 tablespoon each
- New rosemary
- Breadcrumbs
- 1 egg

Guidelines
1. Preheat the Air Fryer to 220ºF.
2. Slash the garlic clove into smidgens. Make the garlic oil by consolidating the garlic and oil. Brush the sheep and flavor with salt and pepper.
3. Slash the nuts to a fine consistency in a bowl and mix in the rosemary and breadcrumbs. Beat/whip the egg in another dish.
4. Dig the meat through the egg combination and coat with the macadamia hull besting.
5. Spot the rack of sheep Noticeable all around Fryer container—setting the clock for 30 minutes.
6. After the time is passed; raise the warmth to 390ºF—setting the ideal opportunity for an extra five minutes.
7. Take the meat from the fryer and let it rest for around ten minutes covered with some aluminum foil.

BEAN STEW PREPARED RIB-EYE STEAK

Cut from the rib region, the rib eye is beautifully marbled, and in view of this additional fat, the taste is astounding. As a result of the fat, make certain to add the tablespoon of water to the lower part of the air fryer. At the point when the fat delivers down, the water will assist with staying away from the fat drippings from smoking.

Active Time: 5 minutes
CookTime: 10 minutes
Fixings | **Serves:**2
- 1 tablespoon water
- ¹/2 teaspoon salt
- ¹/4 teaspoon newly ground dark pepper
- ¹/4 teaspoon garlic powder
- ¹/4 teaspoon stew powder
- ¹/4 teaspoon smoked paprika
- 1 (12-ounce) boneless rib-eye steak, 1" thick
- 1 tablespoon unsalted spread, cut into 2 taps

1. Preheat air fryer at 400°F for 3 minutes. Empty 1 tablespoon water into the lower part of the air fryer.
2. In a little bowl, join salt, pepper, garlic powder, bean stew powder, and paprika.
3. Season rib eye on the two sides with arranged dry rub. Spot steak on fryer container and cook 5 minutes. Flip steak and cook an extra 5 minutes. This should yield a medium-uncommon steak. Because of differences in steak sizes and doneness inclinations, check steak with a meat thermometer to guarantee favored doneness.

4. Move steak to a cutting board and top with two taps of spread. Let rest 5 minutes prior to cutting and serving.

Per serving Calories: 592 | Fat: 46.2 g | Protein: 40.2 g | Sodium: 695 mg | Fiber: 0.3 g | Carbs: 0.8 g | Sugar: 0.1 g

COCOA-CHIPOTLE STRIP STEAK

The air fryer is a straightforward method to yield an ideal steak with a burned outside and a delicious inside. The cocoa powder, chipotle stew powder, and lime juice carry a little Mexico to your steak. Likewise attempt this with chicken, pork, and surprisingly salmon!

Involved Time: 5 minutes
CookTime: 8 minutes
Fixings | **Serves:**2

- 2 teaspoons unsweetened cocoa powder
- 1 teaspoon chipotle bean stew powder
- 1 tablespoon nectar
- $^{1}/2$ teaspoon lime juice
- Squeeze salt
- 1 ($^{3}/4$-pound, $1^{1}/2$"- thick) strip steak

1. In a little bowl, consolidate cocoa powder, stew powder, nectar, lime squeeze, and salt. Brush all over the two sides of steak and refrigerate concealed 30 minutes or to expedite.
2. Preheat air fryer at 400°F for 3 minutes.
3. Spot steak in air fryer container and cook 4 minutes. Flip steak and cook an extra 4 minutes. This should yield a medium-uncommon steak. Because of differences in steak sizes and doneness inclinations, check steak with a meat thermometer to guarantee favored doneness.
4. Move steak to a cutting board and let rest 5 minutes prior to cutting and serving.

Per serving Calories: 479 | Fat: 27.5 g | Protein: 37.4 g | Sodium: 201 mg | Fiber: 2.5 g | Starches: 12.6 g | Sugar: 8.8 g

PORCINI-SCOURED FILETS MIGNONS

Dried mushrooms can be found all things considered strength food merchants or on the web. Additionally, if you can't get your hands on porcinis, attempt different assortments, as they will fill in pleasantly.

Active Time: 15 minutes
CookTime: 12 minutes
Fixings | **Serves:**2

- Porcini Dry Rub
- $^{1}/4$ cup dried porcini mushrooms (about $^{1}/2$ ounce)
- 2 teaspoons sugar
- 2 teaspoons salt
- 2 teaspoons dark peppercorns
- 1 teaspoon smoked paprika
- 1 teaspoon dried minced garlic

Steak
- 2 ($1^{1}/2$"- thick) filet mignon steaks (around 1 pound complete)
- 1 tablespoon unsalted spread, cut into 2 taps

1. Spot Porcini Dry Focus on Fixings a little food processor or zest processor. Heartbeat until powdered. Store in a sealed shut holder until prepared to utilize. This Yields about $^{1}/2$ cup, so you will have extra dry rub for future suppers.
2. Preheat air fryer at 375°F for 3 minutes.
3. Season steaks on the two sides with arranged dry rub. Spot steaks in fryer bin and cook 4 minutes. Flip steaks and cook an extra 4 minutes. Flip steaks once again and cook an extra 4 minutes. This should yield medium-uncommon steaks. Because of differences in steak sizes and doneness inclinations, check steak with a meat thermometer to guarantee favored doneness. Move steaks to a cutting board and top each with a pat of spread. Let rest 5 minutes prior to serving.

Per serving Calories: 431 | Fat: 19.3 g | Protein: 56.3 g | Sodium: 1,304 mg | Fiber: 0.9 g | Carbs: 5.7 g | Sugar: 2.3 g

COWPOKE FLANK STEAK

This flank steak makes certain to put some giddyup in your progression. Furthermore, cowhands realize that a little espresso in your steak rub loans a profound smokiness to the meat. (They likewise know not to crouch wearing spikes, so trust them; cowpokes know things!)

Active Time: 5 minutes
CookTime: 19 minutes

Fixings | **Serves:**4
- $^{1}/4$ cup olive oil
- $^{1}/2$ teaspoon salt
- $^{1}/2$ teaspoon ground cumin

- $1/2$ teaspoon stew powder
- $1/2$ teaspoon garlic powder
- $1/2$ teaspoon moment coffee powder
- (1-pound) flank steak

1. In a medium bowl or gallon plastic resealable sack, consolidate olive oil, salt, cumin, bean stew powder, garlic powder, and coffee powder. Add flank steak, seal, and throw. Refrigerate 30 minutes or up to expedite.
2. Preheat air fryer at 325°F for 3 minutes.
3. Spot steak on fryer container and cook 10 minutes. Flip steak and cook an extra 9 minutes. This should yield a medium-uncommon steak. Because of differences in steak sizes and doneness inclinations, check steak with a meat thermometer to guarantee favored doneness.
4. Move steak to a cutting board. Let rest 5 minutes prior to cutting. Cut daintily contrary to what would be expected for greatest delicacy, then, at that point serve.

Per serving Calories: 253 | Fat: 14.5 g | Protein: 24.8 g | Sodium: 94 mg | Fiber: 0.0 g | Starches: 0.1 g | Sugar: 0.0 g

HAMBURGER WELLINGTON

Hamburger Wellington is a beautiful filet mignon with Dijon mustard and mushroom duxelles wrapped perfectly in puff cake. You'll feel like there is an uncommon minimal present on each plate.

Active Time: 15 minutes
CookTime: 27 minutes
Fixings | Serves:2
- 2 cups hacked shiitake mushrooms (around 4 ounces)
- $1/4$ cup diced yellow onion
- 1 tablespoon new thyme leaves
- 4 teaspoons olive oil, partitioned
- 2 ($1^1/2$"- thick) filet mignon steaks (around 1 pound)
- 4 ounces prosciutto (8 cuts)
- 1 teaspoon Dijon mustard
- $1/4$ cup generally useful flour, isolated
- 1 huge egg, whisked
- 1 sheet puff cake, defrosted to room temperature

1. In a medium skillet over medium-high warmth, pan sear shiitakes, onion, thyme, and 2 teaspoons olive oil. Cook 3–4 minutes until onions are clear and dampness has delivered from mushrooms. Let cool. Move to a little food processor and heartbeat until smooth.
2. In a similar skillet, add staying 2 teaspoons olive oil. Add steaks and burn all sides, 4–5 minutes until sautéed. Put away to rest.
3. On a level, clean surface, place a huge piece of cling wrap. In the wrap cover 4 prosciutto cuts, shaping a square. Spread portion of mushroom combination, or duxelles, over prosciutto. Add a steak to the middle. Brush top with $1/2$ teaspoon Dijon mustard. Utilize the saran wrap to help direct the prosciutto over steak, totally covering the steak. Roll firmly in the wrap and afterward contort finishes of the wrap until a tight seal is shaped. Rehash with outstanding Fixings . Refrigerate 30 minutes to help set the structures.
4. Sprinkle a portion of the flour on level, clean surface. The excess flour can be utilized for your hands and the moving pin. Spot whisked egg in a little bowl close by. Move baked good sheet to $1/4$" thickness. Slice down the middle. Open up steaks and spot one in each piece of puff cake. Wrap steaks with puff cake to cover. Remove any abundance cake. Use egg to seal edges. Brush highest points of Hamburger Wellingtons with egg.
5. Preheat air fryer at 350°F for 3 minutes.
6. Spot Hamburger Wellingtons crease side down in air fryer crate and cook 18 minutes. This should yield a medium-uncommon steak. Because of differences in steak sizes and doneness inclinations, check steak with a meat thermometer to guarantee favored doneness.
7. Move Hamburger Wellingtons to plates. Let rest 5 minutes prior to serving.

Per serving Calories: 764 | Fat: 42.9 g | Protein: 72.8 g | Sodium: 477 mg | Fiber: 2.3 g | Carbs: 18.2 g | Sugar: 2.4 g

KOREAN GOCHUJANG SHORT RIBS

Gochujang, an aged stew glue, isn't exactly pretty much as zesty as sriracha; it has a sweet furthermore, tart segment like ketchup. Slather it on certain ribs with a couple of different flavors, also, these will be the best ribs you'll make this year!

Active Time: 10 minutes
CookTime: 16 minutes
Fixings | **Serves:**2
- $1/4$ cup gochujang sauce
- 2 tablespoons rice vinegar
- 2 tablespoons nectar

- 1 tablespoon soy sauce
- 1 teaspoon ground ginger
- 1 pound boneless meat short ribs
- 1/4 cup cleaved new cilantro

1. In a huge plastic resealable sack, join gochujang sauce, vinegar, nectar, soy sauce, and ginger. Put away 2 tablespoons of combination in a little bowl.
2. Add short ribs to sack, seal, and massage combination into ribs. Refrigerate 30 minutes up to expedite.
3. Preheat air fryer at 325°F for 3 minutes.
4. Spot ribs in air fryer container. Cook 8 minutes. Flip ribs and brush with additional sauce. Cook an extra 8 minutes.
5. Move ribs to a serving plate and enhancement with new cilantro.

Per serving Calories: 404 | Fat: 22.0 g | Protein: 44.1 g | Sodium: 348 mg | Fiber: 0.8 g | Carbs: 6.6 g | Sugar: 4.6 g

BAR-B-QUE SHORT RIBS

Short ribs are taken from the more limited bit of the rib confine. Brimming with meat and fat, they make the best nibbles of the ribs. Cautioning: this isn't exquisite feasting, so bring a pile of napkins!
Involved Time: 10 minutes
CookTime: 16 minutes
Fixings | **Serves:**2

- 1/4 cup ketchup
- 1 teaspoon Worcestershire sauce
- 1 tablespoon unadulterated maple syrup
- 1 teaspoon apple juice vinegar
- 1 teaspoon garlic powder
- 1 tablespoon smoked paprika
- 1 teaspoon ocean salt
- 1 teaspoon newly ground dark pepper
- 1/2 teaspoon cayenne pepper
- 1 pound boneless hamburger short ribs

1. In a huge plastic resealable pack, join ketchup, Worcestershire sauce, syrup, vinegar, garlic powder, paprika, salt, dark pepper, and cayenne pepper. Put away 2 tablespoons of blend in a little bowl.
2. Add short ribs to sack, seal, and massage blend into ribs. Refrigerate 30 minutes or up to expedite.
3. Preheat air fryer at 325°F for 3 minutes.
4. Spot ribs in air fryer bin. Cook 8 minutes. Flip ribs and brush with additional sauce. Cook an extra 8 minutes.

5. Move ribs to a serving plate.

Per serving Calories: 385 | Fat: 20.5 g | Protein: 43.5 g | Sodium: 534 mg | Fiber: 0.6 g | Starches: 7.1 g | Sugar: 5.1 g

SUMMER STEAK SALAD

There is no compelling reason to spend boatloads of money at your neighborhood steakhouse, since this plate of mixed greens will extinguish your hankering. Loaded up with delicious steak strips, radiant greens, energetic blue cheddar, natural nuts and seeds, and new blueberries, this serving of mixed greens is loaded with flavor!
Active Time: 5 minutes
CookTime: 19 minutes
Fixings | **Serves:**4

- 1/4 cup olive oil
- 1 teaspoon salt
- 1/2 teaspoon newly ground dark pepper
- (1-pound) flank steak
- 8 cups blended greens
- 1/4 cup balsamic vinaigrette
- 4 tablespoons disintegrated blue cheddar
- 4 tablespoons pecan pieces
- 4 tablespoons shelled sunflower seeds
- 1 cup blueberries

1. In a medium bowl or gallon plastic resealable sack, consolidate olive oil, salt, and pepper. Add flank steak, seal, and throw. Refrigerate 30 minutes or up to expedite.
2. Preheat air fryer at 325°F for 3 minutes.
3. Spot steak on fryer container and cook 10 minutes. Flip steak and cook an extra 9 minutes. This should yield a medium-uncommon steak. Because of differences in steak sizes and doneness inclinations, check steak with a meat thermometer to guarantee favored doneness.
4. Move steak to a cutting board. Let rest 5 minutes.
5. While steak is resting, add blended greens to a huge blending bowl. Gradually sprinkle in vinaigrette. Throw. Add more and throw once more. Do this until greens are completely dressed. Move to four dishes.
6. Top every plate of mixed greens with blue cheddar, pecans, sunflower seeds, and blueberries.
7. Cut steak meagerly across the grain for greatest delicacy. Top every plate of mixed greens with cut steak. Serve right away.

Per serving Calories: 427 | Fat: 26.0 g | Protein: 30.2 g | Sodium: 269 mg | Fiber: 3.7 g | Carbs: 13.0 g | Sugar: 6.6 g

STEAK ROAD TACOS

Since they're spilling over with flavor, you will think these road tacos fell off an exquisite cuisine truck. Cutting the air-singed flank steak contrary to what would be expected makes this less expensive cut of meat appear as though it is the most extravagant hamburger from the butcher.

Involved Time: 5 minutes
CookTime: 19 minutes
Fixings | Serves:5

- ¼ cup olive oil
- ½ teaspoon salt
- ½ teaspoon ground cumin
- (1-pound) flank steak
- 10 road tacos (4" scaled down flour tortillas)
- 1 cup destroyed red cabbage
- ½ cup Sriracha Mayonnaise (see Section 15)
- ½ cup Pico Guacamole (see Part 15)

1. In a gallon plastic resealable sack, consolidate olive oil, salt, and cumin. Add flank steak, seal, and throw. Refrigerate 30 minutes.
2. Preheat air fryer at 325°F for 3 minutes.
3. Spot steak on fryer container and cook 10 minutes. Flip steak and cook an extra 9 minutes. This should yield a medium-uncommon steak. Because of differences in steak sizes and doneness inclinations, check steak with a meat thermometer to guarantee favored doneness.
4. Move steak to a cutting board. Let rest 5 minutes prior to cutting. Cut daintily contrary to what would be expected for most extreme delicacy.
5. Fabricate road tacos by adding steak cuts to flour tortillas, alongside red cabbage, Sriracha Mayonnaise, and Pico Guacamole. Serve right away.

BURGER CANINES

Turn the exemplary burger and frank on their heads by joining the two. This wiener is really prepared ground meat looking like a sausage and served in a frank bun. You can serve them with your number one burger or wiener Fixings .

Active Time: 10 minutes
CookTime: 6 minutes
Fixings | Serves:4

- ½ pound ground meat
- ¼ teaspoon Worcestershire sauce
- 1 huge egg white
- 2 tablespoons plain bread scraps
- ⅛ teaspoon stew powder
- ¼ teaspoon onion powder
- ¼ teaspoon salt
- 4 top-split wiener buns

1. In a medium bowl, consolidate hamburger, Worcestershire sauce, egg white, bread morsels, stew powder, onion powder, and salt. Structure into four wiener shapes. Move them longer than expected on the grounds that the meat will shrivel some in cooking.
2. Preheat air fryer at 350°F for 3 minutes.
3. Spot burger canines in daintily lubed air fryer container. Cook 3 minutes. Flip. Cook an extra 3 minutes. Move to a paper towel-arranged plate to douse any oil.
4. Spot Cheeseburger Canines in buns and serve.

Per serving Calories: 212 | Fat: 5.1 g | Protein: 14.8 g | Sodium: 423 mg | Fiber: 1.1 g | Carbs: 23.7 g | Sugar: 3.0 g

BULGOGI

Bulgogi, in a real sense deciphered as "fire meat," is a Korean exemplary comprising of slight pieces of marinated hamburger. The air fryer makes fresh edges on the meat strips, which loan added surface to this dish. The ground pear is the clear-cut advantage and quintessential fixing in Bulgogi.

Involved Time: 15 minutes
CookTime: 12 minutes
Fixings | Serves:2

- 2 tablespoons sesame oil
- 2 tablespoons ground pear
- 1 tablespoon soy sauce
- 1 tablespoon earthy colored sugar
- 1 tablespoon gochujang
- 1 teaspoon ground ginger
- 1 clove garlic, minced
- Squeeze salt
- 6 scallions, managed, cut, whites and greens isolated
- 1 (12-ounce) rib-eye steak, 1" thick, meagerly cut
- 2 cups cooked rice
- 2 teaspoons toasted sesame seeds

1. In a gallon plastic resealable pack, join oil, pear, soy sauce, sugar, gochujang, ginger, garlic, salt, and scallion whites. Add daintily cut rib eye, seal, and throw. Refrigerate 30 minutes or up to expedite.
2. Preheat air fryer at 375°F for 3 minutes.
3. Spot steak in air fryer bin and cook 12 minutes, blending at regular intervals. This should yield delicate steak with firm edges.
4. Serve steak more than two dishes of rice. Embellishment with scallion greens and toasted sesame seeds.

Per serving Calories: 627 | Fat: 30.0 g | Protein: 38.0 g | Sodium: 208 mg | Fiber: 1.1 g | Starches: 47.8 g | Sugar: 1.4 g

STEAK AND PEPPERS QUESADILLAS

The air fryer cooks this rib eye like a chief a delicious community with a singed outside. What's more, those peppers and gooey cheddar make these quesadillas basically heavenly. Present with some custom made Pico Guacamole to polish it off!

Involved Time: 15 minutes
CookTime: 29 minutes
Fixings | Serves:4
- 1 (12-ounce) rib-eye steak, 1" thick
- 1/2 teaspoon salt
- 1/4 teaspoon newly ground dark pepper
- 2 teaspoons olive oil
- 1 little red chime pepper, cultivated and cut
- 1 little green chime pepper, cultivated and cut
- 1/2 medium yellow onion, stripped and cut
- 2 teaspoons stew powder
- 3 tablespoons spread, dissolved
- 8 (6") flour tortillas
- 2 cups ground Monterey jack cheddar

1. Preheat air fryer at 400°F for 3 minutes.
2. Season rib eye on the two sides with salt and pepper. Spot steak in air fryer container and cook 5 minutes. Flip steak and cook an extra 5 minutes. This should yield a medium-uncommon steak. Because of differences in steak sizes and doneness inclinations, check steak with a meat thermometer to guarantee favored doneness.
3. Move steak to a cutting board and let rest 5 minutes.
4. While the steak is cooking and resting, sauté olive oil, ringer peppers, onion, and stew powder in a skillet over medium-high warmth 5–7 minutes until peppers are delicate. Put away.

Meagerly cut steak contrary to what would be expected.
5. Lessen heat on air fryer to 350°F.
6. Softly brush dissolved margarine on one side of a tortilla. Spot tortilla spread side down in air fryer crate. Layer 1/4 of the steak on tortilla, followed with 1/4 of the pepper and onion blend, and 1/4 of the cheddar. Top with second tortilla. Gently margarine top of tortilla.

Per serving Calories: 701 | Fat: 44.1 g | Protein: 36.0 g | Sodium: 1,136 mg | Fiber: 3.1 g | Carbs: 35.7 g | Sugar: 4.5 g

BRIE AND FIG JAM SLIDERS

Break out these upscale sliders for a family festivity or for your extravagant visitors! Fig jam and Brie go together like peanut butter and jam. The peppery arugula raises these sliders and will make them return for to an ever increasing extent!

Involved Time: 5 minutes
CookTime: 18 minutes
Fixings | Serves:4
- 1 pound lean ground hamburger
- 1/2 teaspoon dried basil
- 1/2 teaspoon salt
- 8 tablespoons Brie cheddar
- 8 slider buns
- 1/4 cup fig jam
- 1/2 cup arugula

1. In a medium bowl, join meat, basil, and salt. Structure into eight balls.
2. Fold 1 tablespoon of Brie into a ball and press into the center of a hamburger ball. Seal edges and delicately press into a patty. Delicately make a slight space in every patty, as the meat will ascend during warming. Rehash with outstanding meat and Brie.
3. Preheat air fryer at 350°F for 3 minutes.
4. Spot four sliders in delicately lubed air fryer bin or on the air fryer barbecue skillet (adornment). Cook 4 minutes. Flip sliders and cook an extra 5 minutes or until wanted doneness, which can be checked with a meat thermometer. Rehash with outstanding sliders.
5. Move sliders to a plate and serve on buns spread with fig jam and finished off with arugula.

Per serving Calories: 450 | Fat: 14.8 g | Protein: 30.8 g | Sodium: 749 mg | Fiber: 1.5 g | Starches: 42.4 g | Sugar: 13.5 g

REUBEN BURGERS

These burgers have every one of the exemplary kinds of a Reuben sandwich combined with the succulence of the basic cheeseburger. The air-singed corned meat replaces fresh bacon found on certain burgers, and the caraway seeds give a gesture to the conventional rye bread.

Involved Time: 10 minutes
CookTime: 30 minutes
Fixings | Serves:4

- 1 pound lean ground hamburger
- 2 tablespoons minced yellow onion
- 2 teaspoons caraway seeds
- 1 teaspoon salt
- 4 cuts Swiss cheddar
- 8 cuts shop corned meat
- $^1/2$ cup Thousand Island dressing
- 4 burger buns
- 1 cup sauerkraut, depleted

1. Preheat air fryer at 350°F for 3 minutes.
2. Consolidate ground meat, onion, caraway seeds, and salt. Structure into four patties, making a space in the center, as the meat will ascend during warming.
3. Add two patties to delicately lubed fryer crate and cook 6 minutes. Flip burgers and cook an extra 4 minutes. Add a cut of Swiss cheddar to the highest point of the burgers and cook an extra 2 minutes.
4. Move to a serving plate. Rehash with residual burgers. Eliminate when done and allowed them to rest.
5. While burgers are resting, add corned hamburger to air fryer bin. Cook 3 minutes, flip, and cook an extra 3 minutes to accomplish fresh edges.
6. Spread 2 tablespoons dressing on every bun. Spot a burger on every bun and top each with $^1/4$ cup sauerkraut and 2 cuts fresh corned hamburger. Serve warm.

Per serving Calories: 553 | Fat: 25.9 g | Protein: 45.1 g | Sodium: 1,529 mg | Fiber: 2.8 g | Starches: 32.9 g | Sugar: 9.2 g

RED WINE MEAT

Albeit this dinner is essentially made, the Dijon mustard and red wine loan a little acidic chomp that will be valued with the hearty hamburger. Present with potatoes and green beans.

Involved Time: 5 minutes
CookTime: 15 minutes
Fixings | Serves:4

- 1 teaspoon Dijon mustard
- $^1/2$ teaspoon salt
- $^1/4$ cup dry red wine
- $^1/4$ cup tomato glue
- 1 pound meat stew blocks

In a medium bowl, consolidate mustard, salt, wine, and tomato glue. Include meat blocks and throw to join. Add to lower part of cake barrel (embellishment).
Preheat air fryer at 350°F for 3 minutes.
Spot barrel in air fryer crate. Cook 12–15 minutes, mixing twice during cooking.
Eliminate barrel from air fryer and let rest 10 minutes. Spoon into bowls and serve warm.

Per serving Calories: 237 | Fat: 7.2 g | Protein: 25.2 g | Sodium: 396 mg | Fiber: 0.7 g | Starches: 3.6 g | Sugar: 2.1 g

HOISIN HAMBURGER MEATBALLS

Hoisin has an extraordinarily rich flavor, hitting both sweet and pungent preferences. These are incredible straight out of the air fryer however surprisingly better served over rice decorated with scallion greens and eaten with a couple of chopsticks.

Involved Time: 10 minutes
CookTime: 16 minutes
Fixings | Serves:4

- 1 pound lean ground hamburger
- 1 enormous egg
- $^1/2$ cup panko bread morsels
- 4 scallions managed and diced, greens and whites isolated
- 2 tablespoons hoisin sauce
- 1 tablespoon soy sauce
- $^1/2$ teaspoon ground white pepper

1. Preheat air fryer at 350°F for 3 minutes.
2. In a medium bowl, consolidate meat, egg, bread pieces, white pieces of scallions, hoisin sauce, soy sauce, and pepper.

Structure into eighteen meatballs, around 2 tablespoons each.

3. Add half of meatballs to fryer bushel and cook 6 minutes. Flip meatballs. Cook an extra 2 minutes. Move to serving dish.
4. Rehash with outstanding meatballs.
5. Move meatballs to a serving dish. Enhancement with scallion greens.

Per serving Calories: 266 | Fat: 10.0 g | Protein: 25.1 g | Sodium: 450 mg | Fiber: 0.5 g | Starches: 14.4 g | Sugar: 2.9 g

CHERRY-SAGE BEEFBURGERS

The pleasantness from the cherry jam against the solid and exquisite sage makes a flavor combo that will make you screech with enchant. Serve these burgers with no guarantees or with your number one **Fixings** on a high quality cheeseburger bun or in a new lettuce wrap.

Involved Time: 10 minutes
CookTime: 24 minutes
Fixings | **Serves:**4
- 1 pound ground hamburger
- 2 tablespoons minced yellow onion
- 1 enormous egg white
- 1/4 cup panko bread scraps
- 1 tablespoon cherry jam
- 1 tablespoon cleaved new sage leaves
- Squeeze salt

Preheat air fryer at 350°F for 3 minutes.
In a medium bowl, join every one of the **Fixings** and structure into four patties, making a slight space in the center, as the hamburger will ascend during warming.
Add two patties to gently lubed fryer bushel and cook 6 minutes. Flip burgers and cook an extra 6 minutes or until wanted doneness. Rehash with residual burgers.
Move to a plate and serve.

Per serving Calories: 223 | Fat: 8.5 g | Protein: 23.1 g | Sodium: 120 mg | Fiber: 0.3 g | Carbs: 9.3 g | Sugar: 3.0 g

KRAUT CANINES

At the point when you need that barbecue flavor however don't have the opportunity, break out your air fryer, and inside the space of minutes you will be on your own special individual outing. Add some sauerkraut and a little brew mustard and you'll feel like you're at Oktoberfest!

Involved Time: 5 minutes
CookTime: 5 minutes
Fixings | **Serves:**2
- 4 meat wieners
- 4 wiener buns
- 1/2 cup sauerkraut, depleted
- 2 tablespoons brew mustard (or Dijon)

Preheat air fryer at 400°F for 3 minutes.
Add wieners to air fryer bin. Cook 4 minutes.
Eliminate wieners and put in frank buns. Spot once again into the bushel. Cook 1 extra moment.
Move wieners to a plate and topping with sauerkraut and mustard. Serve warm.

Per serving Calories: 580 | Fat: 28.5 g | Protein: 21.0 g | Sodium: 1,721 mg | Fiber: 2.7 g | Starches: 47.4 g | Sugar: 7.2 g

BUFFALO RIB-EYE STEAK

Buffalo is a fantastic wellspring of protein, particularly useful for those after a low-fat, high-protein diet. More slender and somewhat better than meat, buffalo additionally has a more limited cooking time. It is basic that you don't overcook this excellent meat, as it begins to harden past medium-uncommon.

Involved Time: 5 minutes
CookTime: 7 minutes
Fixings | **Serves:**1
- 1/2 teaspoon salt
- 1/4 teaspoon newly ground dark pepper
- 1/8 teaspoon smoked paprika
- 1/8 teaspoon garlic powder
- 1 (8-ounce) buffalo rib-eye steak, 1" thick

1. In a little bowl, consolidate salt, pepper, paprika, and garlic powder.
2. Preheat air fryer at 400°F for 3 minutes.
3. Season rib eye with arranged dry rub on the two sides. Spot in air fryer bin and cook 4 minutes. Flip steak and cook an extra 3 minutes. Check steak with a meat thermometer to guarantee doneness fulfillment.
4. Move steak to a cutting board and let rest 5 minutes prior to serving.

Per serving Calories: 303 | Fat: 8.4 g | Protein: 50.3 g | Sodium: 1,250 mg | Fiber: 0.3 g | Starches: 0.8 g | Sugar: 0.0 g

Normally lean, buffalo is an incredible substitute for hamburger. Since it is more hearty in taste, the blue cheddar kicks up the flavor significantly more with its sharp and impactful flavor. Tempered with lettuce and tomatoes, these wraps consider every contingency.

Involved Time: 10 minutes
CookTime: 7 minutes
Fixings | Serves:2
- 1 (8-ounce) buffalo rib-eye steak, 1" thick
- ¹/2 teaspoon salt
- ¹/4 teaspoon newly ground dark pepper
- 4 tablespoons disintegrated blue cheddar
- ¹/2 cup destroyed lettuce
- 2 medium Roma tomatoes, cultivated and diced
- 4 (6") flour tortillas

1. Preheat air fryer at 400°F for 3 minutes.
2. Season rib eye on the two sides with salt and pepper. Spot in air fryer container and cook 4 minutes. Flip steak and cook an extra 3 minutes. Check steak with a meat thermometer to guarantee doneness inclination.
3. Move steak to a cutting board and let rest 5 minutes prior to cutting. Meagerly cut steak contrary to what would be expected.
4. Gap steak, blue cheddar, lettuce, and tomatoes uniformly among tortillas and fold each into a wrap. Serve.

Per serving Calories: 399 | Fat: 12.2 g | Protein: 34.2 g | Sodium: 1,247 mg | Fiber: 2.5 g | Starches: 34.2 g | Sugar: 4.1 g

J ALAPEÑO B UFFALO M EATBALLS

These buffalo meatballs are made delicate and delicious with the jalapeño jam and onion. Serve this dish for certain pureed potatoes and new vegetables in addition to an additional bit of the jalapeño jam in which to drag your meatballs around for additional flavor.

Involved Time: 10 minutes
CookTime: 16 minutes
Fixings | Serves:4
- 1 pound ground buffalo
- 1 enormous egg
- 2 tablespoons jalapeño jam
- ¹/2 cup plain bread morsels
- ¹/4 cup finely diced yellow onion
- 2 tablespoons cleaved new mint, partitioned
- 1 teaspoon salt
- ¹/2 teaspoon newly ground dark pepper

1. In a medium bowl, join buffalo, egg, jalapeño jam, bread morsels, onion, 1 tablespoon slashed mint, salt, and pepper. Structure into eighteen meatballs, around 2 tablespoons each.
2. Preheat air fryer at 350°F for 3 minutes.
3. Add half of meatballs to fryer container and cook 6 minutes. Flip meatballs. Cook an extra 2 minutes. Move to serving dish.
4. Rehash with residual meatballs.
5. Move meatballs to a serving dish. Enhancement with staying cleaved mint leaves.

Per serving Calories: 301 | Fat: 13.0 g | Protein: 24.3 g | Sodium: 711 mg | Fiber: 0.9 g | Carbs: 15.5 g | Sugar: 5.8 g

B ASIC P ORK F LANK C OOK

The air fryer unquestionably does equity to a delicious pork midsection cook. The inside meat is so exceptionally delicious, and the convection-style cooking does marvels to fresh up the skin. As a result of differing sizes of flank broils, make certain to check the meal with a meat thermometer close to the furthest limit of the cooking cycle.

Active Time: 10 minutes
CookTime: 40 minutes
Fixings | Serves:4
- 1 (2-pound) boneless pork midsection broil
- 3 cloves garlic, split
- 1 tablespoon olive oil
- 1 teaspoon dried rosemary
- 1 teaspoon salt
- ¹/2 teaspoon newly ground dark pepper

1. Preheat air fryer at 350°F for 3 minutes.
2. Cut six arbitrary cuts, around 1" profound, in top of pork midsection. Push a garlic half in each cut.
3. In a little bowl, whisk together olive oil, rosemary, salt, and pepper. Massage into midsection on all sides.
4. Spot pork in air fryer crate. Cook 20 minutes. Flip. Cook 20 minutes more. The inward temperature ought to be at any rate 145°F when checked with a meat thermometer.
5. Allow pork to lay on a cutting board 5 minutes prior to cutting and serving warm.

Per serving **Calories**: 444 | Fat: 23.2 g | Protein: 42.5 g | Sodium: 713 mg | Fiber: 0.2 g | Carbs: 0.4 g | Sugar: 0.0 g

GERMAN MUSTARD PORK MIDSECTION CLEAVES

There are really numerous assortments of mustard in Germany however by and large just a modest bunch of decisions on the racks of American supermarkets. They can go from gentle to very fiery. So take a fast look at the names and pick one that is ideal for your taste buds.

Active Time: 5 minutes
CookTime: 11 minutes
Fixings | Serves:3
1. 3 boneless focus cut pork midsection cleaves, each around 1" thick (around 1 pound absolute)
2. 1 teaspoon salt
3. 1/2 teaspoon newly ground dark pepper
4. 6 teaspoons German mustard
5. Preheat air fryer at 350°F for 3 minutes.
6. Season the two sides of pork cleaves with salt and pepper. Brush the highest point of each cleave with 2 teaspoons mustard.
7. Spot pork on gently lubed air fryer crate with mustard side up. Cook 4 minutes. Flip. Cook 4 minutes more. Flip. Cook an extra 3 minutes. The inside temperature ought to be at any rate 145°F when checked with a meat thermometer.
8. Allow pork to lay on a cutting board 5 minutes prior to serving warm.
    Per serving **Calories**: 313 | Fat: 8.9 g | Protein: 53.7 g | Sodium: 1,696 mg | Fiber: 0.2 g | Carbs: 1.6 g | Sugar: 0.0 g

SALT AND VINEGAR POTATO CHIP PORK FLANK SLASHES

There are a couple of **Fixings** in this formula in light of the fact that the potato chip scraps hit the salt, vinegar, and bland components found in a conventional breading. If you're gutsy, you can choose a different assortment of chip each time you make this formula!

Active Time: 5 minutes
CookTime: 11 minutes
Fixings | Serves:3
*   1 cup squashed salt and vinegar potato chips
*   1 teaspoon dried thyme
*   2 tablespoons margarine, liquefied
*   3 boneless focus cut pork flank slashes, each around 1" thick (around 1 pound absolute)

In a medium bowl, consolidate squashed chips, thyme, and liquefied spread.
Preheat air fryer at 350°F for 3 minutes.
Press chip blend equally over the highest point of every pork cleave.
Spot slashes on daintily lubed air fryer bushel with chip side up. Cook 11 minutes. The interior temperature ought to be in any event 145°F when checked with a meat thermometer.
Allow pork to lay on a cutting board 5 minutes prior to serving warm.

Per serving **Calories**: 306 | Fat: 15.0 g | Protein: 35.7 g | Sodium: 156 mg | Fiber: 0.4 g | Carbs: 5.3 g | Sugar: 0.0 g

SWEET PORK SLASHES

The combination of the peach jam, ketchup, Worcestershire sauce, and lemon juice makes a sweet grill sauce of sorts. The air fryer singes all sides of the hacks while keeping within succulent!

Involved Time: 5 minutes
CookTime: 12 minutes
Fixings | Serves:2
*   2 tablespoons peach jam
*   1 tablespoon ketchup
*   1 teaspoon Worcestershire sauce
*   1 tablespoon lemon juice
*   1 tablespoon olive oil
*   2 (1"- thick) bone-in pork cleaves, roughly 1 pound

1. In a medium bowl, whisk together peach jam, ketchup, Worcestershire sauce, lemon juice, and olive oil. Add pork cleaves and refrigerate covered 30 minutes.
2. Preheat air fryer at 350°F for 3 minutes.
3. Spot pork cleaves in air fryer container. Cook 4 minutes. Flip. Cook 4 minutes more. Flip. Cook an extra 4 minutes. The inward temperature ought to be at any rate 145°F when checked with a meat thermometer.
4. Allow pork to lay on a cutting board 5 minutes prior to serving warm.

Per serving **Calories**: 258 | Fat: 13.5 g | Protein: 27.4 g | Sodium: 73 mg | Fiber: 0.0 g | Starches: 1.2 g | Sugar: 1.1 g

PARMESAN-CRUSTED PORK HACKS

The Parmesan cheddar covering separates these air-seared pork hacks from any others. Done quickly, they can rest while you plate the remainder of your food. When the plate makes it to the table, they will be prepared to eat!

Active Time: 5 minutes
CookTime: 12 minutes
Fixings | **Serves:**2
- 1 huge egg
- 1 tablespoon Dijon mustard
- $1/4$ cup ground Parmesan cheddar
- $1/4$ cup panko bread morsels
- $1/4$ teaspoon newly ground dark pepper
- 2 (1"- thick) bone-in pork slashes, around 1 pound

1. Preheat air fryer at 350°F for 3 minutes.
2. In a little dish, whisk together egg and Dijon mustard. In a shallow dish consolidate Parmesan cheddar, bread morsels, and dark pepper.
3. Plunge pork slashes in egg blend. Dig in bread piece combination.
4. Spot pork on softly lubed air fryer container. Cook 4 minutes. Flip. Cook 4 minutes more. Flip. Cook an extra 4 minutes. The inner temperature ought to be at any rate 145°F when checked with a meat thermometer.
5. Allow pork to lay on a cutting board 5 minutes prior to serving warm.
   Per serving Calories: 376 | Fat: 17.8 g | Protein: 34.3 g | Sodium: 425 mg | Fiber: 0.1 g | Carbs: 12.3 g | Sugar: 0.6 g

PORK SCHNITZEL

Pork schnitzel, or Schweineschnitzel, is pork cutlet that has been beat dainty and breaded. The air fryer cooks all sides to a delicious freshness. Serve this schnitzel with your number one potato dish for a total German feasting experience.

Active Time: 15 minutes
CookTime: 42 minutes
Fixings | **yields** 6 schnitzels
- 6 boneless focus cut pork midsection hacks, each roughly $1/2$" thick (around 1 pound complete)
- $1/2$ cup generally useful flour
- 1 huge egg, whisked
- 1 cup panko bread pieces
- 1 tablespoon ground dry mustard
- 1 teaspoon newly ground dark pepper
- 2 tablespoons lemon juice
- 2 teaspoons salt
- 1 medium lemon, cut into 6 wedges

1. Spot a flank between two bits of material paper. Utilizing the level side of a hammer, hammer out pork until it is $1/8$" thick. Rehash with outstanding flanks. Put away.
2. In a little bowl, add flour. In another bowl, add whisked egg. In a shallow dish, consolidate bread scraps, ground mustard, and dark pepper.
3. Preheat air fryer at 350°F for 3 minutes.
4. Sprinkle every midsection with lemon squeeze and salt on the two sides.
5. Coat every midsection in flour. Shake off overabundance. Plunge in egg and shake off overabundance. Dig in bread scraps.
6. Spot pork on daintily lubed air fryer crate. Cook 4 minutes. Flip. Cook 3 minutes. Rehash with outstanding pork. The inside temperature ought to be in any event 145°F when checked with a meat thermometer.
7. Allow pork to lay on a cutting board 5 minutes prior to serving warm with lemon wedges.

Per serving Calories: 156 | Fat: 3.4 g | Protein: 19.7 g | Sodium: 852 mg | Fiber: 0.3 g | Starches: 11.3 g | Sugar: 0.5 g

STUFFED PORK MIDSECTION CLEAVES

The apple in the stuffing loans a pleasantness to this dish. It additionally gives dampness to hold the pork back from drying out. Present with a prepared yam for a soothing occasion feel to your supper.

Active Time: 5 minutes
CookTime: 11 minutes
Fixings | **Serves:**3
- 3 boneless focus cut pork midsection hacks, each around 1" thick (around 1 pound complete)
- 2 cuts good wheat bread, diced into $1/4$" 3D squares
- $1/4$ cup stripped, cored, and ground Granny Smith apple
- 2 teaspoons finely cleaved new sage leaves
- 1 tablespoon spread, dissolved
- $1/2$ teaspoon salt
- $1/2$ teaspoon newly ground dark pepper

1. Cut a pocket in the thickness of every pork midsection cleave, guaranteeing that the knife doesn't carve entirely through.
2. In a medium bowl, consolidate bread 3D squares, apple, sage, spread, salt, and pepper.
3. Preheat air fryer at 350°F for 3 minutes.
4. Stuff 33% of bread combination into every pork cleave.
5. Spot pork slashes on softly lubed air fryer crate. Cook 11 minutes. The inner temperature ought to be in any event 145°F when checked with a meat thermometer.
6. Allow pork to lay on a cutting board 5 minutes prior to serving warm.

PREPARED PORK

As an additional part to this dish, utilize the pineapple juice from a container of pineapple pieces. Then, at that point throw the pieces in the sauce with the pork toward the finish of this formula. Serve the combination over rice to finish the take-out experience and remember to purchase those fortune treats!

Active Time: 15 minutes
CookTime: 20 minutes

Fixings | **Serves:**4
- 3 tablespoons cornstarch, separated
- 1 tablespoon water
- 2 tablespoons rice vinegar
- 2 tablespoons ketchup
- 1/3 cup pineapple juice
- 2 tablespoons earthy colored sugar
- 2 teaspoons soy sauce
- 1 enormous egg
- 2 tablespoons universally handy flour
- 1 pound boneless pork flank, cut into 1" shapes

1. In a little bowl, make a slurry by whisking together 1 tablespoon cornstarch and water. Put away.
2. In a little pot over medium warmth, consolidate rice vinegar, ketchup, pineapple juice, sugar, and soy sauce. Cook 3 minutes, mixing constantly. Add cornstarch slurry and warmth 1 more moment. Set skillet away from warmth and permit to thicken.
3. In a medium bowl, whisk together egg, flour, and 2 tablespoons cornstarch.
4. Preheat air fryer at 350°F for 3 minutes.

5. Dig pork solid shapes in egg hitter. Shake off any overabundance.
6. Add pork in two clusters to air fryer crate. Cook 4 minutes. Shake tenderly. Cook an extra 4 minutes. Check the pork utilizing a meat thermometer to guarantee the inward temperature is in any event 145°F.
7. Move to a bowl. Add sauce and throw until covered. Serve warm.

Per serving Calories: 227 | Fat: 4.1 g | Protein: 24.5 g | Sodium: 291 mg | Fiber: 0.3 g | Carbs: 20.5 g | Sugar: 10.7 g

FRESH TERIYAKI PORK AND RICE

By meagerly cutting the pork before cooking, you permit the air fryer to give those tasty fresh edges to this delicious meat, which adds another element of flavor and surface to this straightforward dish.

Involved Time: 10 minutes
CookTime: 17 minutes
Fixings | **Serves:**4
- 1 pound pork shoulder, managed and meagerly cut into flimsy 1"- long strips
- 1/2 cup in addition to 1 tablespoon teriyaki sauce
- 2 tablespoons water
- 1 tablespoon nectar
- 2 cups cooked rice
- 1/4 cup slashed new cilantro

1. In a medium bowl, add pork and 1/2 cup teriyaki sauce. Refrigerate covered 30 minutes.
2. Preheat air fryer at 350°F for 3 minutes. Add water to lower part of air fryer.
3. Spot pork in air fryer crate. Cook 5 minutes. Throw. Cook 6 minutes more. Throw. Cook an extra 6 minutes.
4. In a little bowl, whisk together 1 tablespoon teriyaki sauce and nectar. Throw cooked pork in sauce.
5. Serve pork over cooked rice and topping with cilantro.

Per serving Calories: 350 | Fat: 13.4 g | Protein: 23.4 g | Sodium: 909 mg | Fiber: 0.4 g | Starches: 30.1 g | Sugar: 7.5 g

BAR-B-QUE PORK BOWL

Pork, grill sauce, new corn, and pureed potatoes—if there is a route to somebody's heart through their stomach, these four Fixings consolidated ought to get the job done!

Involved Time: 15 minutes
CookTime: 20 minutes
Fixings | Serves:4

- 1 pound pork shoulder, managed and meagerly cut into 1"- long strips
- $^1/2$ cup grill sauce of your decision
- 2 tablespoons water
- 1 cup corn parts
- 2 enormous Chestnut potatoes, stripped and diced into $^1/4$" 3D squares
- 2 tablespoons margarine
- $^1/4$ cup entire milk
- 1 teaspoon salt
- 1 teaspoon newly ground dark pepper
- $^1/4$ cup slashed new parsley

1. In a medium bowl, add pork and grill sauce. Refrigerate covered 30 minutes.
2. Preheat air fryer at 350°F for 3 minutes. Add water to lower part of air fryer.
3. Spot pork in air fryer container. Cook 6 minutes. Throw. Cook 6 minutes more. Add corn and throw. Cook an extra 3 minutes.
4. While pork is cooking, add potatoes to a pot of bubbling salted water and cook 4–5 minutes until fork-delicate. Channel potatoes and move to a medium bowl. Add margarine, milk, salt, and pepper. Pound until smooth.
5. Serve pork and corn over pureed potatoes and trimming with new parsley.

Per serving Calories. 407 | Fat: 19.6 g | Protcin: 23.4 g | Sodium: 1,026 mg | Fiber: 2.8 g | Starches: 32.1 g | Sugar: 9.7 g

ASIAN PORK MEATBALLS

Serve these scrumptious meatballs over rice noodles or lo mein for an Asian play on spaghetti and meatballs! To throw with the noodles, stir up 1 tablespoon soy sauce, 3 minced garlic cloves, $^1/4$ teaspoon coriander, and $^1/4$ teaspoon ground ginger in addition to 1 teaspoon of nectar and 1 teaspoon of hot sauce (sriracha, gochujang, or sambal oelek).

Active Time: 15 minutes
CookTime: 16 minutes
Fixings | Serves:4

- 1 pound lean ground pork
- 1 huge egg
- 1 tcaspoon ground ginger
- $^1/2$ teaspoon ground coriander
- 2 cloves garlic, minced
- 1 teaspoon soy sauce
- $^1/4$ cup plain bread morsels
- 1 scallion, managed and partitioned, white part finely cleaved and green part cut

1. Preheat air fryer at 350°F for 3 minutes.
2. In a medium bowl, consolidate pork, egg, ginger, coriander, garlic, soy sauce, bread morsels, and scallion whites. Structure into sixteen meatballs, around 2 table-spoons each.
3. Add eight meatballs to fryer crate and cook 6 minutes. Flip meatballs. Cook an extra 2 minutes. Move to a plate. Rehash with residual meatballs.
4. Serve warm decorated with scallion greens.

Per serving Calories: 193 | Fat: 5.6 g | Protein: 26.3 g | Sodium: 204 mg | Fiber: 0.5 g | Carbs: 6.1 g | Sugar: 0.5 g

SPAGHETTI AND MEATBALLS

Cooking the meatballs noticeable all around fryer bin prior to covering them with the marinara sauce permits them to get a burn on the outside prior to washing in the sweet-smelling marinara! Top with ground Parmesan cheddar and new parsley, and there will be no disarray why this is a staple on so numerous family tables.

Active Time: 15 minutes
CookTime: 16 minutes
Fixings | Serves:4

- 1 pound dry spaghetti
- 1 pound ground pork
- 1 huge egg
- $^1/4$ cup hacked new basil
- 2 cloves garlic, minced
- $^1/2$ teaspoon salt
- $^1/4$ cup plain bread pieces
- 2 cups marinara sauce
- 4 tablespoons ground Parmesan cheddar
- $^1/4$ cup hacked new parsley

1. Preheat air fryer at 350°F for 3 minutes.
2. In a medium bowl, consolidate pork, egg, basil, garlic, salt, and bread scraps. Structure into sixteen meatballs, around 2 tablespoons each.

3. Add eight meatballs to fryer bin and cook 6 minutes. Move to cake barrel (adornment). Rehash with staying eight meatballs. Pour marinara sauce over meatballs. Spot cake barrel with every one of the meatballs in air fryer crate. Cook an extra 4 minutes.
4. Appropriate spaghetti equally among four dishes. Top each with meatballs and sauce. Trimming with Parmesan cheddar and new parsley. Serve warm.

Per serving Calories: 665 | Fat: 8.6 g | Protein: 43.4 g | Sodium: 797 mg | Fiber: 5.3 g | Carbs: 96.1 g | Sugar: 7.2 g

PORK LETTUCE CUPS

This appears to be an extensive rundown of Fixings , however once you make this formula, you'll need to make it again and again. You'll simply need to recharge the new Fixings each time. The packaged Fixings will be close by as of now!

Active Time: 10 minutes
CookTime: 40 minutes
Fixings | **Serves:**6
- ¹/2 cup rice vinegar
- ¹/4 cup sugar
- Squeeze salt
- 1 huge carrot, stripped and julienned
- 1 medium English cucumber, stripped and diced
- 1 scallion, managed and diced
- 1 (2-pound) boneless pork midsection cook
- 1 teaspoon salt
- ¹/2 teaspoon newly ground dark pepper
- ¹/4 cup soy sauce
- 2 tablespoons nectar
- 1 tablespoon sriracha
- 2 teaspoons fish sauce
- 1 teaspoon ground ginger
- 1 teaspoon ground white pepper
- 12 Bibb lettuce leaves
- ¹/2 cup cleaved new basil

1. In a medium bowl, whisk together vinegar, sugar, and salt. Add carrot, cucumber, and scallion. Throw to cover and refrigerate covered until prepared to utilize.
2. Preheat air fryer at 350°F for 3 minutes.
3. Season cook with salt and dark pepper.
4. Spot pork in air fryer bin. Cook 20 minutes. Flip. Cook 20 minutes more. The inside temperature ought to be at any rate 145°F when checked with a meat thermometer.
5. Allow pork to lay on a cutting board 5 minutes, then, at that point shred pork utilizing two forks.
6. In an enormous bowl, whisk together soy sauce, nectar, sriracha, fish sauce, ginger, and white pepper. Include cut pork and throw to completely cover.
7. Gather lettuce cups by adding an equivalent parts of covered pork to the focal point of every lettuce leaf. Top with vegetable combination and embellishment with new basil.

Per serving Calories: 349 | Fat: 17.2 g | Protein: 29.2 g | Sodium: 1,286 mg | Fiber: 1.1 g | Starches: 14.0 g | Sugar: 11.7 g

BERBERE COUNTRY PORK RIBS

The beautiful Ethiopian flavors of berbere join so well with the sweet maple syrup and citrus squeezed orange, adjusting the kind of these country pork ribs. Also, the air fryer manages its work incredibly by cooking these to delectable flawlessness.

Active Time: 10 minutes
CookTime: 40 minutes

Fixings | **Serves:**4
- 1 tablespoon berbere preparing
- 1 teaspoon salt
- 2 pounds country-style pork ribs
- 2 tablespoons water
- ¹/2 cup newly crushed squeezed orange
- 1 tablespoon maple syrup

1. Massage berbere preparing and salt into ribs.
2. Preheat air fryer at 350°F for 3 minutes. Add water to lower part of air fryer.
3. Add pork to air fryer container. Cook 40 minutes, flipping at regular intervals.
4. In an enormous bowl, whisk together squeezed orange and maple syrup. Add cooked ribs and throw. Serve warm.

Per serving Calories: 421 | Fat: 23.5 g | Protein: 38.3 g | Sodium: 977 mg | Fiber: 0.1 g | Carbs: 7.4 g | Sugar: 5.6 g

LAGER BRATWURST

This German exemplary simply fusses to be presented with your #1 potato dish and a little hot mustard to drag your bratwurst through. If you are against utilizing lager in this formula, substitute meat stock and a scramble or two of Worcestershire sauce. It will be similarly as delectable!

Active Time: 15 minutes
CookTime: 21 minutes
Fixings | Serves:4

- 1 pound uncooked pork bratwurst
- 1 (12-ounce) bottle or container of lager
- 2 cups water
- ¹/2 medium yellow onion, stripped and cut

1. Penetrate every bratwurst multiple times with the prongs of a fork. Add to a medium pot with brew, water, and onion. Heat to the point of boiling. Diminish warmth and stew 15 minutes. Channel.
2. Preheat air fryer at 400°F for 3 minutes.
3. Spot bratwurst and onions in fryer crate. Cook 3 minutes. Flip and cook an extra 3 minutes. Check with a meat thermometer to guarantee an interior temperature of 160°F.
4. Move bratwurst and onions to a plate and serve warm.

Per serving Calories: 309 | Fat: 24.8 g | Protein: 12.6 g | Sodium: 767 mg | Fiber: 0.2 g | Carbs: 4.0 g | Sugar: 0.6 g

MUSTARD SPICE PORK TENDERLOIN

This formula is ideal for family suppers. It's not difficult to prepare, however your visitors could never know it! The mustard accomplishes the work for you, giving a smooth and marginally sweet base for the spice outside layer.

Pantry Staples: Salt, ground dark pepper
Hands On schedule: 5 minutes
Cook Time: 20 minutes
Serves: 6

- ¼ cup mayonnaise
- 2 tablespoons Dijon mustard
- ½ teaspoon dried thyme
- ¼ teaspoon dried rosemary
- (1-pound) pork tenderloin
- ½ teaspoon salt
- ¼ teaspoon ground dark pepper

1. In a little bowl, blend mayonnaise, mustard, thyme, and rosemary. Brush tenderloin with blend on all sides, then, at that point sprinkle with salt and pepper on all sides.
2. Spot tenderloin into ungreased air fryer crate. Change the temperature to 400°F and set the clock for 20 minutes, turning tenderloin partially through cooking. Tenderloin will be brilliant and have an inner temperature of in any event 145°F when done. Serve warm.

Per serving Calories: 158 Protein: 16g Fiber: 0g Net sugars: 1g Fat: 9g Sodium: 557mg Sugars: 1g

BACON-WRAPPED PORK TENDERLOIN

The best part about this dish is that there's bacon in each nibble! Pork can undoubtedly dry out under high warmth, so adding the fat from the bacon secures all the tastiness for a minimal expense dinner that is loaded with flavor.

Pantry Staples: Salt, ground dark pepper, garlic powder
Hands On schedule: 10 minutes
Cook Time: 20 minutes
Serves: 6

- (1-pound) pork tenderloin
- ½ teaspoon salt
- ½ teaspoon garlic powder
- ¼ teaspoon ground dark pepper
- 8 cuts sans sugar bacon

1. Sprinkle tenderloin with salt, garlic powder, and pepper. Fold each piece of bacon over tenderloin and secure with toothpicks.
2. Spot tenderloin into ungreased air fryer bin. Change the temperature to 400°F and set the clock for 20 minutes, turning tenderloin following 15 minutes. When done, bacon will be firm and tenderloin will have an interior temperature of at any rate 145°F.
3. Cut the tenderloin into six even segments and move each to a medium plate and serve warm.

Per serving Calories: 144 Protein: 20g Fiber: 0g Net carbs: 0g Fat: 6g Sodium: 590mg Carbs: 0g

You'll be astonished how consummately air fryers cook pork cleaves. A dull brilliant outside structures on each side, leaving within delicate and damp. Adding your number one flavors can zest things up, yet these are tasty and liquefy in your mouth with simply salt and pepper.

Pantry Staples: Salt, ground dark pepper
Hands On schedule: 5 minutes
Cook Time: 12 minutes
Serves: 4

- (4-ounce) boneless pork cleaves
- ½ teaspoon salt
- ¼ teaspoon ground dark pepper
- 2 tablespoons salted spread, mollified

1. Sprinkle pork cleaves on all sides with salt and pepper. Spot cleaves into ungreased air fryer crate in a solitary layer. Change the temperature to 400°F and set the clock for 12 minutes. Pork hacks will be brilliant and have an inward temperature of at any rate 145°F when done.
2. Use utensils to eliminate cooked pork slashes from air fryer and spot onto an enormous plate. Top each cleave with ½ tablespoon spread and let sit 2 minutes to dissolve. Serve warm.

Per serving
Calories: 278 Protein: 24g Fiber: 0g Net starches: 0g
Fat: 19gSodium: 428mg Starches: 0g Sugar: 0g

BACON AND CHEDDAR STUFFED PORK CLEAVES

Pork cleaves are an incredible spending dinner yet don't generally stand out enough to be noticed they merit. This tasty formula stuffs them with pungent bacon and cheddar for stunning flavor in each nibble. It's a dinner the entire family can appreciate.

Pantry Staples: Salt, ground dark pepper
Hands On schedule: 10 minutes
Cook Time: 12 minutes
Serves: 4

- ½ ounce plain pork skins, finely squashed
- ½ cup destroyed sharp cheddar
- 4 cuts cooked sans sugar bacon, disintegrated
- (4-ounce) boneless pork cleaves
- ½ teaspoon salt
- ¼ teaspoon ground dark pepper
- In a little bowl, blend pork skins, Cheddar, and bacon.

1. Make a 3" cut in the side of every pork cleave and stuff with ¼ pork skin combination. Sprinkle each side of pork slashes with salt and pepper.
2. Spot pork cleaves into ungreased air fryer crate, stuffed side up. Change the temperature to 400°F and set the clock for 12 minutes. Pork cleaves will be carmelized and have an inward temperature of at any rate 145°F when done. Serve warm.

Per serving Calories: 348
Protein: 33g fiber: 0g net sugars: 0g
Fat: 22g sodium: 694mg

PARMESAN-CRUSTED PORK SLASHES

While you may not ordinarily consider cheddar and pork together, this formula may alter your perspective. A delectable thick outside structures on the cheddar and gives the delicious pork significantly more flavor. Add a teaspoon of Italian flavoring for an additional kick. Balance the supper with a side of Bacon-Balsamic Brussels Fledglings

Pantry Staples: Salt, ground dark pepper
Hands On schedule: 5 minutes
Cook Time: 12 minutes
Serves: 4

- 1 huge egg
- ½ cup ground Parmesan cheddar
- (4-ounce) boneless pork hacks
- ½ teaspoon salt
- ¼ teaspoon ground dark pepper

1. Whisk egg in a medium bowl and spot Parmesan in a different medium bowl.
2. Sprinkle pork hacks on the two sides with salt and pepper. Dunk every pork cleave into egg, then, at that point press the two sides into Parmesan.
3. Spot pork hacks into ungreased air fryer bushel. Change the temperature to 400°F and set the clock for 12 minutes, turning cleaves part of the way through cooking. Pork slashes will be brilliant and have an inside temperature of in any event 145°F when done. Serve warm.

Per serving Calories: 298
Protein: 29g fiber: 0g net starches: 2g
Fat: 17g sodium: 626mg starches: 2g sugar: 0g

FIRM PORK PAUNCH

Pork paunch is cut from a similar region as bacon yet is uncured and frequently cut in bigger pieces. Consider it a major chunk of bacon that you can fresh up and eat like a popper. You can make this a dinner or even a superfilling nibble—simply make certain to prepare so the meat has the opportunity to marinate.

Pantry Staples: Salt, ground dark pepper
Hands On schedule: 40 minutes
Cook Time: 20 minutes
Serves: 4

- 1 pound pork paunch, cut into 1" solid shapes
- ¼ cup soy sauce
- 1 tablespoon Worcestershire sauce
- 2 teaspoons sriracha hot bean stew sauce
- ½ teaspoon salt
- ¼ teaspoon ground dark pepper

1. Spot pork gut into a medium sealable bowl or sack and pour in soy sauce, Worcestershire sauce, and sriracha. Seal and let marinate 30 minutes in the fridge.
2. Eliminate pork from marinade, wipe off with a paper towel, and sprinkle with salt and pepper.
3. Spot pork in ungreased air fryer container. Change the temperature to 360°F and set the clock for 20 minutes, shaking the bin partially through cooking. Pork stomach will be done when it has an inner temperature of at any rate 145°F and is brilliant earthy colored.
4. Allow pork to midsection lay on an enormous plate 10 minutes. Serve warm.

Per serving Calories: 588 protein: 11g Fiber: 0g net carbs: 0g fat: 56g Sodium: 423mg carbs: 0g

PORK SPARE RIBS

Cooking delicate, succulent ribs has never been simpler, on account of the air fryer. The sauce in this formula caramelizes to make a thick coating that makes the ideal nibble. Pair with cauliflower rice for a filling family supper.

Pantry Staples: Salt, ground dark pepper, garlic powder
Hands On schedule: 10 minutes
Cook Time: 30 minutes
Serves: 4

- 1 (4-pound) rack pork spare ribs
- 1 teaspoon ground cumin
- 2 teaspoons salt

- 1 teaspoon ground dark pepper
- 1 teaspoon garlic powder
- ½ teaspoon dry ground mustard
- ½ cup low-carb grill sauce

1. Spot ribs on ungreased aluminum foil sheet. Cautiously utilize a knife to eliminate film and sprinkle meat uniformly on the two sides with cumin, salt, pepper, garlic powder, and ground mustard.
2. Cut rack into divides that will fit in your air fryer, and enclose each segment by one layer of aluminum foil, working in clusters if required.
3. Spot ribs into ungreased air fryer bushel. Change the temperature to 400°F and set the clock for 25 minutes.
4. At the point when the clock signals, cautiously eliminate ribs from foil and brush with grill sauce. Get back to air fryer and cook at 400°F for an extra 5 minutes to brown. Ribs will be done when no pink remaining parts and inside temperature is in any event 180°F. Serve warm.

Per serving Calories: 192 Protein: 13g fiber: 0g net sugars: 3g Fat: 12g sodium: 1,374mg starches: 3g

PORK MEATBALLS

This dish is motivated by the kinds of the exemplary egg roll. Ground pork will in general be lean, so make certain to match this formula with a side that is higher in fat to adjust the feast.

Pantry Staples: Salt, garlic powder
Hands On schedule: 10 minutes
Cook Time: 12 minutes
Yields 18 meatballs

- 1 pound ground pork
- 1 huge egg, whisked
- ½ teaspoon garlic powder
- ½ teaspoon salt
- ½ teaspoon ground ginger
- ¼ teaspoon squashed red pepper chips
- 1 medium scallion, managed and cut

1. Consolidate all Fixings in a huge bowl. Spoon out 2 tablespoons blend and fold into a ball. Rehash to shape eighteen meatballs all out.
2. Spot meatballs into ungreased air fryer crate. Change the temperature to 400°F and set the clock for 12 minutes, shaking the bin multiple times all through cooking.

Meatballs will be sautéed and have an inside temperature of at any rate 145°F when done. Serve warm.

Per serving (3 meatballs) calories: 164 Protein: 15g fiber: 0g net sugars: 1g Fat: 10g sodium: 252mg Sugars: 1g

ZEST SCOURED PORK FLANK

The best things about pork are that it's modest and has a gentle flavor that makes it the ideal fresh start for your flavoring. Pair this dish with Simmered Brussels Fledglings for a total dinner that should be possible in a little more than 20 minutes!

Pantry Staples: Salt, ground dark pepper, paprika, garlic powder, coconut oil
Hands On schedule: 5 minutes
Cook Time: 20 minutes

Serves: 6
- 1 teaspoon paprika
- ½ teaspoon ground cumin
- ½ teaspoon bean stew powder
- ½ teaspoon garlic powder
- 2 tablespoons coconut oil
- 1 (1½-pound) boneless pork flank
- ½ teaspoon salt
- ¼ teaspoon ground dark pepper

1. In a little bowl, blend paprika, cumin, stew powder, and garlic powder.
2. Shower coconut oil over pork. Sprinkle pork flank with salt and pepper, then, at that point rub zest combination equally on all sides.
3. Spot pork midsection into ungreased air fryer bin. Change the temperature to 400°F and set the clock for 20 minutes, turning pork partially through cooking. Pork flank will be seared and have an interior temperature of in any event 145°F when done. Serve warm.

Per serving calories: 249 protein: 24g
Fiber: 0g net starches: 1g fat: 16g
Sodium: 278mg starches: 1g sugar: 0g

AIR SINGED PORK HACKS

Planning Time: 5 minutes
Cook Time: 12 minutes

Serves:: 6 **Servings**

Fixings
- 1/3 cup almond flour
- 1/2 pounds pork hacks, boneless
- 1 teaspoon garlic powder
- 1/4 cup parmesan cheddar, ground
- 1 teaspoon paprika
- 1 teaspoon creole flavoring

Strategy
1. Add each fixing into a major ziploc sack, close top and shake until completely covered and consolidated.
2. Take out marinated pork hacks from the ziploc sack and move into your fryer crate in one layer.
3. Cook pork hacks at 380º at 8-12 minutes until all around cooked.
4. Let pork cleaves sit until cooled, serve and appreciate.

Nourishing Data/Serving
Calories 222 kcal, Net Carb 1g, Protein 26g, Dietary Fiber 1g, Carbs 2g, Fat 11g

KETO AIR SINGED BACON

Planning Time: 5 minutes
Cook Time: 10 minutes
Serves:: 4 **Servings**

Fixings
- 6 bacon cuts, no-sugar added
- Technique
- Add cuts of bacon in the fryer bin.
- Secure the top and cook for 5 minutes at 400º.
- Check for doneness and cook until wanted doneness is reached, for 3-5 additional minutes.

Wholesome Data/Serving
Calories 90 kcal, Carbs 0g, Fat 8g, Protein 6g

COCONUT PORK SLASHES

Planning Time: 5 minutes
Cook Time: 15 minutes
Serves:: 2 Servings
Fixings
- 1 tablespoon coconut margarine
- 4 pork slashes
- 2 teaspoon ground garlic cloves
- 1 tablespoon coconut oil
- Salt and pepper, as important
- 2 teaspoon new slashed cilantro

Technique
1. Warmth up air fryer to 350º.
2. Add each preparing fixing into a bowl and join.
3. Add the garlic, margarine and coconut oil into the flavoring combination and blend until entirely joined.
4. Brush and rub pork slashes with the margarine/preparing blend until equally covered.
5. Spot prepared pork slashes in aluminum thwart and refrigerate for 1 hour until marinated.
6. Rub any additional marinade over pork hacks.
7. Spot marinated pork hacks in the fryer container and cook for 7 minutes.
8. Flip pork hacks and cook for 8 additional minutes until very much cooked.
9. Serve and appreciate.

Dietary Data/Serving
Calories 524 kcal, Protein 58g, Dietary Fiber 1g, Complete carbs 2g, All out Fat 29g

DELECTABLY CRISPED PORK TUMMY

Planning Time: 10 minutes
Cook Time: 30 minutes
Serves:: 4 Servings
Fixings
- 3 cups water
- 1 lb. (cut into 3 thick pieces) pork stomach
- 1 tsp pepper
- 1 tsp salt
- 2 cove leaves
- 2 tbsps soy sauce
- 6 garlic cloves

Strategy
1. Add each fixing into an electric pressing factor cooker pot.
2. Cook for 15 minutes at High pressing factor.
3. Delivery pressure normally for 10 minutes and afterward fast delivery cautiously.
4. Cautiously move meat from pressure cooker, utilizing utensils and let sit for 10 minutes until dried and depleted.

5. Cut every pork stomach piece into two long cuts.
6. Add each cut of pork paunch in the fryer bushel.
7. Cook pork paunch cuts until pork stomach is crisped, for 15 minutes at 400º.
8. Serve and appreciate.

Healthful Data/Serving
Calories 594 kcal, Protein 11g, Fat 60g

PORK SLASHES

Planning Time: 5 minutes
Cook Time: 15 minutes
Serves:: 4 Servings
Fixings
- 1/2 teaspoon salt
- 6 boneless pork slashes
- 1 teaspoon smoked paprika
- 1/4 teaspoon pepper
- 1/4 teaspoon bean stew powder
- 1/2 teaspoon onion powder
- 1 cup pork skin morsels
- 2 (beaten) large eggs
- 3 tablespoons parmesan cheddar, ground

Technique
1. For approx. 10 minutes, heat up air fryer to 400º.
2. Sprinkle pepper and salt over pork slashes until equitably prepared on all sides.
3. Add flavors and pork skin morsels into a major bowl and blend well.
4. Add the beaten egg into a subsequent bowl.
5. Drench each and every pork cleave in the egg wash, then, at that point inundate in the pork skin combination prior to moving into the fryer crate.
6. Cook for 12-15 minutes at 400º, contingent upon the thickness of the pork slashes utilized.

Nourishing Data/Serving
Calories 526 kcal, Carbs 5g, Fat 29g, Protein 64g

EXTRA FRESH BACON WITH EGGS

Planning Time: 2 minutes
Cook Time: 8 minutes
Serves:: 5 **Servings**
Fixings
- 5 bacon strips
- 5 (mixed/hardboiled) eggs

Technique
1. Add bacon strips into the fryer bin in a solitary layer.
2. Cook bacon strips for 8 minutes at 375º. Note: Check for doneness from time to time to decide firmness while cooking.
3. Serve crisped bacon with hardboiled/fried eggs

Nourishing Data/Serving
Calories 91 kcal, Protein 2g, Absolute Fat 8g

HERBED SAUSAGE MEATBALL

Planning Time: 10 minutes
Cook Time: 10 minutes
Serves:: 6 (4 meatball)
Fixings
- 4 minced garlic cloves
- 2 tbsps avocado oil
- 1 (delicately beaten) enormous egg
- 1 tsp curry powder
- 1/4 cup disintegrated pork skins
- 1 (4 oz.) container (depleted) diced pimientos
- 1 tbsp minced new tarragon
- 1/4 cup minced new cilantro
- 2 lbs. pork sausage

Strategy
1. Warmth up air fryer to 400º.
2. Add avocado oil into a little skillet over drug heat.
3. Add curry powder and garlic into the hot oil and cook for 1-2 minutes until relaxed.
4. Let sit to cool marginally.
5. Add garlic curry combination, tarragon, cilantro, pork skins, pimientos and egg into a bowl and join.
6. Add pork sausage into the combination and blend well to join.
7. Structure into 24 (1/4") meatballs and move into the fryer bin in one layer. Tip: work in clumps.
8. Cook meatballs, for 7-10 minutes until all around cooked and sautéed delicately.
9. Eliminate meatballs from air fryer and keep warm until prepared to serve.
10. Rehash until no meatball remains.
11. Serve and appreciate.

Dietary Data/Serving
Calories 96 kcal, Protein 4g, Carb 2g, Fat 8g

SMOKED BAR-B-QUE RIBS

Planning Time: 20 minutes
Cook Time: 30 minutes
Serves:: 2 **Servings**
Fixings
- 1 tbsp fluid smoke
- 1 rack (layers on the back eliminated and cut down the middle) spare ribs
- Salt and pepper, as vital
- 2-3 tbsps pork rub
- 1/2 cup low carb grill sauce

Technique
1. Spill ribs with fluid smoke until uniformly covered.
2. Sprinkle pepper, salt and pork rub over ribs until uniformly covered, place top over ribs and let sit for 30 minutes at room temp.
3. Move marinated ribs into the fryer bin, stack and cook at 360º for 15 minutes.
4. Open fryer, turn the ribs and cook for 15 additional minutes.
5. Serve ribs, spilled with grill sauce.

Dietary Data/Serving Calories 333 kcal, Carbs 14g, Fat 25g, Protein 14g

Get ready to dive into a sea of delicious recipes! Fish is one of the best sources of omega-3 fatty acids, which can help fight inflammation and heart disease, and it's a great source of protein to help keep your muscles strong while you're on a ketogenic diet. Still, despite the flavor and health benefits, seafood is not the easiest cuisine to prepare.

Enter the air fryer. The air fryer will be your favorite tool for creating fresh and delicious, perfectly crisp fish and seafood recipes. From Fried Tuna Salad Bites to Firecracker Shrimp, you'll soon be a master of seafood cuisine, creating flavorful dishes your family can't get enough of!

LEMON GARLIC SHRIMP

Lemon and garlic are two amazing flavors to complement any seafood. They're simple but create the most mouthwatering blend of sweet, sour, and savory. Pair this shrimp with a bed of zucchini noodles for a more complete meal.

HandsOn Time: 5 minutes
Cook Time: 6 minutes
Serves 2

- 1 medium lemon
- 8 ounces medium shelled and deveined shrimp
- 2 tablespoons unsalted butter, melted
- 2 teaspoon Old Bay seasoning
- 2 teaspoon minced garlic

Directtions

- ✓ 1 Zest lemon and then cut in half. Place shrimp in a large bowl and squeeze juice from V2 lemon on top of them.
- ✓ 2 Add lemon zest to bowl along with remaining ingredients. Toss shrimp until fully coated.
- ✓ 3 Pour bowl contents into 6" round baking dish. Place into the air fryer basket.
- ✓ 4 Adjust the temperature to 400°F and set the timer for 6 minutes.
- ✓ 5 Shrimp will be bright pink when fully cooked. Serve warm with pan sauce.

Per serving
Calories: 190 Protein: 16.4 g fiber: 0.4 g
Net carbohydrates: 2.5 g fat: 11.8 g Sodium: 812 mg
carbohydrates: 2.9 g sugar: 0.5 g

CAJUN SALMON

Salmon can be a bit plain on its own, but that's something you won't have to worry about with this New Orleans-style recipe! The seasonings bring just the right amount of spice to elevate your fish into an irresistible meal!

HandsOn Time: 5 minutes
Cook Time: 7 minutes
Serves 2

- 2 (4-ounce) salmon fillets, skin removed
- 2 tablespoons unsalted butter, melted
- 1/8 teaspoon ground cayenne pepper
- 2 teaspoon garlic powder
- 1 teaspoon paprika
- 1/4 teaspoon ground black pepper

Directions

- ✓ Brush each fillet with butter.
- ✓ Combine remaining ingredients in a small bowl and then rub onto fish. Place fillets into the air fryer basket.
- ✓ Adjust the temperature to 390°F and set the timer for 7 minutes.
- ✓ When fully cooked, internal temperature will be 145°F. Serve immediately.

Per serving
Calories: 253 Protein: 20.9 g Fiber: 0.4 g Net carbohydrates: 1.0 g fat: 16.6 g Sodium: 46 mg

BLACKENED SHRIMP

This succulent shrimp is just bursting with Cajun flavor. It's a bold and mouthwatering dish that can be eaten on its own or added to a bowl of zucchini noodles for a pasta feel.

HandsOn Time: 5 minutes
Cook Time: 6 minutes
Serves 2

- 8 ounces medium shelled and deveined shrimp
- 2 tablespoons salted butter, melted
- 1 teaspoon paprika
- 2 teaspoon garlic powder
- 4 teaspoon onion powder
- 2 teaspoon Old Bay seasoning

Directions

- ✓ Toss all ingredients together in a large bowl. Place shrimp into the air fryer basket.
- ✓ Adjust the temperature to 400°F and set the timer for 6 minutes.

✓ Turn the shrimp halfway through the cooking time to ensure even cooking. Serve immediately.

Per serving
Calories: 192 Protein: 16.6 g Fiber: 0.5 g
Net carbohydrates: 2.0 g fat: 11.9 g Sodium: 902 mg
Carbohydrates: 2.5 g sugar: 0.2 g

COCONUT SHRIMP

The coconut in this recipe gives the juicy shrimp a sweet, crispy, golden crust. It's the perfect finger food (paired with sriracha) for a summertime barbecue, or it can also be served on a bed of greens for an easy salad.

HandsOn Time: 5 minutes
Cook Time: 6 minutes
Serves 2

- 8 ounces medium shelled and deveined shrimp
- 2 tablespoons salted butter, melted
- 2 teaspoon Old Bay seasoning
- 4 cup unsweetened shredded coconut

Directions
- ✓ In a large bowl, toss the shrimp in butter and Old Bay seasoning.
- ✓ Place shredded coconut in bowl. Coat each piece of shrimp in the coconut and place into the air fryer basket.
- ✓ Adjust the temperature to 400°F and set the timer for 6 minutes.
- ✓ Gently turn the shrimp halfway through the cooking time. Serve immediately.

Per serving Calories: 252 Protein: 16.9 g Fiber: 2.0 g
Net carbohydrates: 1.8 g fat: 17.8 g Sodium: 902 mg
Carbohydrates: 3.8 g sugar: 0.7 g

FOIL-PACKET SALMON

Baking salmon in a foil packet is a great way to steam the meat while locking in the flavors of whichever spices and vegetables you want to cook with it. Typically, this could take up to 30 minutes, but in your air fryer, you'll have perfectly tender salmon in no time!

HandsOn Time: 10 minutes
Cook Time: 12 minutes
Serves 2

- 2 (4-ounce) salmon fillets, skin removed
- 2 tablespoons unsalted butter, melted
- 1/2 teaspoon garlic powder
- 1 medium lemon
- 1/2 teaspoon dried dill

Directions
- ✓ Place each fillet on a 5" x 5" square of aluminum foil. Drizzle with butter and sprinkle with garlic powder.
- ✓ Zest half of the lemon and sprinkle zest over salmon. Slice other half of the lemon and lay two slices on each piece of salmon. Sprinkle dill over salmon.
- ✓ Gather and fold foil at the top and sides to fully close packets. Place foil packets into the air fryer basket.
- ✓ Adjust the temperature to 400°F and set the timer for 12 minutes.
- ✓ Salmon will be easily flaked and have an internal temperature of at least 145°F when fully cooked. Serve immediately.

Per serving
Calories: 252 Protein: 20.9 G Fiber: 0.4 G
Net Carbohydrates: 0.8 G Fat: 16.5 G Sodium: 47 Mg
Carbohydrates: 1.2 G Sugar: 0.2 G

CRISPY FISH STICKS

Say goodbye to store-bought! These fish sticks are easy to make, and even freeze well, and they contain none of the high- carb junk (like wheat flour and cornstarch) you'll find in traditional fish sticks. This is a smart swap you'll be proud to feed to your family!

HandsOn Time: 15 minutes
Cook Time: 10 minutes
Serves 4 (4 sticks per serving)

- 1 ounce pork rinds, finely ground
- 1/4 cup blanched finely ground almond flour
- 1/2 teaspoon Old Bay seasoning
- 1 tablespoon coconut oil 1 large egg
- 1 pound cod fillet, cut into 3/4" strips

Directions
- ✓ Place ground pork rinds, almond flour, Old Bay seasoning, and coconut oil into a large bowl and mix together. In a medium bowl, whisk egg.
- ✓ Dip each fish stick into the egg and then gently press into the flour mixture, coating as fully and evenly as possible. Place fish sticks into the air fryer basket.
- ✓ Adjust the temperature to 400°F and set the timer for 10 minutes or until golden.
- ✓ Serve immediately.

Per serving Calories: 205 Protein: 24.4 g fiber: 0.8 g
Net carbohydrates: 0.8 g fat: 10.7 g sodium: 547 mg
Carbohydrates: 1.6 g sugar: 0.3 g

S A L M O N   P A T T I E S

Salmon Patties, or salmon cakes, are like a fish burger full of heart-healthy omega-3 fatty acids. They're a delicious meal that is best served in a lettuce wrap. You'll want to opt for a wild- caught salmon because this variety helps you to avoid many of the contaminants that farmed salmon often carry.

HandsOn Time: 10 minutes

Cook Time: 8 minutes

Serves 2

- 2 (5-ounce) pouches cooked pink salmon
- 1 large egg
- 1/4 cup ground pork rinds
- 2 tablespoons full-fat mayonnaise
- 2 teaspoons sriracha
- 1 teaspoon chili powder

Directions

- ✓ Mix all ingredients in a large bowl and form into four patties. Place patties into the air fryer basket.
- ✓ Adjust the temperature to 400°F and set the timer for 8 minutes.
- ✓ Carefully flip each patty halfway through the cooking time. Patties will be crispy on the outside when fully cooked.

Per serving Calories: 319 Protein: 33.8 g fiber: 0.5 g Net carbohydrates: 1.4 g fat: 19.0 g Sodium: 843 mg carbohydrates: 1.9 g sugar: 1.3 g

F I R E C R A C K E R   S H R I M P

This dish packs some serious heat! It's perfect for lovers of seafood who can't get enough spice in their life. The secret behind the flavor is hot chili sauce, also known as sriracha. It can be found in any grocery store and has only 1 gram of carbs **Per serving**!

HandsOn Time: 10 minutes

Cook Time: 7 minutes

Serves 4

- 1 pound medium shelled and deveined shrimp
- 2 tablespoons salted butter, melted
- 1/2 teaspoon Old Bay seasoning
- 1/4 teaspoon garlic powder
- 2 tablespoons sriracha
- 1/4 teaspoon powdered erythritol
- 1/4 cup full-fat mayonnaise
- 1/8 teaspoon ground black pepper

Directions

- ✓ In a large bowl, toss shrimp in butter, Old Bay seasoning, and garlic powder. Place shrimp into the air fryer basket.
- ✓ Adjust the temperature to 400°F and set the timer for 7 minutes.
- ✓ Flip the shrimp halfway through the cooking time. Shrimp will be bright pink when fully cooked.
- ✓ In another large bowl, mix sriracha, powdered erythritol, mayonnaise, and pepper. Toss shrimp in the spicy mixture and serve immediately.

Per serving Calories: 143 protein: 16.4 g fiber: 0.0 g Net carbohydrates: 2.8 g sugar alcohol: 0.2 g fat: 6.4 g sodium: 936 mg Carbohydrates: 3.0 g sugar: 1.5 g

C R A B   L E G S

Grab your garlic butter! It'll be perfect for dipping your succulent Crab Legs. This crustaceous creation bakes up beautifully in your air fryer, and you can even use the crabmeat to make the Hot Crab Dip (see recipe in this chapter)!

HandsOn Time: 5 minutes

Cook Time: 15 minutes

Serves: 4

- 1/4 cup salted butter, melted and divided
- 3 pounds crab legs
- 1/4 teaspoon garlic powder Juice
- 1/2 medium lemon

Directions

- ✓ In a large bowl, drizzle 2 tablespoons butter over crab legs. Place crab legs into the air fryer basket.
- ✓ Adjust the temperature to 400°F and set the timer for 15 minutes.
- ✓ Shake the air fryer basket to toss the crab legs halfway through the cooking time.
- ✓ In a small bowl, mix remaining butter, garlic powder, and lemon juice.
- ✓ To serve, crack open crab legs and remove meat. Dip in lemon butter.

Per serving Calories: 123 Protein: 15.7 g fiber: 0.0 g Net carbohydrates: 0.4 g fat: 5.6 g Sodium: 756 mg carbohydrates: 0.4 g sugar: 0.1 g

F O I L - P A C K E T   L O B S T E R   T A I L

Convince anyone you're a master chef or perfectly set the mood for a romantic dinner with this beautifully steamed lobster tail! From a health standpoint, lobster is also rich in vitamin B, which plays a vital role in your body's metabolism.

HandsOn Time: 15 minutes

Cook Time: 12 minutes

Serves 2

- 2 (6-ounce) lobster tails, halved
- 2 tablespoons salted butter, melted
- 1/2 teaspoon Old Bay seasoning Juice of 1/2 medium lemon
- 1 teaspoon dried parsley
-

Directions
- ✓ Place the two halved tails on a sheet of aluminum foil. Drizzle with butter, Old Bay seasoning, and lemon juice.
- ✓ Seal the foil packets, completely covering tails. Place into the air fryer basket.
- ✓ Adjust the temperature to 375°F and set the timer for 12 minutes.
- ✓ Once done, sprinkle with dried parsley and serve immediately.

Per serving Calories: 234 Protein: 28.3 g
Fiber: 0.1 g Net carbohydrates: 0.6 g fat: 11.9 g
Sodium: 951 mg Carbohydrates: 0.7 g sugar: 0.2 g

TUNA ZOODLE CASSEROLE

This is a dish the whole family will love! The spiralized zucchini tossed in three different types of cheese makes this a gooey, delicious, and filling meal. You'll want to choose a spiralizer model based on how frequently you think you'll use it. Handheld spiralizers are great for small portions, but if you make large bowls for the family, then counter-mounted spiralizers with a crank are an excellent option.
HandsOn Time: 15 minutes
Cook Time: 15 minutes
Serves 4
- 2 tablespoons salted butter
- 1/4 cup diced white onion
- 1/4 cup chopped white mushrooms
- 2 stalks celery, finely chopped
- 1/2 cup heavy cream
- 1/2 cup vegetable broth
- 2 tablespoons full-fat mayonnaise
- 1/4 teaspoon xanthan gum
- 1/2 teaspoon red pepper flakes
- 2 medium zucchini, spiralized
- 2 (5-ounce) cans albacore tuna
- 1 ounce pork rinds, finely ground

Directions
- ✓ In a large saucepan over medium heat, melt butter. Add onion, mushrooms, and celery and saute until fragrant, about 3-5 minutes.
- ✓ Pour in heavy cream, vegetable broth, mayonnaise, and xanthan gum. Reduce heat and continue cooking an additional 3 minutes, until the mixture begins to thicken.

- ✓ Add red pepper flakes, zucchini, and tuna. Turn off heat and stir until zucchini noodles are coated.
- ✓ Pour into 4-cup round baking dish. Top with ground pork rinds and cover the top of the dish with foil. Place into the air fryer basket.
- ✓ Adjust the temperature to 370°F and set the timer for 15 minutes.
- ✓ When 3 minutes remain, remove the foil to brown the top of the casserole. Serve warm.

Per serving Calories: 339 Protein: 19.7 g Fiber: 1.8 g
Net carbohydrates: 4.3 g fat: 25.1 g Sodium: 522 mg
Sugar: 4.1 g

SHRIMP SCAMPI

You won't believe how ⬜uickly this succulent and tender Shrimp Scampi comes together. None of the buttery goodness dries out in your air fryer, so you can serve it in the sauce it cooks in!
HandsOn Time: 10 minutes
Cook Time: 8 minutes
Serves 4
- 4 tablespoons salted butter
- 1/2 medium lemon
- 1 teaspoon minced roasted garlic
- 1/4 cup heavy whipping cream
- 1/4 teaspoon xanthan gum
- 1/4 teaspoon red pepper flakes
- 1 pound medium peeled and deveined shrimp
- 1 tablespoon chopped fresh parsley

Directions
- ✓ In a medium saucepan over medium heat, melt butter. Zest the lemon, then squeeze juice into the pan. Add garlic.
- ✓ Pour in the cream, xanthan gum, and red pepper flakes. Whisk until the mixture begins to thicken, about 2-3 minutes.
- ✓ Place shrimp into a 4-cup round baking dish. Pour the cream sauce over the shrimp and cover with foil.
- ✓ Place the dish into the air fryer basket.
- ✓ Adjust the temperature to 400°F and set the timer for 8 minutes.
- ✓ Stir twice during cooking.
- ✓ When done, garnish with parsley and serve warm.

Per serving Calories: 240 protein: 16.7 g fiber: 0.4 g
Net carbohydrates: 2.0 g fat: 17.0 g sodium: 769 mg
Carbohydrates: 2.4 g sugar: 0.6 g

FRIED TUNA SALAD BITES

This is a recipe even the little ones will love! It's a great alternative to fish sticks and is full of nutrients and fiber from the avocado. These bites have all the flavors of a traditional tuna salad with a crunchy outside that will keep the kids coming back for more.

HandsOn Time: 10 minutes
Cook Time: 7 minutes
Yields 12 bites (3 per serving)

- 1 (10-ounce) can tuna, drained
- 1/4 cup full-fat mayonnaise
- 1 stalk celery, chopped
- 1 medium avocado, peeled, pitted, and mashed
- 1/2 cup blanched finely ground almond flour, divided
- 2 teaspoons coconut oil

Directions
- ✓ In a large bowl, mix tuna, mayonnaise, celery, and mashed avocado. Form the mixture into balls.
- ✓ Roll balls in almond flour and spritz with coconut oil. Place balls into the air fryer basket.
- ✓ Adjust the temperature to 400°F and set the timer for 7 minutes.
- ✓ Gently turn tuna bites after 5 minutes. Serve warm.

Per serving Calories: 323 Protein: 17.3 G Fiber: 4.0 G Net Carbohydrates: 2.3 G Fat: 25.4 G Sodium: 311 Mg Carbohydrates: 6.3 G Sugar: 0.8 G

FISH TACO BOWL WITH JALAPENO SLAW

This spicy taco bowl is a great change from beef or chicken. If you've been missing that taco crunch, the slaw will satisfy your craving. The crunchy cabbage paired with a creamy sauce and tart lime make this a memorable dish. If spicy isn't your thing, feel free to omit the jalapenos and add your favorite toppings!

HandsOn Time: 10 minutes
Cook Time: 10 minutes
Serves 2

- 1 cup shredded cabbage
- 1/4 cup full-fat sour cream
- 2 tablespoons full-fat mayonnaise
- 1/4 cup chopped pickled jalapenos
- 2 (3-ounce) cod fillets
- 1 teaspoon chili powder
- 1 teaspoon cumin
- 1/2 teaspoon paprika
- 1/4 teaspoon garlic powder
- 1 medium avocado, peeled, pitted, and sliced
- 1/2 medium lime

Directions
- ✓ In a large bowl, place cabbage, sour cream, mayonnaise, and jalapenos. Mix until fully coated. Let sit for 20 minutes in the refrigerator.
- ✓ Sprinkle cod fillets with chili powder, cumin, paprika, and garlic powder. Place each fillet into the air fryer basket.
- ✓ Adjust the temperature to 370°F and set the timer for 10 minutes.
- ✓ Flip the fillets halfway through the cooking time. When fully cooked, fish should have an internal temperature of at least 145°F.
- ✓ To serve, divide slaw mixture into two serving bowls, break cod fillets into pieces and spread over the bowls, and top with avocado. Squeeze lime juice over each bowl. Serve immediately.

Per serving Calories: 342 Protein: 16.1 g Fiber: 6.4 g Net carbohydrates: 5.3 g fat: 25.2 g Sodium: 587 mg

HOT CRAB DIP

This creamy dip comes together very quickly and is a crowd- pleaser! The hot sauce and jalapenos add a nice kick to this otherwise creamy dip. Serve with sliced cucumbers or pork rinds for dipping.

HandsOn Time: 10 minutes
Cook Time: 8 minutes
Serves 4

- 8 ounces full-fat cream cheese, softened
- 1/4 cup full-fat mayonnaise
- 1/4 cup full-fat sour cream
- 1 tablespoon lemon juice
- 1/2 teaspoon hot sauce
- 1/4 cup chopped pickled jalapenos
- 1/4 cup sliced green onion
- 2 (6-ounce) cans lump crabmeat
- 1/2 cup shredded Cheddar cheese

Directions
- ✓ Place all ingredients into a 4-cup round baking dish and stir until fully combined. Place dish into the air fryer basket.
- ✓ Adjust the temperature to 400°F and set the timer for 8 minutes.
- ✓ Dip will be bubbling and hot when done. Serve warm.

Per serving Calories: 441 Protein: 17.8 g Fiber: 0.6 g Net carbohydrates: 7.6 g fat: 33.8 g Sodium: 791 mg Carbohydrates: 8.2 g sugar: 6.6 g

<u>**A L M O N D   P E S T O   S A L M O N**</u>

Both almonds and salmon are great sources of healthy fat. The almonds add a nice crunch to this dish, and the pesto brings out the natural flavors of the salmon. While basil might not immediately come to your mind when you think of fish, it adds a nice freshness to this warm dish.

HandsOn Time: 5 minutes
Cook Time: 12 minutes
Serves 2

- 1/4 cup pesto 1/4 cup sliced almonds, roughly chopped
- 2 (11/2"-thick) salmon fillets (about 4 ounces each)
- 2 tablespoons unsalted butter, melted

Directions
- ✓ In a small bowl, mix pesto and almonds. Set aside.
- ✓ Place fillets into a 6" round baking dish.
- ✓ Brush each fillet with butter and place half of the pesto mixture on the top of each fillet. Place dish into the air fryer basket.
- ✓ Adjust the temperature to 390°F and set the timer for 12 minutes.
- ✓ Salmon will easily flake when fully cooked and reach an internal temperature of at least 145°F. Serve warm.

Per serving Calories: 433 Protein: 23.3 g fiber: 2.4 g Net carbohydrates: 3.7 g fat: 34.0 g sodium: 341 mg Carbohydrates: 6.1 g sugar: 0.9 g

<u>**C R A B   C A K E S**</u>

These cakes have all the flavor of a traditional crab cake with much fewer carbs. Usually bread crumbs or wheat flour is added as a binder, but this version cuts the carbs by using almond flour. It doesn't change the taste and will make the cakes much easier to flip than completely leaving out a binder would.

HandsOn Time: 10 minutes
Cook Time: 10 minutes
Serves 4

- 2 (6-ounce) cans lump crabmeat
- 1/4 cup blanched finely ground almond flour
- 1 large egg 2 tablespoons full-fat mayonnaise
- 1/2 teaspoon Dijon mustard
- 1/2 tablespoon lemon juice
- 1/2 medium green bell pepper, seeded and chopped
- 1/4 cup chopped green onion
- 1/2 teaspoon Old Bay seasoning

Directions
- ✓ In a large bowl, combine all ingredients. Form into four balls and flatten into patties. Place patties into the air fryer basket.
- ✓ Adjust the temperature to 350°F and set the timer for 10 minutes.
- ✓ Flip patties halfway through the cooking time. Serve warm.

Per serving Calories: 151 protein: 13.4 g fiber: 0.9 g Net carbohydrates: 1.4 g fat: 10.0 g sodium: 467 mg Carbohydrates: 2.3 g sugar: 0.5 g

<u>**C I L A N T R O   L I M E   B A K E D   S A L M O N**</u>

Whether you haven't cooked fish before or have been cooking it for years, this is a great staple recipe. The cilantro adds a freshness that is complemented well by the tartness of the lime. Try this dish with riced cauliflower or steamed veggies and everyone will be asking for seconds.

HandsOn Time: 10 minutes
Cook Time: 12 minutes
Serves 2

- 2 (3-ounce) salmon fillets, skin removed
- 1 tablespoon salted butter, melted
- 1 teaspoon chili powder
- 1/2 teaspoon finely minced garlic
- 1/4 cup sliced pickled jalapenos
- 1/2 medium lime, juiced
- 2 tablespoons chopped cilantro

Directions
- ✓ Place salmon fillets into a 6" round baking pan. Brush each with butter and sprinkle with chili powder and garlic.
- ✓ Place jalapeno slices on top and around salmon. Pour half of the lime juice over the salmon and cover with foil. Place pan into the air fryer basket.
- ✓ Adjust the temperature to 370°F and set the timer for 12 minutes.
- ✓ When fully cooked, salmon should flake easily with a fork and reach an internal temperature of at least 145°F.
- ✓ To serve, spritz with remaining lime juice and garnish with cilantro.

Per serving Calories: 167 protein: 15.8 g fiber: 0.7 g Net carbohydrates: 0.9 g fat: 9.9 g sodium: 248 mg Carbohydrates: 1.6 g sugar: 0.2 g

<u>**S ESAME - C RUSTED T UNA S TEAK**</u>

Tuna is a very mild-tasting fish, which is great for those new to seafood. This dish is very simple to prepare and gives you a much deeper flavor than canned tuna. While some prefer their tuna steaks well-done and flaky, others enjoy a medium-rare tuna steak, which is still safe to eat. Make sure you buy your tuna steak fresh and avoid leaving it uncooked for more than a couple days in the refrigerator.

HandsOn Time: 5 minutes
Cook Time: 8 minutes
Serves 2

- 2 (6-ounce) tuna steaks
- 1 tablespoon coconut oil, melted
- 2 teaspoon garlic powder
- 2 teaspoons white sesame seeds
- 2 teaspoons black sesame seeds

Directions
- ✓ Brush each tuna steak with coconut oil and sprinkle with garlic powder.
- ✓ In a large bowl, mix sesame seeds and then press each tuna steak into them, covering the steak as completely as possible. Place tuna steaks into the air fryer basket.
- ✓ Adjust the temperature to 400°F and set the timer for 8 minutes.
- ✓ Flip the steaks halfway through the cooking time. Steaks will be well-done at 145°F internal temperature. Serve warm.

Per serving Calories: 280 protein: 42.7 g fiber: 0.8 g Net carbohydrates: 1.2 g fat: 10.0 g sodium: 77 mg Carbohydrates: 2.0 g sugar: 0.0 g

<u>**S PICY S ALMON J ERKY**</u>

Jerky isn't just for beef anymore! Salmon jerky is gaining popularity and rightfully so because it's full of so many great nutrients. It's good on the go but can also be used chopped up as a salad topper or served as an appetizer alongside whipped cream cheese.

HandsOn Time: 5 minutes
Cook Time: 4 hours
Serves 4

- 1 pound salmon, skin and bones removed
- 4 cup soy sauce (or li□uid aminos)
- 2 teaspoon li□uid smoke
- 4 teaspoon ground black pepper Juice of V2 medium lime
- 2 teaspoon ground ginger
- 4 teaspoon red pepper flakes

Directions
- ✓ Slice salmon into V4"-thick slices, 4" long.

- ✓ Place strips into a large storage bag or a covered bowl and add remaining ingredients. Allow to marinate for 2 hours in the refrigerator.
- ✓ Place each strip into the air fryer basket in a single layer.
- ✓ Adjust the temperature to 140°F and set the timer for 4 hours.
- ✓ Cool then store in a sealed container until ready to eat.

Per serving Calories: 108 protein: 15.1 g fiber: 0.2 g Net carbohydrates: 0.8 g fat: 4.1 g sodium: 469 mg Carbohydrates: 1.0 g sugar: 0.1 g

<u>**S HRIMP K EBABS**</u>

Everyone loves kebabs, but it's not always barbecue weather outside. The air fryer makes these supersimple and crispy like the grill in no time! You can customize it with your favorite flavors and veggies and even brush with a sugar-free barbecue sauce for an extra kick!

HandsOn Time: 10 minutes
Cook Time: 7 minutes
Serves 2

- 18 medium shelled and deveined shrimp
- 1 medium zucchini, cut into 1" cubes
- 1/2 medium red bell pepper, cut into 1"-thick s□uares
- 1/4 medium red onion, cut into 1"-thick s□uares
- 1/2 tablespoons coconut oil, melted
- 2 teaspoons chili powder
- 1/2 teaspoon paprika
- 1/4 teaspoon ground black pepper

Directions
- ✓ Soak four 6" bamboo skewers in water for 30 minutes. Place a shrimp on the skewer, then a zucchini, a pepper, and an onion. Repeat until all ingredients are utilized.
- ✓ Brush each kebab with coconut oil. Sprinkle with chili powder, paprika, and black pepper. Place kebabs into the air fryer basket.
- ✓ Adjust the temperature to 400°F and set the timer for 7 minutes or until shrimp is fully cooked and veggies are tender.
- ✓ Flip kebabs halfway through the cooking time. Serve warm.

Per serving Calories: 166 protein: 9.5 g fiber: 3.1 g Net carbohydrates: 5.4 g fat: 10.7 g sodium: 391 mg Carbohydrates: 8.5 g sugar: 4.5 g

Even though meats are an easy way to get the protein essential for a healthy ketogenic diet, vegetables are also really important to making sure you're properly nourished. And the air fryer is definitely intended for more than cooking meats! These vegetarian main dishes are great for if you're trying out a Meatless Monday or simply getting your protein from another source than meat.

LOADED CAULIFLOWER STEAK

Cauliflower steaks are a great vegetarian option that have nutrients and flavor. Roasting them with buffalo sauce gives you a light and spicy dish that is totally guilt-free! Serve with crumbled blue cheese or ranch dressing if you need to tone down the spice!

HandsOn Time: 5 minutes
Cook Time: 7 minutes
Serves 4

- 1 medium head cauliflower
- 4 cup hot sauce
- 2 tablespoons salted butter, melted
- 4 cup blue cheese crumbles
- 4 cup full-fat ranch dressing

Directions

- ✓ Remove cauliflower leaves. Slice the head in V2"- thick slices.
- ✓ In a small bowl, mix hot sauce and butter. Brush the mixture over the cauliflower.
- ✓ Place each cauliflower steak into the air fryer, working in batches if necessary.
- ✓ Adjust the temperature to 400°F and set the timer for 7 minutes.
- ✓ When cooked, edges will begin turning dark and caramelized.
- ✓ To serve, sprinkle steaks with crumbled blue cheese. Drizzle with ranch dressing.

Per serving Calories: 122 protein: 4.9 g fiber: 3.0 g Net carbohydrates: 4.7 g fat: 8.4 g sodium: 283 mg Carbohydrates: 7.7 g sugar: 2.9 g

THREE-CHEESE ZUCCHINI

Zucchini is a low-carb vegetable that is high in water content, which means it helps keep you fuller longer, discouraging overeating. This cheesy, handheld dish gives you all of those benefits, plus a nice crunch in each bite that you won't find in many low-carb meals!

HandsOn Time: 15 minutes
Cook Time: 20 minutes
Serves 2

- 2 medium zucchini
- 1 tablespoon avocado oil
- 1/4 cup low-carb, no-sugar-added pasta sauce
- 1/4 cup full-fat ricotta cheese
- 1/4 cup shredded mozzarella cheese
- 1/4 teaspoon dried oregano
- 1/4 teaspoon garlic powder
- 1/2 teaspoon dried parsley
- 2 tablespoons grated vegetarian Parmesan cheese

Directions

- ✓ Cut off 1" from the top and bottom of each zucchini. Slice zucchini in half lengthwise and use a spoon to scoop out a bit of the inside, making room for filling. Brush with oil and spoon 2 tablespoons pasta sauce into each shell.
- ✓ In a medium bowl, mix ricotta, mozzarella, oregano, garlic powder, and parsley. Spoon the mixture into each zucchini shell. Place stuffed zucchini shells into the air fryer basket.
- ✓ Adjust the temperature to 350°F and set the timer for 20 minutes.
- ✓ To remove from the fryer basket, use tongs or a spatula and carefully lift out. Top with Parmesan. Serve immediately.

Per serving Calories: 215 protein: 10.5 g fiber: 2.7 g Net carbohydrates: 6.6 g fat: 14.9 g sodium: 386 mg Carbohydrates: 9.3 g sugar: 5.2 g

PORTOBELLO MINI PIZZAS

This low-calorie alternative to a low-carb pizza really hits the spot! You won't miss out on an ounce of flavor, plus portobello mushrooms are rich in B vitamins that help maintain healthy skin, hair, and eyes!

HandsOn Time: 10 minutes
Cook Time: 10 minutes
Serves 2

- 2 large portobello mushrooms
- 2 tablespoons unsalted butter, melted
- 1/2 teaspoon garlic powder
- 2/3 cup shredded mozzarella cheese
- 4 grape tomatoes, sliced
- 2 leaves fresh basil, chopped
- 1 tablespoon balsamic vinegar

Directions
- ✓ Scoop out the inside of the mushrooms, leaving just the caps. Brush each cap with butter and sprinkle with garlic powder.
- ✓ Fill each cap with mozzarella and sliced tomatoes. Place each mini pizza into a 6" round baking pan. Place pan into the air fryer basket.
- ✓ Adjust the temperature to 380°F and set the timer for 10 minutes.
- ✓ Carefully remove the pizzas from the fryer basket and garnish with basil and a drizzle of vinegar.

Per serving Calories: 244 protein: 10.4 g fiber: 1.4 g Net carbohydrates: 5.4 g fat: 18.5 g sodium: 244 mg Carbohydrates: 6.8 g sugar: 4.3 g

VEGGIE QUESADILLA

This dish uses a simple flatbread instead of a traditional low- carb tortilla. Low-carb tortillas often contain wheat, gluten, and high amounts of fiber, which for some people may cause bloating, weight gain, and trigger an insulin response. This sauteed veggie-filled alternative is so filling and full of nutrients you won't even miss traditional quesadillas.

HandsOn Time: 10 minutes
Cook Time: 5 minutes
Serves 2
- 1 tablespoon coconut oil
- 1/2 medium green bell pepper, seeded and chopped
- 1/4 cup diced red onion
- 1/4 cup chopped white mushrooms
- 4 flatbread dough tortillas
- 2/3 cup shredded pepper jack cheese
- 1/2 medium avocado, peeled, pitted, and mashed
- 1/4 cup full-fat sour cream
- 1/4 cup mild salsa

Directions
- ✓ In a medium skillet over medium heat, warm coconut oil. Add pepper, onion, and mushrooms to skillet and saute until peppers begin to soften, 3-5 minutes.
- ✓ Place two tortillas on a work surface and sprinkle each with half of cheese. Top with sauteed veggies, sprinkle with remaining cheese, and place remaining two tortillas on top. Place quesadillas carefully into the air fryer basket.
- ✓ Adjust the temperature to 400°F and set the timer for 5 minutes.

- ✓ Flip the quesadillas halfway through the cooking time. Serve warm with avocado, sour cream, and salsa.

Per serving Calories: 795 protein: 34.5 g fiber: 6.5 g Net carbohydrates: 12.9 g fat: 61.3 g sodium: 1,051 mg Carbohydrates: 19.4 g sugar: 7.4 g

ROASTED VEGGIE BOWL

Vegetables are a very important part of a keto diet. Equally important is deciding which vegetables to eat. This bowl is made up of a combination of very low-carb and high-fiber veggies to feed your body tons of nutrients while satisfying your palate.

HandsOn Time: 10 minutes
Cook Time: 15 minutes
Serves: 2
- 1 cup broccoli florets
- 1 cup quartered Brussels sprouts
- 1/2 cup cauliflower florets
- 1/4 medium white onion, peeled and sliced
- 1/4" thick 1/2 medium green bell pepper, seeded and sliced
- 1/4" thick 1 tablespoon coconut oil
- 2 teaspoons chili powder
- 1/2 teaspoon garlic powder
- 1/2 teaspoon cumin

Directions
- ✓ Toss all ingredients together in a large bowl until vegetables are fully coated with oil and seasoning.
- ✓ Pour vegetables into the air fryer basket.
- ✓ Adjust the temperature to 360°F and set the timer for 15 minutes.
- ✓ Shake two or three times during cooking. Serve warm.

Per serving Calories: 121 Protein: 4.3 g fiber: 5.2 g Net carbohydrates: 7.9 g fat: 7.1 g sodium: 112 mg Carbohydrates: 13.1 g sugar: 3.8 g

SPINACH ARTICHOKE CASSEROLE

This casserole boosts one of your favorite dips to the next level. With the same warm creaminess, but with more nutrients and substance than the original dip, you'll be happy to make this meatless meal a part of your regular rotation!

HandsOn Time: 15 minutes
Cook Time: 15 minutes
Serves 4
- 1 tablespoon salted butter, melted
- 1/4 cup diced yellow onion

- 8 ounces full-fat cream cheese, softened
- 1/3 cup full-fat mayonnaise
- 1/3 cup full- fat sour cream
- 1/4 cup chopped pickled jalapenos
- 2 cups fresh spinach, chopped
- 2 cups cauliflower florets, chopped
- 1 cup artichoke hearts, chopped

Directions
- ✓ In a large bowl, mix butter, onion, cream cheese, mayonnaise, and sour cream. Fold in jalapenos, spinach, cauliflower, and artichokes.
- ✓ Pour the mixture into a 4-cup round baking dish. Cover with foil and place into the air fryer basket.
- ✓ Adjust the temperature to 370°F and set the timer for 15 minutes.
- ✓ In the last 2 minutes of cooking, remove the foil to brown the top. Serve warm.

Per serving Calories: 423 Protein: 6.7 g fiber: 5.3 g Net carbohydrates: 6.8 g fat: 36.3 g sodium: 495 mg Carbohydrates: 12.1 g sugar: 4.4 g

CHEESY ZOODLE BAKE

This is a dish the whole family will love! The spiralized zucchini tossed in two different types of cheese make this a gooey and delicious and filling meal.

HandsOn Time: 10 minutes
Cook Time: 8 minutes
Serves 4 2 tablespoons salted butter
- 1/4 cup diced white onion
- 1/2 teaspoon minced garlic
- 1/2 cup heavy whipping cream
- 2 ounces full-fat cream cheese
- 1 cup shredded sharp Cheddar cheese
- 2 medium zucchini, spiralized

Directions
- ✓ In a large saucepan over medium heat, melt butter. Add onion and saute until it begins to soften, 1-3 minutes. Add garlic and saute 30 seconds, then pour in cream and add cream cheese.
- ✓ Remove the pan from heat and stir in Cheddar. Add the zucchini and toss in the sauce, then put into a 4- cup round baking dish. Cover the dish with foil and place into the air fryer basket.
- ✓ Adjust the temperature to 370°F and set the timer for 8 minutes.
- ✓ After 6 minutes remove the foil and let the top brown for remaining cooking time. Stir and serve.

Per serving Calories: 337 protein: 9.6 g fiber: 1.2 g Net carbohydrates: 4.7 g fat: 28.4 g sodium: 298 mg Carbohydrates: 5.9 g sugar: 4.3 g

GREEK STUFFED EGGPLANT

Perfectly roasted and filled with nutrient-rich veggies, stuffed eggplant is a perfect fresh and fibrous meal even if you're not vegetarian! This meatless masterpiece is bursting with succulent Greek flavors to keep you satisfied!

HandsOn Time: 15 minutes
Cook Time: 20 minutes
Serves 2
- 1 large eggplant
- 2 tablespoons unsalted butter
- 1/4 medium yellow onion, diced
- 1/4 cup chopped artichoke hearts
- 1 cup fresh spinach
- 2 tablespoons diced red bell pepper
- 1/2 cup crumbled feta

Directions
- ✓ Slice eggplant in half lengthwise and scoop out flesh, leaving enough inside for shell to remain intact. Take eggplant that was scooped out, chop it, and set aside.
- ✓ In a medium skillet over medium heat, add butter and onion. Saute until onions begin to soften, about 3-5 minutes. Add chopped eggplant, artichokes, spinach, and bell pepper. Continue cooking 5 minutes until peppers soften and spinach wilts. Remove from the heat and gently fold in the feta.
- ✓ Place filling into each eggplant shell and place into the air fryer basket.
- ✓ Adjust the temperature to 320°F and set the timer for 20 minutes.
- ✓ Eggplant will be tender when done. Serve warm.

Per serving Calories: 291 protein: 9.4 g fiber: 10.8 g Net carbohydrates: 11.8 g fat: 18.7 g sodium: 374 mg Carbohydrates: 22.6 g sugar: 12.5 g

ROASTED BROCCOLI SALAD

Broccoli takes on a different taste when roasted, and in this salad it creates the perfect hint of sweet. The almonds add a nice crunch for contrast, not to mention a burst of healthy fats. Almonds are a great addition to salads and taste even better when roasted. You can even roast almonds in the air fryer while you prepare a meal (see Ranch Roasted Almonds in Chapter 3)!

HandsOn Time: 10 minutes
Cook Time: 7 minutes
Serves: 2

- 3 cups fresh broccoli florets
- 2 tablespoons salted butter, melted
- 1/4 cup sliced almonds
- 1/2 medium lemon

Directions

- ✓ Place broccoli into a 6" round baking dish. Pour butter over broccoli. Add almonds and toss. Place dish into the air fryer basket.
- ✓ Adjust the temperature to 380°F and set the timer for 7 minutes.
- ✓ Stir halfway through the cooking time.
- ✓ When timer beeps, zest lemon onto broccoli and s□ueeze juice into pan. Toss. Serve warm.

Per serving Calories: 215 protein: 6.4 g fiber: 5.0 g Net carbohydrates: 7.1 g fat: 16.3 g sodium: 136 mg Carbohydrates: 12.1 g sugar: 3.0 g

WHOLE ROASTED LEMON CAULIFLOWER

This is a bright and refreshing entree with plenty of substance for a meal, or in smaller portions it can be served as a nutritious side dish with just the right amount of tang. The options for dressing up cauliflower are endless, and this recipe proves it.

HandsOn Time: 5 minutes
Cook Time: 15 minutes
Serves 4

- 1 medium head cauliflower
- 2 tablespoons salted butter, melted
- 1 medium lemon
- 1/2 teaspoon garlic powder
- 1 teaspoon dried parsley

Directions

- ✓ Remove the leaves from the head of cauliflower and brush it with melted butter. Cut the lemon in half and zest one half onto the cauliflower. S□ueeze the juice of the zested lemon half and pour it over the cauliflower.
- ✓ Sprinkle with garlic powder and parsley. Place cauliflower head into the air fryer basket.
- ✓ Adjust the temperature to 350°F and set the timer for 15 minutes.
- ✓ Check cauliflower every 5 minutes to avoid overcooking. It should be fork tender.
- ✓ To serve, s□ueeze juice from other lemon half over cauliflower. Serve immediately.

Per serving Calories: 91 Protein: 3.0 g fiber: 3.2 g Net carbohydrates: 5.2 g fat: 5.7 g Sodium: 90 mg carbohydrates: 8.4 g sugar: 3.1 g

CHEESY CAULIFLOWER PIZZA CRUST

Cauliflower pizza crust is a trendy alternative to regular crust, and for a good reason! It's full of nutrients and tastes amazing! Load this pizza up with cheese and even your favorite low-carb veggies for a fresh and filling vegetarian meal!

HandsOn Time: 15 minutes
Cook Time: 11 minutes
Serves 2

- 1 (12-ounce) steamer bag cauliflower
- 1/2 cup shredded sharp Cheddar cheese
- 1 large egg
- 2 tablespoons blanched finely ground almond flour
- 1 teaspoon Italian blend seasoning

Directions

- ✓ Cook cauliflower according to package instructions. Remove from bag and place into cheesecloth or paper towel to remove excess water. Place cauliflower into a large bowl.
- ✓ Add cheese, egg, almond flour, and Italian seasoning to the bowl and mix well.
- ✓ Cut a piece of parchment to fit your air fryer basket. Press cauliflower into 6" round circle. Place into the air fryer basket.
- ✓ Adjust the temperature to 360°F and set the timer for 11 minutes.
- ✓ After 7 minutes, flip the pizza crust.
- ✓ Add preferred toppings to pizza. Place back into air fryer basket and cook an additional 4 minutes or until fully cooked and golden. Serve immediately.

Per serving Calories: 230 protein: 14.9 g fiber: 4.7 g Net carbohydrates: 5.3 g fat: 14.2 g sodium: 257 mg Carbohydrates: 10.0 g sugar: 4.2 g

QUICHE-STUFFED PEPPERS

Add some excitement to your crustless □uiche by baking it right in a pepper! These easy □uiches will help you get more vegetables in your day, and there's no limit to the different ways you can customize them!

HandsOn Time: 5 minutes
Cook Time: 15 minutes
Serves 2

- 2 medium green bell peppers

- 3 large eggs
- 1/4 cup full-fat ricotta cheese
- 1/4 cup diced yellow onion
- 1/2 cup chopped broccoli
- 1/2 cup shredded medium Cheddar cheese

Directions

- ✓ Cut the tops off of the peppers and remove the seeds and white membranes with a small knife.
- ✓ In a medium bowl, whisk eggs and ricotta.
- ✓ Add onion and broccoli. Pour the egg and vegetable mixture evenly into each pepper. Top with Cheddar. Place peppers into a 4-cup round baking dish and place into the air fryer basket.
- ✓ Adjust the temperature to 350°F and set the timer for 15 minutes.
- ✓ Eggs will be mostly firm and peppers tender when fully cooked. Serve immediately.

Per serving Calories: 314 Protein: 21.6 g fiber: 3.0 g
Net carbohydrates: 7.8 g fat: 18.7 g
Sodium: 325 mg carbohydrates: 10.8 g sugar: 4.5 g

ROASTED GARLIC WHITE ZUCCHINI ROLLS

This recipe turns those lasagna layers into perfectly portioned zucchini rolls! It also swaps out the meat for mushrooms, resulting in a lower-calorie dish.

HandsOn Time: 20 minutes
Cook Time: 20 minutes
Serves 4

- 2 medium zucchini
- 2 tablespoons unsalted butter
- 4 white onion, peeled and diced
- 2 teaspoon finely minced roasted garlic
- 4 cup heavy cream
- 2 tablespoons vegetable broth
- 1/8 teaspoon xanthan gum
- 2 cup full-fat ricotta cheese
- 1/4 teaspoon salt
- 1/2 teaspoon garlic powder
- 1/4 teaspoon dried oregano
- 2 cups spinach, chopped
- 1/2 cup sliced baby portobello mushrooms
- 3/4 cup shredded mozzarella cheese, divided

Directions

- ✓ Using a mandoline or sharp knife, slice zucchini into long strips lengthwise. Place strips between paper towels to absorb moisture. Set aside.
- ✓ In a medium saucepan over medium heat, melt butter. Add onion and saute until fragrant. Add garlic and saute 30 seconds.
- ✓ Pour in heavy cream, broth, and xanthan gum. Turn off heat and whisk mixture until it begins to thicken, about 3 minutes.
- ✓ In a medium bowl, add ricotta, salt, garlic powder, and oregano and mix well. Fold in spinach, mushrooms, and V2 cup mozzarella.
- ✓ Pour half of the sauce into a 6" round baking pan. To assemble the rolls, place two strips of zucchini on a work surface. Spoon 2 tablespoons of ricotta mixture onto the slices and roll up. Place seam side down on top of sauce. Repeat with remaining ingredients.
- ✓ Pour remaining sauce over the rolls and sprinkle with remaining mozzarella. Cover with foil and place into the air fryer basket.
- ✓ Adjust the temperature to 350°F and set the timer for 20 minutes.
- ✓ In the last 5 minutes, remove the foil to brown the cheese. Serve immediately.

Per serving Calories: 245 Protein: 10.5 g Fiber: 1.8 g
Net carbohydrates: 5.3 g Fat: 18.9 g
Sodium: 346 mg

SPICY PARMESAN ARTICHOKES

Artichokes are a versatile food that are rich in vitamin B12, which helps maintain the health of nerve cells as well as aiding in digestion and heart health. They bake perfectly in your air fryer, and with just a bit of cheese and seasoning they're transformed into an absolutely delicious dish!

HandsOn Time: 10 minutes
Cook Time: 10 minutes
Serves 4

- 2 medium artichokes, trimmed and quartered, center removed
- 2 tablespoons coconut oil
- 1 large egg, beaten
- 1/2 cup grated vegetarian Parmesan cheese
- 1/4 cup blanched finely ground almond flour
- 1/2 teaspoon crushed red pepper flakes

Directions

- ✓ In a large bowl, toss artichokes in coconut oil and then dip each piece into the egg.
- ✓ Mix the Parmesan and almond flour in a large bowl. Add artichoke pieces and toss to cover as completely as possible, sprinkle

with pepper flakes. Place into the air fryer basket.
- ✓ Adjust the temperature to 400°F and set the timer for 10 minutes.
- ✓ Toss the basket two times during cooking. Serve warm.

Per serving Calories: 189 protein: 7.9 g fiber: 4.2 g Net carbohydrates: 5.8 g fat: 13.5 g sodium: 294 mg Carbohydrates: 10.0 g sugar: 0.9 g

ZUCCHINI CAULIFLOWER FRITTERS

These fritters are a crispy way to make sure your kids are getting their vegetables! Your air fryer gives them a crispy outside and a flavor-filled middle, meaning sinking your teeth into them will always put a smile on your face! For a nice creamy addition, scoop a dollop of full-fat sour cream on top!

HandsOn Time: 15 minutes
Cook Time: 12 minutes
Serves 2

- 1 (12-ounce) cauliflower steamer bag
- 1 medium zucchini, shredded
- 1/4 cup almond flour
- 1 large egg
- 1/2 teaspoon garlic powder
- 1/4 cup grated vegetarian Parmesan cheese

Directions
- ✓ Cook cauliflower according to package instructions and drain excess moisture in cheesecloth or paper towel. Place into a large bowl.
- ✓ Place zucchini into paper towel and pat down to remove excess moisture. Add to bowl with cauliflower. Add remaining ingredients.
- ✓ Divide the mixture evenly and form four patties. Press into 1/4"-thick patties. Place each into the air fryer basket.
- ✓ Adjust the temperature to 320°F and set the timer for 12 minutes.
- ✓ Fritters will be firm when fully cooked. Allow to cool 5 minutes before moving. Serve warm.

Per serving
Calories: 217 protein: 13.7 g fiber: 6.5 g Net carbohydrates: 8.5 g fat: 12.0 g sodium: 263 mg Carbohydrates: 16.1 g sugar: 6.8 g

BASIC SPAGHETTI SQUASH

Spaghetti squash can be used to create a wide variety of dishes from savory Italian dinners to breakfast boats. Your air fryer can help you get the perfect bake on your squash, and you'll be on your way to enjoying all of its versatile qualities in no time!

HandsOn Time: 10 minutes
Cook Time: 45 minutes
Serves 2

- 1/2 large spaghetti squash
- 1 tablespoon coconut oil
- 2 tablespoons salted butter, melted
- 1/2 teaspoon garlic powder
- 1 teaspoon dried parsley

Directions
- ✓ Brush shell of spaghetti squash with coconut oil. Place the skin side down and brush the inside with butter. Sprinkle with garlic powder and parsley.
- ✓ Place squash with the skin side down into the air fryer basket.
- ✓ Adjust the temperature to 350°F and set the timer for 30 minutes.
- ✓ When the timer beeps, flip the squash so skin side is up and cook an additional 15 minutes or until fork tender. Serve warm.

Per serving Calories: 182 protein: 1.9 g Fiber: 3.9 g Net carbohydrates: 14.3 g fat: 11.7 g sodium: 134 mg Carbohydrates: 18.2 g sugar: 7.0 g

SPAGHETTI SQUASH ALFREDO

Spaghetti squash is a great alternative to regular pasta. It's right there in the name! Especially if you're someone who cares about texture, you'll love this smart swap and all the yummy Alfredo sauce it's baked in!

HandsOn Time: 10 minutes
Cook Time: 15 minutes
Serves 2

- 1/2 large cooked spaghetti squash
- 2 tablespoons salted butter, melted
- 1/2 cup low-carb Alfredo sauce
- 1/4 cup grated vegetarian Parmesan cheese
- 1/2 teaspoon garlic powder
- 1 teaspoon dried parsley
- 1/4 teaspoon ground peppercorn
- 1/2 cup shredded Italian blend cheese

Directions
- ✓ Using a fork, remove the strands of spaghetti squash from the shell. Place into a large bowl with butter and Alfredo sauce.

Sprinkle with Parmesan, garlic powder, parsley, and peppercorn.
- ✓ Pour into a 4-cup round baking dish and top with shredded cheese. Place dish into the air fryer basket.
- ✓ Adjust the temperature to 320°F and set the timer for 15 minutes.
- ✓ When finished, cheese will be golden and bubbling. Serve immediately.

Per serving Calories: 375 Protein: 13.5 g fiber: 4.0 g Net carbohydrates: 20.1 g fat: 24.2 g sodium: 950 mg Carbohydrates: 24.1 g sugar: 8.0 g

CAPRESE EGGPLANT STACKS

These stacks are a warm twist on the classic fresh caprese salad.
HandsOn Time: 5 minutes
Cook Time: 12 minutes
Serves 4

- 1 medium eggplant, cut into 1/4" slices
- 2 large tomatoes, cut into 1/4" slices
- 4 ounces fresh mozzarella, cut into 1/2-ounce slices
- 2 tablespoons olive oil
- 1/4 cup fresh basil, sliced

Directions
- ✓ In a 6" round baking dish, place four slices of eggplant on the bottom. Place a slice of tomato on top of each eggplant round, then mozzarella, then eggplant. Repeat as necessary.
- ✓ Drizzle with olive oil. Cover dish with foil and place dish into the air fryer basket.
- ✓ Adjust the temperature to 350°F and set the timer for 12 minutes.
- ✓ When done, eggplant will be tender. Garnish with fresh basil to serve.

Per serving Calories: 195 Protein: 8.5 g Fiber: 5.2 g Net carbohydrates: 7.5 g fat: 12.7 g Sodium: 184 mg Carbohydrates: 12.7 g sugar: 7.5 g

Desserts are usually the toughest thing for anybody to give up on any kind of diet. Thankfully, there are a ton of keto-friendly options to keep you on track while keeping your sweet tooth satisfied! With your air fryer, you're able to create a wide range of perfectly portioned goodies that always hit the spot! As an added bonus, with the smaller cooking chamber than a traditional oven, these treats will also cook in practically no time! From Chocolate Espresso Mini Cheesecake to Caramel Monkey Bread, this chapter has enough sweet treats to make sure you never feel deprived!

ALMOND BUTTER COOKIE BALLS

These cookie balls are a poppable version of a warm and gooey chocolate chip cookie! Be sure to use an almond butter that has two ingredients maximum (almonds and salt); many brands enhance the flavor with ingredients like sugar and honey, adding a ton of carbs you don't need.

HandsOn Time: 5 minutes
Cook Time: 10 minutes
Yields 10 balls (1 ball per serving)

- 1 cup almond butter 1 large egg
- 1 teaspoon vanilla extract
- 1/4 cup low-carb protein powder
- 1/4 cup powdered erythritol
- 1/4 cup shredded unsweetened coconut
- 1/4 cup low-carb, sugar-free chocolate chips
- 1/2 teaspoon ground cinnamon

Directions
- ✓ In a large bowl, mix almond butter and egg. Add in vanilla, protein powder, and erythritol.
- ✓ Fold in coconut, chocolate chips, and cinnamon. Roll into 1" balls. Place balls into 6" round baking pan and put into the air fryer basket.
- ✓ Adjust the temperature to 320°F and set the timer for 10 minutes.
- ✓ Allow to cool completely. Store in an airtight container in the refrigerator up to 4 days.

Per serving Calories: 224 protein :11.2g fiber: 3.6 g net carbohydrates 13g

CINNAMON SUGAR PORK RINDS

You might not have ever thought you'd be eating pork rinds for dessert, but this recipe is a true game changer. Pork rinds not only give you a protein boost, but they also give you a crunch that you just can't get from other low-carb snacks. The sweetness in this recipe will mask any meaty flavor, and your air fryer will make sure of that by baking the taste right in!

HandsOn Time: 5 minutes
Cook Time: 5 minutes
Serves 2

- 2 ounces pork rinds
- 2 tablespoons unsalted butter, melted
- 2 teaspoon ground cinnamon
- 4 cup powdered erythritol

Directions
- ✓ 1 In a large bowl, toss pork rinds and butter. Sprinkle with cinnamon and erythritol, then toss to evenly coat.
- ✓ 2 Place pork rinds into the air fryer basket.
- ✓ 3 Adjust the temperature to 400°F and set the timer for 5 minutes.
- ✓ 4 Serve immediately.

Per serving Calories: 264 Protein: 16.3 g fiber: 0.4 g Net carbohydrates: 0.1 g sugar alcohol: 18.0 g fat: 20.8 g Sodium: 467 mg carbohydrates: 18.5 g

PECAN BROWNIES

These fudgy brownies are a dense and decadent dream. Finally, a chocolate-heavy, guilt-free dessert you can happily indulge in! And the pecans really hit the spot!

HandsOn Time: 10 minutes
Cook Time: 20 minutes
Serves: 6

- 1/2 cup blanched finely ground almond flour
- 1/2 cup powdered erythritol
- 2 tablespoons unsweetened cocoa powder
- 1/2 teaspoon baking powder
- 1/4 cup unsalted butter, softened
- 1 large egg
- 1/4 cup chopped pecans
- 1/4 cup low-carb, sugar-free chocolate chips

Directions
- ✓ 1 In a large bowl, mix almond flour, erythritol, cocoa powder, and baking powder. Stir in butter and egg.
- ✓ 2 Fold in pecans and chocolate chips. Scoop mixture into 6" round baking pan. Place pan into the air fryer basket.
- ✓ 3 Adjust the temperature to 300°F and set the timer for 20 minutes.
- ✓ 4 When fully cooked a toothpick inserted in center will come out clean. Allow 20 minutes to fully cool and firm up.

Per serving

Calories: 215 protein: 4.2 g Fiber: 2.8 g Net carbohydrates: 2.3 g sugar alcohol: 16.7 g fat: 18.9 g sodium: 53 mg Carbohydrates: 21.8 g sugar: 0.6 g

MINI CHEESECAKE

This is the base of all keto-friendly cheesecakes you'll make in your air fryer. It's the classic vanilla cheesecake, but it can be customized so many different ways. From its crunchy walnut crust to its creamy center, this 15-minute cheesecake will quickly become a new favorite!

HandsOn Time: 10 minutes

Cook Time: 15 minutes

Serves 2

- 1/2 cup walnuts
- 2 tablespoons salted butter
- 2 tablespoons granular erythritol
- 4 ounces full-fat cream cheese, softened
- 1 large egg
- 1/2 teaspoon vanilla extract
- 1/8 cup powdered erythritol

Directions

- ✓ Place walnuts, butter, and granular erythritol in a food processor. Pulse until ingredients stick together and a dough forms.
- ✓ Press dough into 4" springform pan then place the pan into the air fryer basket.
- ✓ Adjust the temperature to 400°F and set the timer for 5 minutes.
- ✓ When timer beeps, remove the crust and let cool.
- ✓ In a medium bowl, mix cream cheese with egg, vanilla extract, and powdered erythritol until smooth.
- ✓ Spoon mixture on top of baked walnut crust and place into the air fryer basket.
- ✓ Adjust the temperature to 300°F and set the timer for 10 minutes.
- ✓ Once done, chill for 2 hours before serving.

Per serving Calories: 531 protein: 11.4 g fiber: 2.3 g Net carbohydrates: 5.1 g sugar alcohol: 24.0 g fat: 48.3 g sodium: 333 mg Carbohydrates: 31.4 g sugar: 2.9 g

CHOCOLATE ESPRESSO MINI CHEESECAKE

This cheesecake definitely gives off major mocha vibes. Perfect for any sweet tooth out there that loves to enjoy a cup of coffee after dinner, this dessert is subtly rich and incredibly luscious.

HandsOn Time: 5 minutes

Cook Time: 15 minutes

Serves: 2

- 1/2 cup walnuts
- 2 tablespoons salted butter
- 2 tablespoons granular erythritol
- 4 ounces full-fat cream cheese, softened
- 1 large egg
- 1/2 teaspoon vanilla extract
- 2 tablespoons powdered erythritol
- 2 teaspoons unsweetened cocoa powder
- 1 teaspoon espresso powder

Directions

- ✓ Place walnuts, butter, and granular erythritol in a food processor. Pulse until ingredients stick together and a dough forms.
- ✓ Press dough into 4" springform pan and place into the air fryer basket.
- ✓ Adjust the temperature to 400°F and set the timer for 5 minutes.
- ✓ When timer beeps, remove crust and let cool.
- ✓ In a medium bowl, mix cream cheese with egg, vanilla extract, powdered erythritol, cocoa powder, and espresso powder until smooth.
- ✓ Spoon mixture on top of baked walnut crust and place into the air fryer basket.
- ✓ Adjust the temperature for 300°F and set the timer for 10 minutes.
- ✓ Once done, chill for 2 hours before serving.

Per serving Calories: 535 protein: 11.6 g fiber: 7.2 g Net carbohydrates: 5.9 g sugar alcohol: 24.0 g fat: 48.4 g sodium: 336 mg Carbohydrates: 37.1 g sugar: 5.9 g

MINI CHOCOLATE CHIP PAN COOKIE

This Quick dessert can bake before you even finish dinner! It's a very soft, chewy cookie thanks to the gelatin. To make this dessert even more special for a family treat, add a drizzle of low-carb chocolate syrup, your favorite roasted chopped nuts, and a dollop of sugar-free whipped cream!

HandsOn Time: 10 minutes

Cook Time: 7 minutes

Serves 4

- 1/2 cup blanched finely ground almond flour
- 1/4 cup powdered erythritol
- 2 tablespoons unsalted butter, softened
- 1 large egg
- 1/2 teaspoon unflavored gelatin
- 1/2 teaspoon baking powder
- 1/2 teaspoon vanilla extract
- 2 tablespoons low-carb, sugar-free chocolate chips

Directions

- ✓ In a large bowl, mix almond flour and erythritol. Stir in butter, egg, and gelatin until combined.
- ✓ Stir in baking powder and vanilla and then fold in chocolate chips. Pour batter into 6" round baking pan. Place pan into the air fryer baske
- ✓ Adjust the temperature to 300°F and set the timer for 7 minutes.
- ✓ When fully cooked, the top will be golden brown and a toothpick inserted in center will come out clean. Let cool at least 10 minutes
  .

Per serving Calories: 188 protein: 5.6 g fiber: 2.0 g Net carbohydrates: 2.3 g sugar alcohol: 12.5 g Fat: 15.7 g Sodium: 80 mg Carbohydrates: 16.8 g

BLACKBERRY CRISP

You can enjoy certain fruits on a low-carb diet. Blackberries have one of the lowest glycemic indexes compared to other berries and are perfect to incorporate into a keto diet. This dessert is tart, fruity, and perfect for warm summer evenings! You can even top with a low-carb ice cream for extra decadence!

HandsOn Time: 5 minutes
Cook Time: 15 minutes
Serves 4

- 2 cups blackberries
- 1/3 cup powdered erythritol
- 2 tablespoons lemon juice
- 1/4 teaspoon xanthan gum
- 1 cup Crunchy Granola

Directions

- ✓ In a large bowl, toss blackberries, erythritol, lemon juice, and xanthan gum.
- ✓ Pour into 6" round baking dish and cover with foil. Place into the air fryer basket.
- ✓ Adjust the temperature to 350°F and set the timer for 12 minutes.
- ✓ When the timer beeps, remove the foil and stir.

- ✓ Sprinkle granola over mixture and return to the air fryer basket.
- ✓ Adjust the temperature to 320°F and set the timer for 3 minutes or until top is golden.
- ✓ Serve warm.

Per serving Calories: 496 protein: 9.2 g fiber: 12.5 g Net carbohydrates: 9.7 g sugar alcohol: 21.8 g fat: 42.1 g sodium: 5 mg Carbohydrates: 44.0 g sugar: 5.7 g

PROTEIN POWDER DOUGHNUT HOLES

You can't forget about the doughnut holes . . . some would argue they're the best part! These poppable cake doughnut balls are great for breakfast or for dessert!

HandsOn Time: 25 minutes
Cook Time: 6 minutes
Yields 12 holes (2 per serving)

- 2 cup blanched finely ground almond flour
- 2 cup low-carb vanilla protein powder
- 2 cup granular erythritol
- 2 teaspoon baking powder
- 1 large egg
- 5 tablespoons unsalted butter, melted
- 2 teaspoon vanilla extract

Directions

- ✓ Mix all ingredients in a large bowl. Place into the freezer for 20 minutes.
- ✓ Wet your hands with water and roll the dough into twelve balls.
- ✓ Cut a piece of parchment to fit your air fryer basket. Working in batches as necessary, place doughnut holes into the air fryer basket on top of parchment.
- ✓ Adjust the temperature to 380°F and set the timer for 6 minutes.
- ✓ Flip doughnut holes halfway through the cooking time.
- ✓ Let cool completely before serving.

Per serving Calories: 221 protein: 19.8 g fiber: 1.7 g Net carbohydrates: 1.5 g sugar alcohol: 20.0 g fat: 14.3 g sodium: 160 mg carbohydrates: 23.2 g sugar: 0.4 g

Layered Peanut Butter Cheesecake Brownies

This layered dessert is decadent, creamy, and perfect for a special occasion! Your guests won't even know it's low-carb. The rich chocolaty brownies make a great base for the fluffy peanut butter cheesecake layer. Add an extra drizzle of chocolate over the top for an extra special presentation.

HandsOn Time: 20 minutes
Cook Time: 35 minutes
Serves 6

- 2 cup blanched finely ground almond flour
- 1 cup powdered erythritol, divided
- 2 tablespoons unsweetened cocoa powder
- 1/2 teaspoon baking powder
- 1/4 cup unsalted butter, softened 2 large eggs, divided
- 8 ounces full-fat cream cheese, softened
- 1/4 cup heavy whipping cream
- 1 teaspoon vanilla extract
- 2 tablespoons no-sugar-added peanut butter

Directions

- ✓ In a large bowl, mix almond flour, V2 cup erythritol, cocoa powder, and baking powder. Stir in butter and one egg.
- ✓ Scoop mixture into 6" round baking pan. Place pan into the air fryer basket.
- ✓ Adjust the temperature to 300°F and set the timer for 20 minutes.
- ✓ When fully cooked a toothpick inserted in center will come out clean. Allow 20 minutes to fully cool and firm up.
- ✓ In a large bowl, beat cream cheese, remaining V2 cup erythritol, heavy cream, vanilla, peanut butter, and remaining egg until fluffy.
- ✓ Pour mixture over cooled brownies. Place pan back into the air fryer basket.
- ✓ Adjust the temperature to 300°F and set the timer for 15 minutes.
- ✓ Cheesecake will be slightly browned and mostly firm with a slight jiggle when done. Allow to cool, then refrigerate 2 hours before serving.

Per serving Calories: 347 Protein: 8.3 g Fiber: 2.0 g Net carbohydrates: 3.8 g sugar alcohol: 24.0 g fat: 30.9 g Sodium: 207 mg

Pumpkin Spice Pecans

These are a great addition to salads and desserts and your snack drawer as well! Pecans are a perfect fit for a ketogenic diet because they have high-fat, moderate-protein, and low-carb content. These pecans also taste great with a little cream cheese sandwiched between them as a treat!

HandsOn Time: 5 minutes
Cook Time: 6 minutes
Serves: 4

- 1 cup whole pecans
- 4 cup granular erythritol
- 1 large egg white
- 2 teaspoon ground cinnamon
- 2 teaspoon pumpkin pie spice
- 2 teaspoon vanilla extract

Directions

- ✓ Toss all ingredients in a large bowl until pecans are coated. Place into the air fryer basket.
- ✓ Adjust the temperature to 300°F and set the timer for 6 minutes.
- ✓ Toss two to three times during cooking.
- ✓ Allow to cool completely. Store in an airtight container up to 3 days.

Per serving Calories: 178 Protein: 3.2 g fiber: 2.6 g Net carbohydrates: 1.4 g sugar alcohol: 15.0 g fat: 17.0 g Sodium: 13 mg carbohydrates: 19.0 g sugar: 1.1 g

Coconut Flour Mug Cake

Coconut flour is a great substitute for almond flour in ketogenic baking. It has a sweeter taste and is more absorbent than almond flour, so you'll need only about a third as much when swapping it in. It's also the perfect trade when you're trying to avoid nut allergies!

HandsOn Time: 5 minutes
Cook Time: 25 minutes
Serves 1

- 1 large egg
- 2 tablespoons coconut flour
- 2 tablespoons heavy whipping cream
- 2 tablespoons granular erythritol
- 4 teaspoon vanilla extract
- 4 teaspoon baking powder

Directions

- ✓ In a 4" ramekin, whisk egg, then add remaining ingredients. Stir until smooth. Place into the air fryer basket.
- ✓ Adjust the temperature to 300°F and set the timer for 25 minutes. When done a toothpick

should come out clean. Enjoy right out of the ramekin with a spoon. Serve warm.

Per serving Calories: 237 Protein: 9.9 g fiber: 5.0 g net carbohydrates: 5.7 g sugar alcohol: 30.0 g fat: 16.4 g Sodium: 213 mg carbohydrates: 40.7 g sugar: 4.2 g

PUMPKIN COOKIE WITH CREAM CHEESE FROSTING

This cookie is filled with the perfect flavors for fall. The soft spiced cookie complements the creamy frosting and makes a quick and slightly savory treat.

HandsOn Time: 10 minutes
Cook Time: 7 minutes
Serves 6

- 1/2 cup blanched finely ground almond flour
- 1/2 cup powdered erythritol, divided
- 2 tablespoons butter, softened
- 1 large egg
- 1/2 teaspoon unflavored gelatin
- 1/2 teaspoon baking powder
- 1/2 teaspoon vanilla extract
- 1/2 teaspoon pumpkin pie spice
- 2 tablespoons pure pumpkin puree
- 1/2 teaspoon ground cinnamon, divided
- 1/4 cup low-carb, sugar-free chocolate chips
- 3 ounces full-fat cream cheese, softened

Directions

- ✓ In a large bowl, mix almond flour and V4 cup erythritol. Stir in butter, egg, and gelatin until combined.
- ✓ Stir in baking powder, vanilla, pumpkin pie spice, pumpkin puree, and V4 teaspoon cinnamon, then fold in chocolate chips.
- ✓ Pour batter into 6" round baking pan. Place pan into the air fryer basket.
- ✓ Adjust the temperature to 300°F and set the timer for 7 minutes.
- ✓ When fully cooked, the top will be golden brown and a toothpick inserted in center will come out clean. Let cool at least 20 minutes.
- ✓ To make the frosting: mix cream cheese, remaining V4 teaspoon cinnamon, and remaining V4 cup erythritol in a large bowl. Using an electric mixer, beat until it becomes fluffy. Spread onto the cooled cookie. Garnish with additional cinnamon if desired.

Per serving Calories: 199 protein: 4.8 g fiber: 1.9 g Net carbohydrates: 2.9 g sugar alcohol: 16.7 g fat: 16.2 g sodium: 105 mg carbohydrates: 21.5 g sugar: 1.1 g

TOASTED COCONUT FLAKES

If you love a crunchy topping on your low-carb ice cream or yogurt, these flakes are perfect! They add a little sweetness and a big crunch to any meal and take just a few minutes to prepare! They're also delicious as a snack on the go. Store them in a hard container such as a small glass mason jar while you're on the go so they don't get crushed.

HandsOn Time: 5 minutes
Cook Time: 3 minutes
Serves 4

- 1 cup unsweetened coconut flakes
- 2 teaspoons coconut oil
- 4 cup granular erythritol
- 1/8 teaspoon salt

Directions

- ✓ Toss coconut flakes and oil in a large bowl until coated. Sprinkle with erythritol and salt.
- ✓ Place coconut flakes into the air fryer basket.
- ✓ Adjust the temperature to 300°F and set the timer for 3 minutes.
- ✓ Toss the flakes when 1 minute remains. Add an extra minute if you would like a more golden coconut flake.
- ✓ Store in an airtight container up to 3 days.

Per serving Calories: 165 protein: 1.3 g fiber: 2.7 g Net carbohydrates: 2.6 g sugar alcohol: 15.0 g fat: 15.5 g sodium: 76 mg Carbohydrates: 20.3 g sugar: 0.5 g

CHOCOLATE-COVERED MAPLE BACON

Sweet and salty just go together. And this Chocolate-Covered Maple Bacon is an easy way to get in protein and fat while satisfying your sweet tooth! For added crunch, try sprinkling on some crushed almonds after you dip the bacon in chocolate!

HandsOn Time: 5 minutes
Cook Time: 12 minutes
Serves 2 8 slices sugar-free bacon

- 1 tablespoon granular erythritol
- 1/3 cup low-carb, sugar-free chocolate chips
- 1 teaspoon coconut oil
- 1/2 teaspoon maple extract

Directions

- ✓ Place bacon into the air fryer basket and sprinkle with erythritol.
- ✓ Adjust the temperature to 350°F and set the timer for 12 minutes.
- ✓ Turn bacon halfway through the cooking time. Cook to desired doneness, checking at

9 minutes. (Smaller air fryers will cook much faster.)

- ✓ When bacon is done, set aside to cool.
- ✓ In a small microwave-safe bowl, place chocolate chips and coconut oil. Microwave for 30 seconds and stir. Add in maple extract.
- ✓ Place bacon onto a sheet of parchment. Drizzle chocolate over bacon and place in refrigerator to cool and harden, about 5 minutes.

Per serving Calories: 379 protein: 15.3 g fiber: 2.7 g Net carbohydrates: 3.0 g sugar alcohol: 26.1 g fat: 25.9 g sodium: 649 mg Carbohydrates: 31.8 g sugar: 0.2 g

VANILLA POUND CAKE

This simple vanilla cake is a moist and delicious dessert that can also be used as a base for other cake flavors. Add fresh strawberries to the batter for a strawberry cake or even fresh lime juice for a citrus feel!

Hands On Time: 10 minutes
Cook Time: 25 minutes
Serves 6

- 1 cup blanched finely ground almond flour
- 1/4 cup salted butter, melted
- 1/2 cup granular erythritol
- 1 teaspoon vanilla extract
- 1 teaspoon baking powder
- 1/2 cup full-fat sour cream
- 1 ounce full-fat cream cheese, softened 2 large eggs

Directions
- ✓ In a large bowl, mix almond flour, butter, and erythritol.
- ✓ Add in vanilla, baking powder, sour cream, and cream cheese and mix until well combined. Add eggs and mix.
- ✓ Pour batter into a 6" round baking pan. Place pan into the air fryer basket.
- ✓ Adjust the temperature to 300°F and set the timer for 25 minutes.
- ✓ When the cake is done, a toothpick inserted in center will come out clean. The center should not feel wet.

Allow it to cool completely, or the cake will crumble when moved.

Per serving Calories: 253 Protein: 6.9 G Fiber: 2.0 G Net Carbohydrates: 3.2 G Sugar Alcohol: 20.0 G Fat: 22.6 G Sodium: 191 Mg cCarbohydrates: 25.2 G Sugar: 1.5 G

CHOCOLATE MAYO CAKE

You'll be in chocolate heaven with this simple yet decadent chocolate cake. It stays mouthwateringly moist in the middle, thanks to the mayonnaise, making this cake the perfect tool for con□uering your chocolate cravings!

• HandsOn Time: 10 minutes • **Cook Time**: 25 minutes
Serves 6

- 1 cup blanched finely ground almond flour
- 1/4 cup salted butter, melted
- 1/2 cup plus 1 tablespoon granular erythritol
- 1 teaspoon vanilla extract
- 1/4 cup full-fat mayonnaise
- 1/4 cup unsweetened cocoa powder
- 2 large eggs

Directions
- ✓ In a large bowl, mix all ingredients until smooth.
- ✓ Pour batter into a 6" round baking pan. Place into the air fryer basket.
- ✓ Adjust the temperature to 300°F and set the timer for 25 minutes.
- ✓ When done, a toothpick inserted in center will come out clean. Allow cake to cool completely, or it will crumble when moved.

Per serving Calories: 270 protein: 7.0 g fiber: 3.3 g Net carbohydrates: 3.0 g sugar alcohol: 22.5 g fat: 25.1 g sodium: 143 mg Carbohydrates: 28.8 g

RASPBERRY DANISH BITES

These bites are great for those who love shortbread cookies. The cookies themselves are fluffy and moist, and paired with the raspberry preserves they are the perfect snack. Feel free to use your favorite flavor of fruit preserves, just be sure to check the labels to make sure there are no added sugars or high-glycemic sweeteners.

HandsOn Time: 30 minutes
Cook Time: 7 minutes
Serves: 10

- 1 cup blanched finely ground almond flour
- 1 teaspoon baking powder
- 3 tablespoons granular Swerve
- 2 ounces full-fat cream cheese, softened
- 1 large egg
- 10 teaspoons sugar-free raspberry preserves

Directions
- ✓ Mix all ingredients except preserves in a large bowl until a wet dough forms.

- ✓ Place the bowl in the freezer for 20 minutes until dough is cool and able to roll into a ball.
- ✓ Roll dough into ten balls and press gently in the center of each ball. Place 1 teaspoon preserves in the center of each ball.
- ✓ Cut a piece of parchment to fit your air fryer basket. Place each Danish bite on the parchment, pressing down gently to flatten the bottom.
- ✓ Adjust the temperature to 400°F and set the timer for 7 minutes.
- ✓ Allow to cool completely before moving, or they will crumble.

Per serving Calories: 96 protein: 3.4 g fiber: 1.3 g Net carbohydrates: 4.0 g sugar alcohol: 4.5 g fat: 7.7 g sodium: 76 mg Carbohydrates: 9.8 g sugar: 2.4 g

CREAM CHEESE DANISH

This Danish can double as a dessert or a sweet treat for breakfast! It's easy to make and pairs well with your favorite low-carb fruits. It tastes especially good alongside coffee or tea!

HandsOn Time: 20 minutes
Cook Time: 15 minutes
Serves 6

- 3/4 cup blanched finely ground almond flour
- 1 cup shredded mozzarella cheese
- 5 ounces full-fat cream cheese, divided
- 2 large egg yolks
- 3/4 cup powdered erythritol, divided
- 2 teaspoons vanilla extract, divided

Directions

- ✓ In a large microwave-safe bowl, add almond flour, mozzarella, and 1 ounce cream cheese. Mix and then microwave for 1 minute.
- ✓ Stir and add egg yolks to the bowl. Continue stirring until soft dough forms. Add V2 cup erythritol to dough and 1 teaspoon vanilla.
- ✓ Cut a piece of parchment to fit your air fryer basket. Wet your hands with warm water and press out the dough into a V4"-thick rectangle.
- ✓ In a medium bowl, mix remaining cream cheese, erythritol, and vanilla. Place this cream cheese mixture on the right half of the dough rectangle. Fold over the left side of the dough and press to seal. Place into the air fryer basket.
- ✓ Adjust the temperature to 330°F and set the timer for 15 minutes.
- ✓ After 7 minutes, flip over the Danish.

- ✓ When the timer beeps, remove the Danish from parchment and allow to completely cool before cutting.

Per serving Calories: 185 protein: 7.4 g fiber: 0.5 g Net carbohydrates: 2.3 g sugar alcohol: 18.0 g Fat: 14.5 g Sodium: 205 mg Carbohydrates: 20.8 g Sugar: 1.3 g

CARAMEL MONKEY BREAD

This isn't your mama's monkey bread! Packed with protein and low on carbs, this caramel monkey bread is so delicious your non-keto friends will be asking for the recipe! Although erythritol doesn't caramelize in the same way sugar traditionally does, it still creates a flavorful and sticky alternative that will have you forgetting all about the sugar.

HandsOn Time: 15 minutes
Cook Time: 12 minutes
Serves 6 (2 pieces per serving)

- 1/2 cup blanched finely ground almond flour
- 1/2 cup low-carb vanilla protein powder
- 3/4 cup granular erythritol, divided
- 1/2 teaspoon baking powder
- 8 tablespoons salted butter, melted and divided
- 1 ounce full-fat cream cheese, softened
- 1 large egg
- 1/4 cup heavy whipping cream
- 1/2 teaspoon vanilla extract

Directions

- ✓ In a large bowl, combine almond flour, protein powder, V2 cup erythritol, baking powder, 5 tablespoons butter, cream cheese, and egg. A soft, sticky dough will form.
- ✓ Place the dough in the freezer for 20 minutes. It will be firm enough to roll into balls. Wet your hands with warm water and roll into twelve balls. Place the balls into a 6" round baking dish.
- ✓ In a medium skillet over medium heat, melt remaining butter with remaining erythritol. Lower the heat and continue stirring until mixture turns golden, then add cream and vanilla. Remove from heat and allow it to thicken for a few minutes while you continue to stir.
- ✓ While the mixture cools, place baking dish into the air fryer basket.
- ✓ Adjust the temperature to 320°F and set the timer for 6 minutes.
- ✓ When the timer beeps, flip the monkey bread over onto a plate and slide it back into

the baking pan. Cook an additional 4 minutes until all the tops are brown.
- ✓ Pour the caramel sauce over the monkey bread and cook an additional 2 minutes. Let cool completely before serving.

Per serving Calories: 322 Protein: 20.4 g Fiber: 1.7 g Net carbohydrates: 2.0 g sugar alcohol: 30.0 g fat: 24.5 g Sodium: 301 mg Carbohydrates: 33.7 g sugar: 0.9 g

CINNAMON CREAM PUFFS

This recipe is perfect for Sunday brunch! The sweet dough is loaded with protein to keep you going while the inside has fragrant cinnamon to make this treat even more delicious! If you want a chocolate filling instead, simply add a tablespoon of cocoa powder to the filling!

HandsOn Time: 15 minutes
Cook Time: 6 minutes
- Yields 8 puffs (1 per serving)
- 1/2 cup blanched finely ground almond flour
- 1/2 cup low-carb vanilla protein powder
- 1/2 cup granular erythritol
- 1/2 teaspoon baking powder
- 1 large egg
- 5 tablespoons unsalted butter, melted 2 ounces full-fat cream cheese
- 1/4 cup powdered erythritol
- 1/4 teaspoon ground cinnamon
- 2 tablespoons heavy whipping cream
- 1/2 teaspoon vanilla extract

Directions
- ✓ Mix almond flour, protein powder, granular erythritol, baking powder, egg, and butter in a large bowl until a soft dough forms.
- ✓ Place the dough in the freezer for 20 minutes. Wet your hands with water and roll the dough into eight balls.
- ✓ Cut a piece of parchment to fit your air fryer basket. Working in batches as necessary, place the dough balls into the air fryer basket on top of parchment.
- ✓ Adjust the temperature to 380°F and set the timer for 6 minutes.
- ✓ Flip cream puffs halfway through the cooking time.

- ✓ When the timer beeps, remove the puffs and allow to cool.
- ✓ In a medium bowl, beat the cream cheese, powdered erythritol, cinnamon, cream, and vanilla until fluffy.
- ✓ Place the mixture into a pastry bag or a storage bag with the end snipped. Cut a small hole in the bottom of each puff and fill with some of the cream mixture.
- ✓ Store in an airtight container up to 2 days in the refrigerator.

Per serving Calories: 178 Protein: 14.9 g Fiber: 1.3 g Net carbohydrates: 1.3 g sugar alcohol: 19.5 g Fat: 12.1 g Sodium: 121 mg Carbohydrates: 22.1 g Sugar: 0.4 g

PAN PEANUT BUTTER COOKIES

Sometimes you just need a good peanut butter cookie. These four-ingredient treats can conquer your cravings in minutes! Thanks to the air fryer's small cooking chamber, you'll get an even, all around bake in no time for the perfect cookies!

HandsOn Time: 5 minutes
Cook Time: 8 minutes
Serves 8
- 1 cup no-sugar-added smooth peanut butter
- 3 cup granular erythritol
- 1 large egg
- 1 teaspoon vanilla extract

Directions
- ✓ In a large bowl, mix all ingredients until smooth. Continue stirring for 2 additional minutes, and the mixture will begin to thicken.
- ✓ Roll the mixture into eight balls and press gently down to flatten into 2" round disks.
- ✓ Cut a piece of parchment to fit your air fryer and place it into the basket. Place the cookies onto the parchment, working in batches as necessary.
- ✓ Adjust the temperature to 320°F and set the timer for 8 minutes. Flip the cookies at the 6-minute mark. Serve completely cooled.

THREE-CHEDDAR PIZZA FRITTATA

Fixings

- ½ (10-ounce) pack frozen spinach, defrosted
- 6 huge eggs
- 2 tablespoons olive oil
- ½ teaspoon dried Italian flavoring
- Salt and pepper
- ¼ cup ricotta cheddar
- ¼ cup ground parmesan cheddar
- 2 ½ ounces destroyed mozzarella cheddar
- 1 ounce cut pepperoni

Directions

1. Preheat the stove to 375°F and oil a pie plate with cooking shower.
2. Thaw out the frozen spinach in the microwave for 4 minutes at that point crush out the water.
3. Whisk together the eggs, olive oil, Italian flavoring, salt and pepper in a bowl.
4. Mix in the ricotta cheddar, parmesan cheddar, and depleted spinach until very much joined.
5. Empty the combination into the pie plate and top with mozzarella and pepperoni.
6. Heat for 35 to 40 minutes until the egg is set and the cheddar softly cooked. Makes 4 Servings.

MOZZARELLA FISH LIQUEFY

Fixings

- 1 tablespoon olive oil
- ½ cup diced yellow onion
- 8 ounces canned fish
- ¼ cup mayonnaise
- 2 enormous eggs, whisked
- 2 ounces destroyed mozzarella cheddar
- Salt and pepper
- 1 green onion, cut slight

Guidelines

1. Heat the oil in a skillet over medium heat.
2. Add the onion and cook until clear, around 5 minutes.
3. Channel the fish at that point piece it into the skillet and mix in the leftover Fixings .

4. Season with salt and pepper and cook for 2 minutes or until the cheddar dissolves.
5. Spoon into a bowl and top with cut green onion to serve. Makes 2 Servings.

AVOCADO EGG AND SALAMI SANDWICHES

Fixings

- 4 Simple Cloud Buns
- 1 teaspoon spread
- 4 huge eggs
- 1 medium tomato, cut into 4 cuts
- 1 ounce new mozzarella, cut slender
- 1 little avocado, cut flimsy
- 2 ounces cut salami
- Salt and pepper

Directions

1. Toast the cloud buns on a preparing sheet in the stove until brilliant earthy colored.
2. Heat the spread in a huge skillet over medium heat.
3. Break the eggs into the skillet and season with salt and pepper.
4. Cook the eggs until done to the ideal level at that point place one on each cloud bun.
5. Top the buns with cut tomato, mozzarella, avocado and salami. Makes 2 Servings.

MUSHROOM SOUP WITH SEARED EGG

Fixings

- 1 teaspoon olive oil
- 4 white mushrooms, cut slim
- 100 grams cauliflower, riced
- 1 cup vegetable stock
- 3 tablespoons substantial cream
- 2 tablespoons destroyed cheddar
- 1 teaspoon spread
- 1 huge egg

Directions

1. Heat the oil in a little pan over medium heat.
2. Add the mushrooms and cook until they are delicate, around 6 minutes.
3. Mix in the riced cauliflower, vegetable stock, and weighty cream.
4. Season with salt and pepper at that point mix in the cheddar.
5. Stew the soup until it thickens to the ideal level at that point eliminate from heat.
6. Fry the egg in the spread until cooked to the ideal level at that point serve over the soup.

Fixings

- 3 tablespoons low-carb marinara sauce
- 1 little zucchini (60g), cut dainty into adjusts
- 2 tablespoons ricotta cheddar
- 3 ounces destroyed mozzarella
- Dried oregano

Directions

1. Spoon 1 tablespoon marinara sauce into a microwave-safe bowl.
2. Spread 33% of the zucchini cuts over the sauce at that point cover with a tablespoon of ricotta.
3. Repeat the layers of sauce, zucchini, and ricotta.
4. Top with the excess zucchini and the last tablespoon of marinara.
5. Sprinkle with mozzarella at that point microwave for 3 to 4 minutes until the whole blend is heated through and the cheddar is liquefied.
6. Sprinkle with dried oregano and serve hot.

F I R M C H I P O T L E C H I C K E N T H I G H S

Fixings

- ½ teaspoon chipotle stew powder
- ¼ teaspoon garlic powder
- ¼ teaspoon onion powder
- ¼ teaspoon ground coriander
- ¼ teaspoon smoked paprika
- 12 ounces boneless chicken thighs
- Salt and pepper
- 1 tablespoon olive oil
- 3 cups new child spinach

Directions

1. Consolidate the chipotle stew powder, garlic powder, onion powder, coriander, and smoked paprika in a little bowl.
2. Hammer the chicken thighs out level at that point season with salt and pepper on the two sides.
3. Slice the chicken thighs down the middle and heat the oil in a weighty skillet over medium-high heat.
4. Add the chicken thighs skin-side-down to the skillet and sprinkle with the flavor blend.
5. Cook the chicken thighs for 8 minutes at that point flip and cook on the opposite side for 3 to 5 minutes.

6. During the most recent 3 minutes, add the spinach to the skillet and cook until shriveled.
7. Serve the fresh chicken thighs on a bed of withered spinach. Makes 2 Servings.

P E P P E R O N I , H A M A N D C H E D D A R S T R O M B O L I

Fixings

- 1 ¼ cups destroyed mozzarella cheddar
- ¼ cup almond flour
- 3 tablespoons coconut flour
- 1 teaspoon dried Italian flavoring
- Salt and pepper
- 1 huge egg, whisked
- 6 ounces cut shop ham
- 2 ounces cut pepperoni
- 4 ounces cut cheddar
- 1 tablespoon dissolved spread
- 6 cups new plate of mixed greens

Directions

1. Preheat the stove to 400°F and fix a heating sheet with material.
2. Liquefy the mozzarella cheddar in a microwave-safe bowl until it very well may be mixed smooth.
3. In a different bowl, mix together the almond flour, coconut flour, and dried Italian flavoring.
4. Empty the dissolved cheddar into the flour combination and work it along with some salt and pepper.
5. Add the egg and work it into a mixture at that point turn out onto a piece of material.
6. Lay a piece of material on top and carry the mixture out into an oval.
7. Utilize a blade to cut corner to corner cuts along the edges, leaving the center 4 inches immaculate.
8. Layer the ham and cheddar cuts in the mixture at that point overlap the strips up and over.
9. Brush the top with spread at that point heat for 15 to 20 minutes until the batter is carmelized.
10. Cut the Stromboli and present with a little plate of mixed greens. Makes 3 Servings.

Spring Salad with Steak and Sweet Dressing

Fixings
- 2 cuts thick-cut bacon
- 2 tablespoons white wine vinegar
- 2 tablespoons olive oil
- 2 tablespoons new raspberries
- Fluid stevia, to taste
- 4 cups crisp spring greens
- 1 ounce toasted pine nuts
- 1 tablespoon spread
- 7 ounces meat flank steak

Directions
1. Cook the bacon in a skillet over medium-high heat until fresh then cleave fine.
2. Join the white wine vinegar, olive oil, raspberries, and fluid stevia in a blender.
3. Mix the Fixings until smooth and very much consolidated.
4. Join the spring greens, simmered pine nuts, and disintegrated bacon in an enormous bowl.
5. Throw with the dressing at that point split between two plates.
6. Dissolve the margarine in a weighty skillet over medium-high heat at that point add the steak.
7. Season with salt and pepper at that point burn on one side, around 3 to 4 minutes.
8. Flip the steak and cook to the ideal level at that point rest for 5 minutes.
9. Cut the steak and split it between the Servings of mixed greens. Makes 2 Servings.

Stunning Low Carb Keto Bread Formula

Fixings :
- 7 enormous eggs
- ½ cup dissolved ghee
- 2 cups almond flour
- 1 t preparing powder
- ¼ t ocean salt

Directions
1. Preheat the stove to 350°F and fix a portion skillet with material paper covering the sides.
2. In a huge blending bowl, beat the eggs utilizing a hand blender on fast for 1 moment. Add the dissolved ghee and beat until just fused.

3. Decrease the speed to low and continuously add the leftover Fixings until totally blended and the player is thick.
4. Empty the hitter into the pre-arranged dish and spread with a spatula. Heat for 40-45 minutes, or until light brilliant earthy colored on top.
5. Cool the bread on a cooling rack for 10 minutes prior to cutting.

Tip: This bread likewise copies as heavenly flavorful or sweet biscuits. Mix in blueberries to make blueberry biscuits (remember, nonetheless, that the carb tally will go up) or hacked jalapeños and wholesome yeast for a fiery biscuit with a messy bend.

Simple Low Carb Keto Noatmeal

Fixings
- ⅓ cups full-fat coconut milk
- ½ cup riced cauliflower
- 1 T hemp hearts
- 1 T chia seeds
- 1 T unsweetened coconut chips
- 2 t cut almonds
- ½ t cinnamon
- ½ t Stevia
- 3 raspberries (for embellish)

Directions
1. Heat coconut milk over low heat until steaming, around 3 minutes.
2. Add cauliflower rice and heat 3-4 minutes.
3. Eliminate from heat and mix in the remainder of the Fixings . Let stand 3-4 minutes to thicken.
4. Fill a bowl and trimming with new raspberries.

"Messy" Broccoli Lunch Biscuits

Fixings
- 2 t ghee, relaxed + extra for lubing
- 1 cup broccoli florets, finely slashed
- 2 cups almond flour
- 2 enormous field raised eggs
- 1 cup unsweetened almond milk
- 2 T wholesome yeast
- 1 t heating powder
- ½ t ocean salt

Guidelines

1. Preheat the broiler to 350°F and oil a huge biscuit tin with ghee.
2. Mix together every one of the Fixings in an enormous blending bowl until very much joined.
3. Spoon the blend into the biscuit tins. Heat for 30 minutes until a toothpick embedded in the middle tells the truth.

Tip: Coconut flour can be fill in for almond meal in this formula, yet decline the sum to a large portion of a cup.

DAIRY FREE COCONUT YOGURT

Fixings

- 2 15 oz. jars natural coconut cream, chilled in the cooler 4 hours
- 2 without dairy probiotic pills with bacterial strains L. bulgaricus, S. thermophilus and L. casei
- 1 T nectar

Directions

1. Open coconut cream and separate the fluid from the cream.
2. In a food processor or high velocity blender, add the cream with the probiotic pills and nectar. Cycle on high for 3 minutes until pills are separated.
3. Check the consistency of the yogurt. On the off chance that it's excessively thick, add a tad bit of the coconut water and mix.
4. Move the yogurt to a glass container and seal with cover.
5. Preheat the stove to 100°F. Spot the glass container in the broiler for 24 hours to mature.
6. Once matured, eliminate from the stove, cool and mix the yogurt. Chill in the fridge for in any event 2 hours.

HOT AND FIRM CAULIFLOWER SQUANDERS

Ingredients

- 1 huge head of cauliflower, broken into florets
- 2 eggs
- ⅔ cup almond flour
- 1 T nourishing yeast
- ½ t turmeric
- ½ t ocean salt
- ¼ t dark pepper
- 1-2 T ghee

Directions

1. Add the cauliflower to a huge pot shrouded in water. Heat to the point of boiling and boil for 8 minutes. Strain. Add the florets into a food processor and heartbeat until riced.
2. Add cauliflower, eggs, almond flour, nourishing yeast, turmeric, salt and pepper to a blending bowl. Mix well to join. Structure into patties.
3. Heat the ghee over medium heat in a skillet. Scoop about a large portion of the blend into three squanders and cook until brilliant earthy colored on each side, 3-4 minutes. Put away until the remainder of the squanders are cooked. Serve hot.

SHRIMP AND CAULIFLOWER "CORN MEAL"

Fixings

For Shrimp:
- 1 pound enormous shrimp, stripped/deveined (defrosted whenever frozen)
- 1 T grass-took care of margarine (or ghee)
- 2 garlic cloves, minced
- 2 t paprika
- ½ t onion powder
- ½ t dried thyme
- ¼ t cayenne pepper
- ¼ t ocean salt

For Cauliflower Corn meal:
- 1 head of cauliflower, broken into florets
- ½ cup almond milk, unsweetened
- 1 T grass-took care of margarine (or ghee)
- 1 T nourishing yeast
- ¼ t ocean salt

Discretionary Garnishes:
- Green onion, finely cleaved
- Lemon wedges
- Hot sauce

Guidance
1. Start by setting cauliflower florets in a huge pot with 1 cup water. Bring to a low boil and cover. Boil 20 minutes or until cauliflower is fork delicate.
2. Channel florets and spot into a blender with ½ cup almond milk, 1 tablespoon spread,

nourishing yeast and ocean salt. Heartbeat until smooth.

3. To cook shrimp, soften grass-took care of margarine in an enormous skillet over medium heat. Mix in shrimp and flavors and cook 6 minutes, mixing at times.

4. Pour corn meal onto serving plate and top with shrimp and sauce combination. Get done with hot sauce, green onion and a crush of lemon.

AVOCADO CHOCOLATE BROWNIES

Fixings

- ⅔ cup crude cacao powder
- 2 eggs
- 2 avocados, pounded
- ¼ cup coconut oil, softened
- ⅓ cup sans dairy dull chocolate chips, dissolved
- 2 T stevia
- 1 t heating powder
- Ocean salt

Guidelines

1. Preheat the broiler to 325°F and oil a 8x8 stove safe skillet with coconut oil.
2. In a blending bowl, join the dry Fixings . In a different blending bowl, mix together eggs and squashed avocado until just consolidated.
3. Slowly add the dry Fixings to the wet, followed by liquefied coconut oil and dissolved dull chocolate. Mix well.
4. Utilize a spatula to equitably spread the player into the pre-arranged container. Heat for 30-35 minutes. Cool the brownies to room temperature prior to cutting.

3-LAYER KETO COOLER TIDBITS

Fixings

- ⅓ cup crude cacao glue
- ¼ cup coconut oil
- ⅓ cup coconut margarine
- ⅓ cup cashew margarine
- 9 crude cashews

Guidelines

1. Add the cacao glue and coconut oil to a pan and bring to a low stew, mixing until smooth.

2. Eliminate from the heat and let cool totally. Gap the fluid uniformly between the nine depressions of an ice block plate, and freeze for 10 minutes.

3. Spoon the coconut margarine uniformly ridiculous base, and freeze for an additional 10 minutes.

4. Spoon the cashew margarine uniformly over the highest point of each fat tidbit, and top with one cashew each. Freeze for an additional 10 minutes or until strong.

5. Pop the fat snacks out of the ice block plate by running a little spatula around the edges.

KETO "PB&J" CUPS

Fixings

- 3 T water
- ⅓ cup new raspberries
- 1 t stevia
- ½ t grass-took care of gelatin
- ½ cup coconut oil
- ½ cup smooth almond spread

Directions

1. In a pot over low heat, consolidate water and raspberries. Bring to boil, lessen heat and stew 5 minutes. Squash raspberries with a fork and eliminate from heat.
2. Mix in stevia and progressively sprinkle in gelatin as you mix. Fill a little container and cool in fridge 30 minutes.

3. Liquefy coconut oil and almond spread in a twofold boiler. Mix until smooth.
4. Line 6 biscuit tins with liners and pour 2 tablespoons of almond spread blend in every biscuit tin. Spot in cooler 15 minutes to set.
5. Add a stacking teaspoon of jam to each tin followed by outstanding almond margarine combination on top. Spot in cooler 15 minutes prior to appreciating. Store in the cooler.

AVOCADO CREAM AND ZOODLES

Fixings

- 1 zucchini
- 1/2 avocado (100g)
- 20 basil leaves
- 1.5 tablespoon olive oil
- 3 earthy colored mushrooms (30g)
- 1 garlic clove
- 1 teaspoon lemon juice
- 1/4 teaspoon salt

Directions

1. Spiralize your zucchini. Cut the mushrooms into equal parts.
2. In a stick blender cup, add the avocado, basil, 1 tablespoon olive oil, garlic, lemon squeeze and salt. Press the catch on the stick blender for about a moment until everything is really velvety and heavenly.
3. Add 1/2 tablespoon of olive oil in a griddle and cook the mushrooms until delicate. Add the zucchini noodles and cook only briefly or so until they get hot.
4. Add the avocado cream, combine everything as one and serve.

CHICKEN CUTLET AND CAULI RICE

Fixings

- 1 little cauliflower (300g)
- 2 tablespoon sesame oil
- 1 tablespoon coconut aminos
- 1 teaspoon dashi powder
- 1/4 teaspoon salt + pepper
- 1 skinless chicken bosom (260g)
- squeeze salt + pepper
- 1 egg
- 4 tablespoon almond flour
- 40g pork skins
- squeeze salt + pepper
- browning oil (refined coconut oil/fat/meat tallow)

Directions

1. Rice the cauliflower in a food processor or by utilizing a cheddar grater. In a wok, heat the sesame oil and add the riced cauliflower. A few minutes, add the coconut aminos, dashi, salt and pepper, and blend until joined. Fry until the cauliflower is delicate and crunchy.
2. Pulverize the pork skins utilizing a food processor/espresso processor/or your hands. Blend the skins in with the almond flour, salt and pepper. Add the egg in a little bowl and whisk.
3. Cut the chicken bosom in 2 length ways. Sprinkle the salt and pepper on the two sides and dunk in it the whisked egg. Coat the chicken with the breading on the two sides.
4. Fry the cutlet in 150C/300F preheated oil and fry until the inward temperature of the chicken cutlet registers to 65C/150F. Present with the cauli rice. Save half for another meal.

BLT LETTUCE BOATS

Fixings

- 2 lettuce leaves
- 2 cuts bacon
- 1/2 avocado
- 1/4 tomato
- 1 tablespoon mayo

Directions

1. Fry the bacon in a skillet until firm.
2. Cut the tomato into a couple of cuts. Cut the avocado.
3. Spoon 1/2 tablespoon of mayo over every lettuce leaf and cover with the bacon, tomato and avocado.

ROSEMARY CHICKEN AND BROCCOLI

Fixings

- 1 boneless chicken leg (125g)
- 1/3 broccoli head (100g)
- 1/4 teaspoon salt
- 1/4 teaspoon dark pepper
- 1/2 teaspoon rosemary
- 1 tablespoon olive oil
- 2 tablespoon water

Guidelines

1. Cut the chicken leg into reduced down pieces. Sprinkle the salt and pepper on top of it. Separate the broccoli into florets.
2. In a cast iron skillet, heat the olive oil and add the chicken skin side down to the container alongside the rosemary. Fry 3 minutes to fresh up the skin and turn the chicken around.
3. Add the broccoli florets and cook briefly combining everything as one. Add the water, cover and let the steam of the water cook the broccoli for 2 minutes. Reveal and serve.

SIDE CAESAR SALAD 2

Fixings

- 4 lettuce leaves
- 30g prosciutto
- 1 egg
- 1 tomato
- 1 tablespoon caesar dressing

Directions

1. Put some water to boil and add the egg. Boil for 7 minutes precisely, move to a bowl loaded up with ice water. Strip it.

2.   Cut the egg in four. Tear the lettuce leaves.
3.   Combine everything as one with the caesar dressing and eat with the extra pork broil.

ZUCCHINI SALAD W/FLAME BROILED CHICKEN THIGH

Fixings
- 1/4 zucchini
- 1/4 red pepper
- 50g swiss chard
- 1/4 tomato
- 5 basil leaves
- 1 tablespoon olive oil
- 1 teaspoon vinegar
- 1 garlic clove
- 1/4 teaspoon salt and pepper
- 1 chicken thigh with skin (75g)
- 1 tablespoon olive oil
- 1/2 teaspoon salt and pepper

Directions
1. Utilizing a peeler, strip the zucchini lenght-wise to make long strips. Cut the red pepper and cut down the middle. Dice the tomato. Cleave the swiss chard. Mince the basil leaves and garlic cloves.
2. Blend the entirety of the above with the olive oil, vinegar and salt and pepper together in a bowl and put on a plate.
3. Sprinkle the salt and pepper over the chicken thigh. Preheat the oil in a cast iron skillet and spot chicken bosom skin-side down and cook until firm. Turn it around, cook a couple of more minutes until cooked through. Spot on the plate with the serving of mixed greens.

ROSEMARY SHRIMPS AND RADISHES

Fixings
- 5 radishes (85g)
- 10 shrimps (100g)
- 3 broccoli florets (60g)
- 1 tablespoon rosemary
- 1 tablespoon olive oil
- 1/2 teaspoon salt, pepper

Directions
1. Put some water to boil in a pot and add the broccoli. Cook until delicate.
2. In a skillet, heat the oil and add the radishes aside and the shrimps to another. Sprinkle the salt, pepper and rosemary and cook for a couple of moments. The radishes ought to be delicate and crunchy, and the shrimps ought to be orange.
3. Put everything on a plate and appreciate!

CHICKEN BROCHETTES AND SIMPLE SERVING OF MIXED GREENS

Fixings
- 3 chicken brochettes
- 5 lettuce leaves
- 1/4 red pepper
- 1 cut tomato
- 1 tablespoon sesame dressing

Guidelines
1. Tear the lettuce into scaled down pieces. Cut the red pepper and tomato. Add the sesame dressing and coat well.
2. Add the brochettes to a plate alongside the serving of mixed greens.

CHICKEN BROCHETTES AND SESAME SALAD

Fixings
- 3 chicken and veggie brochettes
- 3 lettuce leaves
- 1 tomato cut
- 1/4 avocado
- 1 tablespoon sesame dressing

Guidelines
1. Tear the lettuce into reduced down pieces. Scoop out the avocado and 3D square it, cut the tomato cut in a couple of pieces. Add the sesame dressing and coat well.
2. Add the brochettes to a plate alongside the serving of mixed greens.

CUSHIONED OMELET AND VEGGIES

Fixings
- 1/2 zucchini (100g)
- 1/2 little cucumber
- 1/2 cup new spinach
- 1 hard-boiled egg
- 1 serving basil vinaigrette

Guidelines
1. Utilizing a cabbage shredder, meagerly cut the zucchini and cucumber.
2. Slash the spinach and cut the egg in 4.
3. Spot everything on a plate and pour the dressing over.

Fixings
- 1 segment caesar dressing
- 1 enormous kale leaf (50g)
- 1/2 avocado
- 1/2 tomato
- 1/8 red onion
- 100g meagerly cut meat
- 1 tablespoon olive oil
- 1/4 teaspoon salt, pepper, garlic powder

Guidelines
1. Cautiously trim the stem of the kale leaf so you can roll the leaf to make a sandwich.
2. Cut the avocado, red onion and tomato.
3. Heat the olive oil in a skillet and add the cut meat. Sprinkle the salt, pepper and garlic powder and cook until cooked through, 1-2 minutes.
4. Spoon the caesar dressing over the whole leaf. Toward one side, add the entirety of the garnishes and cautiously fold the leaf into a wrap. You can utilize aluminum foil to hold it back from carrying out.

CHICKEN MEATBALL LETTUCE CUPS

Fixings
- 4 lettuce leaves
- 2 chicken meatballs
- 1/4 tomato
- 1/2 avocado
- 1/2 tablespoon mayo
- 1/2 tablespoon dijon
- touch of parsley

Directions
1. Dice the tomato and avocado. Cut the meatballs into four pieces. Spot two lettuce leaves on top of one another.
2. Blend the mayo and dijon in a little bowl. Spread half on each cup.
3. Add a large portion of the meatballs, tomato and avocado to every lettuce cup. Add a touch of cleaved parsley over everything.

CHICKEN MEATBALL LETTUCE CUPS

Fixings
- 4 lettuce leaves
- 2 chicken meatballs
- 1/4 tomato
- 1/2 avocado
- 1/2 tablespoon mayo
- 1/2 tablespoon dijon
- touch of parsley

Directions
1. Dice the tomato and avocado. Cut the meatballs into four pieces. Spot two lettuce leaves on top of one another.
2. Blend the mayo and dijon in a little bowl. Spread half on each cup.
3. Add a large portion of the meatballs, tomato and avocado to every lettuce cup. Add a touch of cleaved parsley over everything.

CHICKEN MEATBALLS AND ARUGULA SALAD

Fixings
- 2 chicken meatballs
- 40g arugula
- 1 tablespoon cut dark olives
- 1/4 avocado
- 1/2 tomato
- 1 serving caesar dressing

Directions
1. Cut the avocado, tomato and chicken meatballs. Put everything on a plate and shower the caesar dressing over everything.

AIR SEARED HOT BROCCOLI

Fixings
- 1/2 tablespoons avocado oil
- 1 pound (cut into florets) broccoli
- Salt
- 1 tablespoon minced garlic
- 2 teaspoons fluid stevia
- 2 tablespoons soy sauce, decreased sodium
- 1 teaspoon rice vinegar
- 2 teaspoons sriracha
- Lemon juice
- 1/3 cup salted almonds, simmered

Technique
1. Add garlic, avocado oil, broccoli and salt into a major bowl and throw until combination is joined and the florets are completely covered.

Add combination into the air fryer crate and spread equally in one layer for cooking.

2. Cook the broccoli combination for around 15-20 minutes, until fresh and brilliant earthy colored, at 400ºF. Mix combination halfway while cooking. Note: Leave however much space as could reasonably be expected between the florets.

3. Meanwhile, add rice vinegar, sriracha, soy sauce and stevia into a little broiler safe bowl, mix to join and heat in a microwave until combination dissolves together, for 10 15 seconds.

4. Move the air singed broccoli combination into a serving bowl and top with the stevia-sauce. Throw combination until covered and sprinkle with more salt as important. Top with lemon squeeze and cooked almonds and mix until consolidated.

GOUDA BACON BURGER

Fixings
- 2 tablespoons stevia
- 2 tablespoons vanilla concentrate
- ¾ pound. (80% lean) ground hamburger
- 3 strips (divided) bacon
- 2 tablespoons bar-b-que sauce
- 1 tablespoon onion, minced
- Newly ground dark pepper, to taste
- ½ teaspoon salt
- 2 gouda cheddar cuts

Sauce
- 2 tablespoons mayo
- 2 tablespoons bar-b-que sauce
- Newly ground dark pepper, to taste
- ¼ teaspoon ground paprika

Serving
- 2 keto moves/buns
- Tomato
- Lettuce

Technique
1. Heat up air fryer to 390ºF. Add little sum water into the cabinet of the air fryer. Add stevia and vanilla concentrate not a bowl and join. Add pieces of bacon into the wire crate of the air fryer and coat with the stevia-vanilla combination.

2. Cook bacon for 4 minutes at 390ºF. Turn, cover with additional stevia-vanilla combination and cook until crisped, for 4 additional minutes. Meanwhile, add pepper, salt, bar-b-que sauce, onion and ground hamburger into a major bowl and join.

3. Structure ground meat blend into 2 patties. Spot patties into the wire container of your air fryer and cook until wanted doneness is reached, for 15-20 minutes at 370ºF. Turn burgers halfway while air searing.

4. Add dark pepper, paprika, mayo and bar-b-que sauce into a bowl and consolidate for the sauce. Add a gouda cheddar cut over every burger patty and cook until cheddar is dissolved, for 1 more moment noticeable all around fryer.

5. Spread sauce inside keto buns or rolls and top with burger, tomato lettuce and vanilla cooked bacon.

CRISPED PECORINO AUBERGINES

Fixings
- 1/2 cup pork skin pieces
- 1 (cut coarsely into 1/2" cuts) eggplant, huge
- Salt, as fundamental
- 3 tablespoons pecorino romano cheddar, finely ground
- 3 tablespoons almond flour
- 1 teaspoon Italian flavoring
- Avocado oil
- 1 tablespoon water + 1 egg
- 1/4 cup mozzarella cheddar, ground
- 1 cup marinara sauce
- 2 tablespoons cilantro

Strategy
1. Sprinkle eggplant cuts with salt, focus on and let sit for around 15 minutes. Meanwhile, add water and egg into a bowl and blend. Include the almond flour and blend until a hitter consistency is reached.

2. Add salt, Italian flavoring, pecorino Romano cheddar and pork skins into an average level lined bowl and mix well until consolidated. Dunk eggplant cuts into the hitter until uniformly covered. Submerge covered eggplant cuts into the pork skin combination until entirely covered.

3. Move eggplant cuts into a platter and coat equitably with avocado oil. Heat up air fryer to 360ºF. Add the breaded eggplant cuts on the air fryer container and cook for 8 minutes. Add mozzarella cheddar and 1 tablespoon marinara sauce over eggplant cuts and cook until cheddar is liquefied, for 1-2 additional minutes.

4. Fill in as wanted and delve in.

AIR SINGED LASAGNA

Fixings
- 1 (cut into slight long cuts) zucchini
- 1 cup marinara sauce

Sausage Layer
- 1 teaspoon garlic, minced
- 1 cup white onion, diced
- 1/2 pound. gentle Italian sausage

Cheddar Layer
- 1/2 cup mozzarella cheddar, destroyed
- 1/2 cup ricotta cheddar
- 1 egg
- 1/2 cup (partitioned) parmesan, destroyed
- 1/2 teaspoon dried Italian flavoring
- 1/2 teaspoon minced garlic
- 1/2 teaspoon dark pepper

Technique
1. Splash avocado oil into 7" springform container. Lay zucchini cuts into the pre-arranged dish in meeting layers. Top zucchini cuts with 1/4 cup marinara sauce and spread until layer is covered uniformly.
2. Add Italian sausage, garlic and onions into a major bowl and join. Lay sausage over marinara layer and spread until layer is covered equally. Top layer with the excess marinara sauce and spread until layer is covered equally.
3. Add 1/4 cup parmesan cheddar, and the mozzarella cheddar and ricotta into a spotless bowl and join. Top meat/marinara layer with cheddar blend and spread until layer is covered uniformly.
4. Add the leftover parmesan cheddar over cheddar layer. Spot a foil top over spring structure container and move into the fryer crate. Cook lasagna for 20 minutes at 350º. Dispose of the foil, cook until effervescent and the top gets carmelized at 350º, for 8-10 minutes.
5. Let sit for 10 minutes until cooled prior to eliminating from the container.

NO-NOODLE CHEDDAR LASAGNA

Fixing
- 8 oz of mozzarella cut
- 1 (25 ounces) container marinara sauce
- 1 enormous egg
- 1/2 cup of Parmesan cheddar
- 1/2 cups of ricotta cheddar

- 1 little onion
- 2 minced cloves garlic
- 1 pounds of ground meat

Directions
1. Push the sauté work on your Moment Pot for medium heat, earthy colored the ground hamburger in addition to the onion and garlic.
2. In the interim, consolidate together in a little blending bowl the Parmesan, ricotta cheddar with egg.
3. When the searing is finished, channel oil from the pot and eliminate hamburger combination.
4. Blend marinara sauce with meat combination in a medium size bowl (Put half cup away for the top).
5. Layer 1/2 lasagna meat with mozzarella and finally ricotta cheddar blend in a spring structure container fixed with aluminum foil that finds a way into your pressing factor cooker. Repeat stages a subsequent time. Add half cup of the leftover marinara sauce. Orchestrate a sling over rack in the Pot and include some water.
6. Spot spring structure dish in the pot and cover top freely utilizing aluminum foil. Cover with the top and keep secure. Cook for 9 minutes on high pressing factor. When the time is finishes, speedy delivery, eliminate the cover and serve.

EGG CHOMPS STRAIGHTFORWARD CHEDDAR

Fixings
- 1 tablespoon of avocado oil
- ¼ cup of hefty cream
- ¼ cup of natural cottage cheddar
- 4 oz of destroyed natural cheddar
- 6 enormous fed eggs

Guidelines
1. In your pressing factor cooker, add two cups of water. Organize rack in the foundation of the pot. Brush avocado oil on the Egg Nibble shape.
2. Mix the eggs, cheddar, hefty cream and cottage cheddar in a powerful blender on high, for 30 seconds.
3. Fill the wells of the Egg Nibble shape with the egg combination, about ¾ full. Top with bacon press or a level plate (Don't utilize plastic).
4. Cover and keep top secure, set valve to fixing. Set physically for 8 minutes. When the time total, eliminate the form from Pot. Eliminate the egg nibbles with a spoon.